Diffusion Imaging: From Head to Toe

Guest Editor

L. CELSO HYGINO CRUZ Jr, MD

MAGNETIC RESONANCE IMAGING CLINICS OF NORTH AMERICA

www.mri.theclinics.com

Consulting Editors
VIVIAN S. LEE, MD, PhD, MBA
LYNNE STEINBACH, MD
SURESH MUKHERJI, MD

February 2011 • Volume 19 • Number 1

SAUNDERS an imprint of ELSEVIER, Inc.

W.B. SAUNDERS COMPANY
A Division of Elsevier Inc.

1600 John F. Kennedy Boulevard • Suite 1800 • Philadelphia, Pennsylvania 19103-2899

http://www.theclinics.com

MRI CLINICS OF NORTH AMERICA Volume 19, Number 1
February 2011 ISSN 1064-9689, ISBN 13: 978-1-4557-0466-8

Editor: Joanne Husovski
Developmental Editor: Natalie Whitted

Magnetic Resonance Imaging Clinics of North America (ISSN 1064-9689) is published quarterly by Elsevier Inc., 360 Park Avenue South, New York, NY 10010-1710. Months of issue are February, May, August, and November. Business and Editorial Offices: 1600 John F. Kennedy Blvd., Ste. 1800, Philadelphia, PA 19103-2899. Customer Service Office: 3251 Riverport Lane, Maryland Heights, MO 63043. Periodicals postage paid at New York, NY and additional mailing offices. Subscription prices are $309.00 per year (domestic individuals), $501.00 per year (domestic institutions), $158.00 per year (domestic students/residents), $345.00 per year (Canadian individuals), $628.00 per year (Canadian institutions), $448.00 per year (international individuals), $628.00 per year (international institutions), and $228.00 per year (international and Canadian students/residents). International air speed delivery is included in all *Clinics* subscription prices. All prices are subject to change without notice. **POSTMASTER:** Send address changes to *Magnetic Resonance Imaging Clinics*, Elsevier Health Sciences Division, Subscription Customer Service, 3251 Riverport Lane, Maryland Heights, MO 63043. Customer Service (orders, claims, online, change of address): Elsevier Health Sciences Division, Subscription Customer Service, 3251 Riverport Lane, Maryland Heights, MO 63043. Tel:1-800-654-2452 (U.S. and Canada); 314-447-8871 (outside U.S. and Canada). Fax: 314-447-8029. E-mail: journalscustomerservice-usa@elsevier.com (for print support); journalsonlinesupport-usa@elsevier.com (for online support).

Reprints. For copies of 100 or more of articles in this publication, please contact the Commercial Reprints Department, Elsevier Inc., 360 Park Avenue South, New York, NY 10010-1710. Tel.: 212-633-3812; Fax: 212-462-1935; E-mail: reprints@elsevier.com.

Magnetic Resonance Imaging Clinics of North America is covered in the *RSNA Index of Imaging Literature, MEDLINE/PubMed (Index Medicus),* and *EMBASE/Excerpta Medica.*

Printed and bound by CPI Group (UK) Ltd, Croydon, CR0 4YY

Transferred to Digital Print 2011

GOAL STATEMENT

The goal of *Magnetic Resonance Imaging Clinics of North America* is to keep practicing physicians up to date with current clinical practice by providing timely articles reviewing the state of the art in patient care.

ACCREDITATION

The *Magnetic Resonance Imaging Clinics of North America* is planned and implemented in accordance with the Essential Areas and Policies of the Accreditation Council for Continuing Medical Education (ACCME) through the joint sponsorship of the University of Virginia School of Medicine and Elsevier. The University of Virginia School of Medicine is accredited by the ACCME to provide continuing medical education for physicians.

The University of Virginia School of Medicine designates this educational activity for a maximum of 15 *AMA PRA Category 1 Credits*™ for each issue, 60 credits per year. Physicians should only claim credit commensurate with the extent of their participation in the activity.

The American Medical Association has determined that physicians not licensed in the US who participate in this CME activity are eligible for a maximum of 15 *AMA PRA Category 1 Credits*™ for each issue, 60 credits per year.

Credit can be earned by reading the text material, taking the CME examination online at http://www.theclinics.com/home/cme, and completing the evaluation. After taking the test, you will be required to review any and all incorrect answers. Following completion of the test and evaluation, your credit will be awarded and you may print your certificate.

FACULTY DISCLOSURE/CONFLICT OF INTEREST

The University of Virginia School of Medicine, as an ACCME accredited provider, endorses and strives to comply with the Accreditation Council for Continuing Medical Education (ACCME) Standards of Commercial Support, Commonwealth of Virginia statutes, University of Virginia policies and procedures, and associated federal and private regulations and guidelines on the need for disclosure and monitoring of proprietary and financial interests that may affect the scientific integrity and balance of content delivered in continuing medical education activities under our auspices.

The University of Virginia School of Medicine requires that all CME activities accredited through this institution be developed independently and be scientifically rigorous, balanced and objective in the presentation/discussion of its content, theories and practices.

All authors/editors participating in an accredited CME activity are expected to disclose to the readers relevant financial relationships with commercial entities occurring within the past 12 months (such as grants or research support, employee, consultant, stock holder, member of speakers bureau, etc.). The University of Virginia School of Medicine will employ appropriate mechanisms to resolve potential conflicts of interest to maintain the standards of fair and balanced education to the reader. Questions about specific strategies can be directed to the Office of Continuing Medical Education, University of Virginia School of Medicine, Charlottesville, Virginia.

The faculty and staff of the University of Virginia Office of Continuing Medical Education have no financial affiliations to disclose.

The authors/editors listed below have identified no professional or financial affiliations for themselves or their spouse/partner:

Leonardo K. Bittencourt, MD; Arthur F.N.G. Borgonovi, BSc; Pilar Caro, MD; Flávia Martins Costa, MD; Antonio C. Coutinho Jr, MD; L. Celso Hygino Cruz Jr, MD (Guest Editor); Claudio de Carvalho Rangel, MD; Eduard de Lange, MD (Test Author); Raquel de Vasconcellos Carvalhaes de Oliveira, MD; Romeu Cortes Domingues, MD; Thomas M. Döring, MSc; Elisa Carvalho Ferreira, MD; Emerson L. Gasparetto, MD, PhD; Alexander R. Guimarães, MD, PhD; Joanne Husovski (Acquisitions Editor); Dow-Mu Koh, MD, MRCP, FRCR; Arun Krishnaraj, MD, MPH; Vivian S. Lee, MD, PhD, MBA (Consulting Editor); Antonio Luna, MD; Gabriela Martins, MD; Celso Matos, MD; Fernanda Philadelpho Arantes Pereira, MD; Cintia E. Pires, MD; James Schafer, MD; Ashok Srinivasan, MD; Lynne Steinbach, MD (Consulting Editor); Tatiana Chinem Takayassu, MD; Evandro Miguelote Vianna, MD.

The authors/editors listed below identified the following professional or financial affiliations for themselves or their spouse/partner:

Eduardo H.M.S.G. de Figueiredo, BSc is employed by GE Healthcare.
Suresh Mukherji, MD (Consulting Editor) is a consultant for Philips.
Anwar R. Padhani, MBBS, FRCP, FRCR is on the Speakers' Bureau for Siemens Healthcare.
Javier Sanchez-Gonzalez, PhD is employed by Philips Healthcare.

Disclosure of Discussion of non-FDA approved uses for pharmaceutical products and/or medical devices:

The University of Virginia School of Medicine, as an ACCME provider, requires that all faculty presenters identify and disclose any "off label" uses for pharmaceutical and medical device products. The University of Virginia School of Medicine recommends that each physician fully review all the available data on new products or procedures prior to instituting them with patients.

TO ENROLL

To enroll in the Magnetic Resonance Imaging Clinics of North America Continuing Medical Education program, call customer service at 1-800-654-2452 or visit us online at www.theclinics.com/home/cme. The CME program is available to subscribers for an additional fee of $196.00.

Contributors

CONSULTING EDITORS

VIVIAN S. LEE, MD, PhD, MBA
Professor of Radiology, Physiology, and
Neurosciences; Vice-Dean for Science; and
Senior Vice-President and Chief Scientific
Officer at New York University Langone
Medical Center, New York, New York

LYNNE STEINBACH, MD
Professor of Clinical Radiology and Orthopaedic
Surgery at the University of California San
Francisco, San Francisco, California

SURESH MUKHERJI, MD
Professor and Chief of Neuroradiology
and Head and Neck Radiology;
Professor of Radiology, Otolaryngology
Head Neck Surgery, Radiation Oncology,
Oral Medicine, and Periodontics
at the University of Michigan Health System,
Ann Arbor, Michigan

GUEST EDITOR

L. CELSO HYGINO CRUZ Jr, MD
Radiologist, Clínicas de Diagnóstico
Por Imagem (CDPI), Multi-Imagem,
IRM-Ressonância Magnética; Department
of Radiology, Federal University of Rio de
Janeiro, Brazil; Research Scholar, Division
of Neuroradiology, Department of Radiology,
Duke University, Durham, North Carolina

AUTHORS

ARTHUR F.N.G. BORGONOVI, BSc
HC, Hospital das Clínicas; HCor, Hospital
do Coração, São Paulo, Brazil

LEONARDO K. BITTENCOURT, MD
Clínica de Diagnóstico por Imagem, Carlos
Bittencourt Diagnóstico por Imagem and
Department of Radiology, Rio de Janeiro
Federal University, Rio de Janeiro, Brazil

PILAR CARO, MD
MR Unit, DADISA, Health Time Group, Cadiz, Spain

FLÁVIA MARTINS COSTA, MD
Radiologist, Clínica de Diagnóstico por
Imagem, Clínica Multi Imagem e Ressonância,
Rio de Janeiro, Brazil

ANTONIO C. COUTINHO Jr, MD
Clínica de Diagnóstico por Imagem, Centro de
Diagnostico por Imagem da Casa de Saude
N. Sra. de Fatima (Fatima Digittal), Rio de
Janeiro, Brazil

L. CELSO HYGINO CRUZ Jr, MD
Radiologist, Clínicas de Diagnóstico Por
Imagem (CDPI), Multi-Imagem, IRM -
Ressonância Magnética; Department of
Radiology, Federal University of Rio de
Janeiro, Brazil; Research Scholar, Division of
Neuroradiology, Department of Radiology,
Duke University, Durham, North Carolina

**RAQUEL DE VASCONCELLOS
CARVALHAES DE OLIVEIRA, MSc**
Statistician; Public Health Researcher,
Clinic Epidemiology Department,
Instituto de Pesquisa Evandro Chagas,
Fundação Oswaldo Cruz (Fiocruz),
Manguinhos, Rio de Janeiro, Brazil

CLAUDIO DE CARVALHO RANGEL, MD
Clínica de Diagnóstico por Imagem, Barra da
Tijuca; IRM–Ressonância Magnética, Botafogo;
Chairman, Department of Radiology, Hospital
Central da Policia Militar, Rio de Janeiro, Brazil

EDUARDO H.M.S.G. DE FIGUEIREDO, BSc
GE Healthcare, São Paulo, Brazil

ROMEU CORTES DOMINGUES, MD
Chairman, Clínica de Diagnóstico por Imagem, Barra da Tijuca; Chairman, Clínica Multi-Imagem, Ipanema, Rio de Janeiro, Brazil

THOMAS M. DORING, MSc
Federal University of Rio de Janeiro; Clínica de Diagnóstico por Imagem, Rio de Janeiro, Brazil

ELISA CARVALHO FERREIRA, MD
Radiologist, Clínica de Diagnóstico por Imagem, Clínica Multi Imagem e Ressonância, Rio de Janeiro, Brazil

EMERSON L. GASPARETTO, MD, PhD
Clínica de Diagnóstico por Imagem, Barra da Tijuca; Clínica Multi-Imagem, Ipanema; Department of Radiology, Federal University of Rio de Janeiro, Rio de Janeiro, Brazil

ALEXANDER R. GUIMARÃES, MD, PhD
Assistant Professor; Associate Director – Clinical Fellowship, Division of Abdominal Imaging and Interventional Radiology, Department of Radiology, Massachusetts General Hospital, Harvard Medical School, Boston; Director of Abdominal Imaging, Martinos Center for Biomedical Imaging, Department of Radiology, Massachusetts General Hospital, Harvard Medical School, Massachusetts Institute of Technology, Charlestown, Massachusetts

DOW-MU KOH, MD, MRCP, FRCR
Consultant Radiologist, Department of Radiology, Royal Marsden Hospital, Sutton, Surrey, United Kingdom

ARUN KRISHNARAJ, MD, MPH
Division of Abdominal Imaging and Interventional Radiology, Department of Radiology, Massachusetts General Hospital, Harvard Medical School, Boston, Massachusetts

ANTONIO LUNA, MD
Chief of MRI Section, MR Unit, SERCOSA, Health Time Group, Clinica las Nieves, Jaén, Spain

GABRIELA MARTINS, MD
Medical Doctor Specialized in Breast Imaging, Department of Breast Imaging, Clínica de Diagnóstico por Imagem, Leblon; Department of Breast Imaging, Multi-imagem Ressonância Magnética, Ipanema, Rio de Janeiro, Brazil

CELSO MATOS, MD
Associate Professor, Department of Radiology, Hospital Erasme, Université Libre de Bruxelles, Brussels, Belgium

SURESH MUKHERJI, MD
Professor and Chief of Neuroradiology and Head and Neck Radiology; Professor of Radiology, Otolaryngology Head Neck Surgery, Radiation Oncology, Oral Medicine, and Periodontics at the University of Michigan Health System, Ann Arbor, Michigan

ANWAR R. PADHANI, MBBS, FRCP, FRCR
Consultant Radiologist, Paul Strickland Scanner Centre, Mount Vernon Cancer Center, Northwood, Middlesex, United Kingdom

FERNANDA PHILADELPHO ARANTES PEREIRA, MD
Medical Doctor Specialized in Breast Imaging, Department of Breast Imaging, Clínica de Diagnóstico por Imagem, Leblon; Department of Radiology, Federal University of Rio de Janeiro, Rio de Janeiro, Brazil

CINTIA E. PIRES, MD
Clínica de Diagnóstico por Imagem, Rio de Janeiro, Brazil

JAVIER SÁNCHEZ-GONZALEZ, PhD
MR Clinical Scientist, Philips Healthcare, Maria de Portugal, Madrid, Spain

JAMES SCHAFER, MD
Division of Neuroradiology, Department of Radiology, University of Michigan Health System, Ann Arbor, Michigan

ASHOK SRINIVASAN, MD
Assistant Professor, Division of Neuroradiology, Department of Radiology, University of Michigan Health System, Ann Arbor, Michigan

TATIANA CHINEM TAKAYASSU, MD
Clínica de Diagnóstico por Imagem, Barra da Tijuca, Rio de Janeiro, Brazil

EVANDRO MIGUELOTE VIANNA, MD
Radiologist, Clínica de Diagnóstico por Imagem, Clínica Multi Imagem e Ressonância, Rio de Janeiro, Brazil

Contents

> MR image contrast is based on intrinsic tissue properties and specific pulse sequences and parameter adjustments. A growing number of MRI imaging applications are based on diffusion properties of water. To better understand MRI diffusion-weighted imaging, a brief overview of MR physics is presented in this article followed by physics of the evolving techniques of diffusion MR imaging and diffusion tensor imaging.

> Diffusion-weighted imaging has been used extensively in clinical practice for the early diagnosis of central nervous system conditions that restrict the diffusion of water molecules because it provides information about tumor cellularity or abscesses containing viscous fluid. DTI can detect brain lesions before any conventional imaging. Even though the role of these modalities is well defined for many neurologic lesions that affect the brain, its clinical application in spinal cord diseases is increasing. This article discusses the several central nervous system conditions that may be diagnosed with diffusion imaging.

> Diffusion weighting (DW) represents a magnetic resonance imaging contrast distinct from T1 and T2 in terms of imaging physics and its relationship to underlying physiology and pathophysiology. DW imaging has become a sine qua non of neuroimaging because of its exquisite sensitivity to the molecular motion of water that is altered in many pathologic conditions including acute ischemia. This article reviews the physical principles of DW imaging in the head and neck and describes how it can help to solve this and several other related problems.

> Diffusion-weighted imaging (DWI) is feasible in the chest with currently available MR imaging scanners, although it is technically demanding. Although there is scarce clinical experience, the use of DWI has shown promising results in the characterization of pulmonary nodules, in lung cancer characterization and staging, and in the evaluation of mediastinal and pleural pathology. Ongoing research opens a door to noninvasive evaluation of heart fibers by means of diffusion-tensor imaging. Another area under investigation is the use of DWI of hyperpolarized gases as an early biomarker of pulmonary disease.

> Several studies have investigated the role of advanced magnetic resonance imaging
> (MRI) techniques, such as diffusion-weighted imaging (DWI), to improve the speci-
> ficity of MRI for the evaluation of breast lesions. Potential roles for DWI and the
> apparent diffusion coefficient in characterizing breast tumors and distinguishing
> malignant from benign tissues have been reported. This article discusses the clinical
> applications of breast DWI, including literature results, technical issues and limita-
> tions, and the potential applications. The analysis of DWI at our institution is also dis-
> cussed. The establishment of standard DWI protocols and diagnostic criteria is
> necessary to ensure accuracy and reproducibility at different centers.

> Recent technological achievements have enabled the transposition of diffusion-
> weighted imaging (DWI) with good diagnostic quality into other body regions, espe-
> cially the abdomen and pelvis. Many emerging and established applications are now
> being evaluated on the upper abdomen, the liver being the most studied organ. This
> article discusses imaging strategies for DWI on the upper abdomen, describes the
> clinical protocol, and reviews the most common clinical applications of DWI on solid
> abdominal organs.

> Diffusion-weighted imaging (DWI) is a powerful imaging technique in neuroimaging;
> its value in abdominal and pelvic imaging has only recently been appreciated as a re-
> sult of improvements in magnetic resonance imaging technology. There is growing
> interest in the use of DWI for evaluating pathology in the pelvis. Its ability to nonin-
> vasively characterize tissues and to depict changes at a cellular level allows DWI
> to be an effective complement to conventional sequences of pelvic imaging, espe-
> cially in oncologic patients. The addition of DWI may obviate contrast material in
> those with renal insufficiency or contrast material allergy.

> Conventional MR imaging provides low specificity in the differential diagnosis of
> musculoskeletal (MSK) tumors and is unable to offer information about the extent
> of tumoral necrosis and the presence of viable cells, information crucial to assess
> treatment response and prognosis. Therefore, diffusion-weighted imaging (DWI) is
> now used with conventional MR imaging to improve diagnostic accuracy and
> treatment evaluation. This article discusses the technical aspects of DWI, partic-
> ularly the quantitative and qualitative interpretation of images in MSK tumors.
> The clinical application of DWI for tumor detection, characterization, differentiation
> of tumor tissue from others, and assessment of treatment response are
> emphasized.

Functional imaging techniques are increasingly being used to monitor response to therapies, often predicting the success of therapy before conventional measurements are changed. This review focuses on magnetic resonance imaging (MRI) depicted water diffusivity as a tumor response parameter. Response assessments are undertaken by noting changes in signal intensity on high b-value images or by using measurements of apparent diffusion coefficient values. The different diffusion-weighted (DW)-MRI appearances in response to treatment of soft tissue disease and bone metastases are discussed. DW-MRI changes observed in response to cytotoxics, radiotherapy, antiangiogenics, embolization, and thermocoagulation are detailed.

Magnetic Resonance Imaging Clinics of North America

FORTHCOMING ISSUES

Cartilage Imaging
Richard Kijowski, MD,
Guest Editor

MRI of the Newborn
Claudia Hillenbrand, PhD and
Thierry Huisman, MD,
Guest Editors

RECENT ISSUES

November 2010

Normal Variants and Pitfalls in Musculoskeletal MRI
William B. Morrison, MD and
Adam C. Zoga, MD,
Guest Editors

August 2010

MRI of the Liver
Alisha Qayyum, MD,
Guest Editor

May 2010

Breast MRI
Linda Moy, MD and
Cecilia L. Mercado, MD,
Guest Editors

RELATED INTEREST

Emergency Neuroradiology
Alexander J. Nemeth, MD, and Matthew T. Walker, MD, *Guest Editors*
Radiologic Clinics of North America, January 2011

THE CLINICS ARE NOW AVAILABLE ONLINE!

Access your subscription at:
www.theclinics.com

Preface
Diffusion Imaging: From Head to Toe

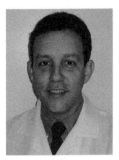

L. Celso Hygino Cruz Jr, MD
Guest Editor

Imaging methods are part of doctors' daily practice. As a result, MRI was ranked the top medical innovation by physicians in a recent study. The authors of that study believe that it might provide an impetus for further research aimed at understanding the socioeconomic factors that contribute to the perceived value of innovations, and much is being done to reach this importance. There is an urge for changes, and technical improvements are continuously released.

Regarding the advances made by MRI in recent years, one special "senior" advanced sequence has had a continuous improvement of its applications: diffusion imaging. Diffusion-weighted imaging was first used for acute stroke in the early to mid 1990s, what had changed and revolutionized the management of those patients. Over the following years, its application in neuroradiology improved, and acquisition techniques have evolved since then alongside the implementation of more powerful, homogeneous, and linear gradients with greater stability, which provide a higher quality of diffusion imaging. New insights have been added to diffusion imaging, which enable us to get functional and even microstructural information through new forms of acquisition and postprocessing of the diffusion imaging, such as diffusion tensor imaging and tractography. Thus, the clinical applications have been increased not only in the clinical role of neuroimaging but also

in the analysis of other parts of the body, including the spine, breast, body, bones, and even the thorax and the heart.

These fundamental assumptions were determined for the selection of the theme. The intent of this issue of *Magnetic Resonance Imaging Clinics of North America* is to provide the readers with an updated view of the current clinical applications of diffusion imaging, or those that may soon have mainstream clinical application. Thus, the topics were chosen in order to provide an overview of the technical and clinical issues related to the role of diffusion imaging. Furthermore, we also point out exciting new applications in the main body systems.

From the data presently available, one may conclude that diffusion imaging is able to provide information with regards to diagnosis, staging of the disease, treatment planning, response to treatment, as well as management of patients. Nevertheless, there are many challenges still unresolved. It is precisely these challenges that place and sharpen the human intelligence to seek answers and technological advances.

The topics herein published are devoted to the acquisition of information that could benefit physicians in different clinical practices and also in the academic field. The articles adhered to conquer this meaning by following this ideal, trying to cover

Magn Reson Imaging Clin N Am 19 (2011) xi–xii
doi:10.1016/j.mric.2010.11.002

all the body systems, starting with some information regarding imaging techniques. Therefore, we will follow the journey from the neurological, and head and neck applications going through the thorax, including heart and breast, as well as the abdomen and pelvis. Finally, the musculoskeletal system and a special topic addressing monitoring treatment response are also included. I hope that the readers will find the articles informative, entertaining, and provocative, helping them in their daily questions.

I wish to express my sincere gratitude to all the authors, who range from well-known to young and brilliant radiologists, for their invaluable contribution, allowing this project to become a reality. I would also like to thank Romeu Domingues, MD, for his encouragement and enormous contribution to my career. I do not have words to express my thankfulness to Suresh Mukherji, MD, Consulting Editor, for the privilege of being chosen and for placing his trust in me to captain this project.

I have tried hard to make you proud of the results coming from all the sweat deposited on these pages. Thanks must also be given to Barton Dudlick and Joanne Husovski, series editors, for their guidance, patience, and encouraging support throughout the process of preparation of this issue.

Last, and by no means least, I want to dedicate this conquest to my parents, Luiz Celso and Leonice, as well as to my wife, Simone, for their support and understanding during all the processes of making this work.

L. Celso Hygino Cruz Jr, MD
CDPI and IRM - Ressonância Magnética
Rua Capitão Salomão, 44
Botafogo, Rio de Janeiro
CEP 22290-240, Brazil

E-mail address:
celsohygino@hotmail.com

Basic Concepts of MR Imaging, Diffusion MR Imaging, and Diffusion Tensor Imaging

Eduardo H.M.S.G. de Figueiredo, BSc[a],*,
Arthur F.N.G. Borgonovi, BSc[b,c], Thomas M. Doring, MSc[d,e]

KEYWORDS
- Magnetic resonance imaging • Diffusion-weighted imaging
- Diffusion tensor imaging

BASIC PHYSICS OF MAGNETIC RESONANCE

Magnetic resonance (MR) imaging stems from the application of nuclear magnetic resonance (NMR) to radiological imaging. The adjective "magnetic" refers to the use of magnetic fields and "resonance" refers to the need of matching the frequency of an oscillating electromagnetic field to the "precessional" frequency of the spin of some nuclei in a tissue molecule.[1]

Interest in medical diagnostic possibilities of NMR began in 1971, with the study by Damadian[2] of the differences in relaxation times T1 and T2, among different tissues, and between normal and cancerous tissues.[3] In 1973, the imaging area for MR started with pioneering articles published by Lauterbur[4] and Mansfield and Grannell,[5] when the idea of spatial varying magnetic fields to give the localization information was first introduced.

The phenomenon of magnetic resonance is based on the interaction between external magnetic fields and nuclei, which have a nonzero magnetic moment. According to classical theory of electromagnetism, individual nuclear moments called spins in a static magnetic field B_0 precess with Larmor frequency w_0 about B_0. A bulk of spins forms the net magnetization vector pointing along B_0. When radiofrequency (RF) is applied in this system at Larmor frequency, the spins absorb the radiofrequency energy and the net magnetization vector flips by a certain angle in relation to B_0. The net magnetization vector can be decomposed into 2 components, a longitudinal component parallel to B_0 and a transversal component perpendicular to B_0. As the transversal component precesses around a receiver coil, it induces a current in that coil, in accordance with Faraday's law of induction. This current becomes the MR signal.[6]

After stopping sending RF to the spins system, the MR signal decays mainly via 2 processes: loss of phase between spins and energy release to the environment. The loss of phase between spins can occur due to interaction spin-spin, and this process is described as T2 relaxation, or it can occur due to B_0 inhomogeneities, described as T2* relaxation. In both ways, the transverse component of net magnetization vector decreases and even though there is energy in the system, the

[a] GE Healthcare, Avenida das Nações Unidas, 8501, 3 andar, 05425-070, São Paulo, São Paulo, Brazil
[b] Hospital das Clínicas, Avenida Dr. Enéas de Carvalho Aguiar, 255, 3 andar, 05403-900, São Paulo, São Paulo, Brazil
[c] Hospital do Coração, Avenida Dr. Enéas de Carvalho Aguiar, 255, 3 andar, 05403-900, São Paulo, São Paulo, Brazil
[d] Federal University of Rio de Janeiro, Avenida das Américas, 4666, grupo302A, Barra da Tijuca, Rio de Janeiro, Rio de Janeiro, Brazil
[e] Clínica de Diagnóstico por Imagem, Avenida das Américas, 4666, grupo302A, Barra da Tijuca, Rio de Janeiro, Rio de Janeiro, Brazil
* Corresponding author.
E-mail address: eduardo.figueiredo@ge.com

Magn Reson Imaging Clin N Am 19 (2011) 1–22
doi:10.1016/j.mric.2010.10.005

mri.theclinics.com

MR signal decays. The interaction between spins and the environment they insert, called spin-lattice interaction and described as T1 relaxation, causes the spins that form the net magnetization vector to release their energy, and its longitudinal component grows back along the B_0 direction.

The tissue relaxation characteristics are expressed in image contrast and are controlled by the pulse sequence chosen. The "pulse sequence" is a sequence of RF pulses, magnetic field gradient pulses, signal sampling, and time periods between them. RF pulses are basically responsible for excitation of spins and their manipulation to obtain a signal echo. Magnetic field gradients are responsible for selecting the slice to be imaged, spatially encoding the signal induced in receiver coils, using frequency and phase as location information and in some pulse sequences, gradients also control the image contrast. Spin echo and gradient echo are examples of pulse sequences that control image contrast, by applying RF pulses or gradient pulses, respectively.

Although tissue relaxation characteristics are the main source of contrast information, MR images can represent other aspects of the biologic architecture. Random thermal motion of spins in a gradient field causes a phase shift of their transverse magnetization with respect to static spins, and can be used as a source of contrast using proper pulse sequence. To better understand this mechanism of image acquisition, a brief overview of MR physics is presented in this article.

Magnetic Resonance Concepts

MR imaging works because, in the presence of an external magnetic field, one can measure the interaction between protons in human body and the external magnetic field itself. Protons interact with the external magnetic field, due to an intrinsic magnetic characteristic called spin. The classical view of spin is the effect of one charged particle—a proton, for example—spinning around itself, which creates a magnetic moment pointing perpendicularly toward a spinning axis (**Fig. 1**). In the presence of an external magnetic field, this proton behaves similarly to a magnetic bar, tending to align to the field and precesses around it.

When we are dealing with individual protons, we need to look at them through "quantum mechanical glasses," and "not-so-intuitive" thoughts are permitted under this treatment. A not-intuitive behavior is that this proton can align in either a parallel or an antiparallel orientation to the external magnetic field. There is a difference of energy between a parallel and an antiparallel state, and if this exact amount of energy is matched by an

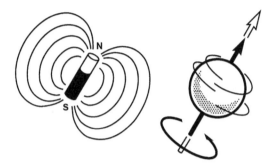

Fig. 1. In the classical view, a charged particle with spin can be compared as a magnetic dipole such as a bar magnet. (*Courtesy of* GE Healthcare, São Paulo, Brazil.)

incident radiation and is delivered to the proton, it absorbs this energy and changes from one state to another. This phenomenon is called magnetic resonance. The difference of energy states depends on the magnitude of the external magnetic field B_0 where this proton is inserted, and is expressed in terms of the Larmor equation (1) as:

$$w_0 = yB_0 \qquad \textbf{(1)}$$

In equation (1), w_0 is the frequency needed from the incident electromagnetic field to match the energy difference between states of nuclei, with the gyromagnetic constant y in the presence of an external magnetic field of amplitude B_0. The gyromagnetic constant y is an important nucleus characteristic. Human body abundance and proper gyromagnetic constant make hydrogen nuclei (H^+) the best choice for magnetic resonance imaging.

But in MR imaging, we are not dealing with a single spin and instead of a quantum mechanics view, a classical treatment can be used to understand MR imaging physics. In a classical mechanics view, spins in the presence of an external magnetic field B_0 start to precess around B_0, with an angular frequency w_0 (**Fig. 2**). The precessional frequency is given by the same relationship expressed in quantum mechanics treatment, the Larmor equation.

The sum of many spins rotating around B_0 forms the magnetization vector M that points in the same direction as B_0. When RF wave in resonance frequency w_0 irradiates the bulk of spins, the quantum effect of states transition is analogous to flip the vector M by a certain angle in relation to B_0. If RF in resonance frequency is applied by a certain time that flips the vector M 90°, this RF pulse is said to be a "90° RF pulse." The same nomenclature applies to a "180° RF pulse."

Consider the following experiment: a bulk of spins in the presence of external magnetic field B_0. At this time, the equilibrium time, vector M,

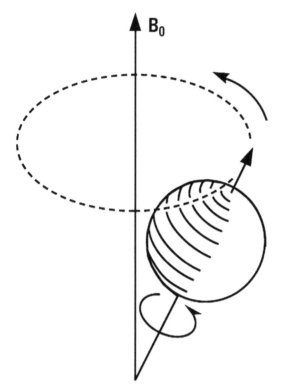

Fig. 2. Precession of spin axis around B_0. (*Courtesy of GE Healthcare, São Paulo, Brazil.*)

possesses only the longitudinal component M_z. A 90° RF pulse is applied. After turning RF off, vector M has only the transversal component M_{xy} and under the influence of B_0 starts to precess around it. At this time, vector M induces current in the receiver coil, according to Faraday's law of induction, and generates the MR signal (**Fig. 3**). When it passes through the receiver coil a maximum signal is obtained, and when it is the farthest from the coil a minimal signal is obtained. Plotting signal versus time, a sinusoidal function is to be expected.

But instead of a simple sinusoidal function, a sinusoidal function with amplitude decrease over time is obtained (**Fig. 4**). The signal represented in **Fig. 4** is called FID (free induction decay), which decays due to a process known as relaxation.

Relaxation Effects

Signal relaxation is a result of loss of phase between spins and energy release to the environment where spins are inserted. Immediately after a 90° RF pulse, all spins that form the M_{xy} vector are pointing in the same direction, and they are said to be "in phase." Turning RF off, they are set free to precess around B_0, and they precess with an angular frequency according to the Larmor equation. The first problem is that not all spins feel the same static field, due to B_0 inhomogeneities, and as they feel differently, they precess with different frequencies. This difference causes a loss of phase between them and after some time carrying out vector addition, it can be understood why the signal vanishes (**Fig. 5**). This process is called T2* decay or T2* relaxation, and effects of this nature can be restored once it is not a random effect but a scanner characteristic.

The same loss of phase described here can happen even though scanner B_0 homogeneity is perfect. Spins that form vector M_{xy} can interact with each other, feeling the tiny magnetic field of neighboring spins, in addition to B_0, and each spin starts to precess with a different frequency, resulting in the same loss of phase caused by B_0 inhomogeneities. The central difference is that this loss of phase cannot be recovered once thermal motion of spins is random. This process is called T2 relaxation or T2 decay. T2* and T2 decay express exponential behavior (see **Fig. 4**) and are modeled in terms of transversal components of vector M.

Another source of signal decay is spins giving up energy, which are absorbed by an RF pulse to the

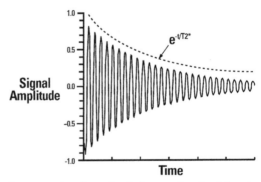

Fig. 4. MR signal amplitude (proportional to M vector magnitude) as function of time. The exponential damped sine function is called FID and is characterized by relaxation effect. (*Courtesy of* GE Healthcare, São Paulo, Brazil.)

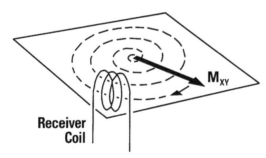

Fig. 3. In the transversal plane, rotating magnetization vector M induces current in receiver coil according to Faraday's law of induction. (*Courtesy of* GE Healthcare, São Paulo, Brazil.)

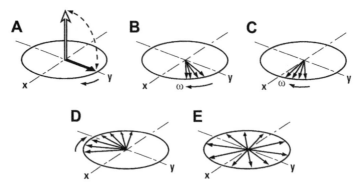

Fig. 5. Signal loss due to dephasing between spins, caused by T2* and T2 relaxation. (*Courtesy of* GE Healthcare, São Paulo, Brazil.)

environment. In terms of magnetization vectors, vector M_{xy} decreases and M_z increases over time, until all energy has been released and the vector M has only a longitudinal component (**Fig. 6**), returning to equilibrium. The energy exchange is governed by the interaction between spins and the lattice, and it is called T1 decay or T1 relaxation.

T1, T2, and T2* are tissue properties, and are measured in seconds (T2* carries B_0 inhomogeneities information, caused by the tissue and the scanner). T1 is the time needed for M_z to achieve approximately 63% of its initial value, after a 90° RF pulse. T2 and T2* are the times taken for M_{xy} to achieve approximately 37% of its initial value, after a 90° RF pulse, T2* being measured taking into account inhomogeneity effects and T2 being measured taking into account only spin-spin interactions. Image contrast contains all relaxation effects, but usually they are weighted in one effect, meaning that differences in the gray scale mostly represent differences in tissue relaxation

properties. Image weighting is controlled by pulse sequences.

Pulse Sequences

In the circumstance whereby the external magnetic field is not particularly uniform, dephasing between spins caused by field inhomogeneities are the main source of signal loss. Fortunately, this effect can be reversed by a well-known RF pulse sequence called the "spin echo method."

The spin echo sequence is based on the application of 2 RF pulses: a 90° RF pulse (or excitation pulse) followed by a 180° RF pulse (or refocusing pulse). The 90° RF pulse tips all spins that form the vector M into a transversal plane and immediately after they reach the plane, they are in phase and M_{xy} has its maximum amplitude. After turning the RF pulse off, spins start to precess and lose phase by T2* relaxation effects. The 180° RF pulse is applied after a time t, defined as t = TE/2 (t is set equal to 0 at the time the first 90° RF pulse is applied), rotating the spins by 180° in relation to the position they were in. At the end of refocusing the pulse application, the spins localization remains in the transversal plane, but "faster" spins with higher precessional frequency are put behind "slower" spins with lower precessional frequency. The accumulated phase between spins caused by field inhomogeneities through the time from t = 0 seconds to t = TE/2 seconds is compensated after a 180° RF pulse at the time t = TE seconds (called echo time), TE/2 seconds after refocusing pulse. The whole picture is better understood in **Figs. 7** and **8**.

The realignment of spins is called spin echo. It is possible to apply many refocusing pulses after a 90° RF pulse, collecting many spin echoes as shown in **Fig. 8**. B_0 inhomogeneities are canceled in this method, because they are static in time, and

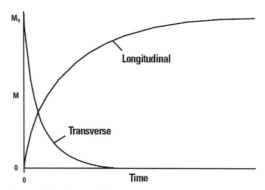

Fig. 6. The decay of transverse magnetization occurs by means of T2 and T2* effects, while recovery of longitudinal magnetization reflects energy transference to the environment. (*Courtesy of* GE Healthcare, São Paulo, Brazil.)

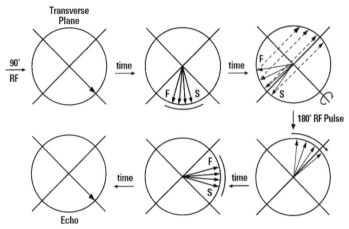

Fig. 7. The mechanism of spin echo with application of 180° RF pulse. (*Courtesy of* GE Healthcare, São Paulo, Brazil.)

the same B_0 inhomogeneity that spins feel before refocusing pulse they also experience after it. But spin-spin interactions are not static in time and T2 decay cannot be avoided. The longer the time a spin echo is collected, the stronger a T2 relaxation effect is presented.

Another important figure in pulse sequence is the repetition time TR, the time between 2 excitation pulses. In the spin echo sequence, TR is the time between 2 90° RF pulses applied in the same location.

TR and TE are the main parameters in spin echo sequence used to control contrast image weighting. Signal is acquired in echo time t = TE, and according to parameters set in the sequence, the spin echo received in the receiver coil will express differences among tissues, regarding proton density (PD), and T2 or T1 relaxation.

Consider 2 different magnetization vectors, M_a and M_b, possessing different PD, T1, and T2 properties. At equilibrium state, M vector magnitude depends on PD available in the tissue. A 90° RF pulse is applied in the system, and M_a and M_b relay into the transversal plane. Dephase between spins starts at different rates, and a refocusing pulse is applied at TE/2 to provide a spin echo at TE. If

TE is short enough, T2 differences will not be relevant and the signal induced in the receiver coil will mostly represent PD properties. To fulfill this requisite, TR must be kept long enough, to allow M vectors to recover all their longitudinal magnetization and so that T1 differences will not influence M_{xy} vector after the next excitation pulse (**Fig. 9**). Therefore, PD-weighted images acquired with a spin echo sequence are obtained by using long TR and short TE.

If a T2-weighted image is desired, a long TR is needed to avoid T1 influence through excitation pulse repetitions, but TE must be adequate to reflect T2 relaxation differences in signal amplitudes acquired (**Fig. 10**). The optimal TE to optimize contrast between M_a and M_b is the time when the difference between transverse magnetization of M_a and M_b is larger. Therefore, T2-weighted images acquired with a spin echo sequence are obtained by using long TR and adequate TE.

To acquire T1-weighted images, a short TE is needed for a signal echo not to reflect T2 differences. After applying the first excitation pulse, M_a and M_b remain in a transversal plane and dephasing between spins is caused by T2*

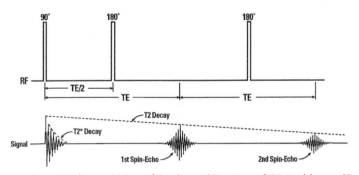

Fig. 8. A spin echo experiment with acquisition of 2 echoes. (*Courtesy of* GE Healthcare, São Paulo, Brazil.)

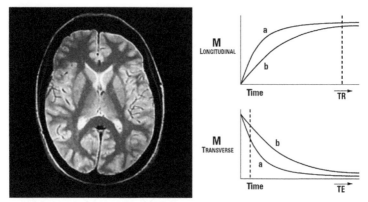

Fig. 9. Proton density—weighted image acquired using long TR and short TE. (*Courtesy of* GE Healthcare, São Paulo, Brazil.)

relaxation effects. The refocusing pulse is applied at a short TE/2 time and the first echo acquired represents PD differences. Then, T1 relaxation effects become significant and M_z recovery starts to M_a and M_b. In order that all the following echoes represent T1 differences, TR must be adequate and optimize T1 image contrast between M_a and M_b, and the next excitation pulse must be applied at the time when longitudinal magnetization M_a and M_b is larger (**Fig. 11**). Therefore, T1-weighted images acquired with spin echo sequences are obtained by using adequate TR and short TE.

Gradient echo (GRE) is another important pulse sequence that, instead of using RF pulses to refocus spins, uses a gradient pulse, referring to a controlled linear change of magnetic field strength during a short period. The gradient is characterized by its amplitude, representing how much field strength has changed in a certain distance, and its polarity, representing the direction of the change in field strength.

In a GRE experiment, an excitation and 2 gradient pulses are applied with different polarities and duration. The first gradient pulse is applied after the excitation pulse. While the first gradient is turned on the magnetic field amplitude changes regarding spatial location, and spins precess at different frequencies according to the Larmor equation, causing a certain phase accumulation between them, and the signal diminishes. The first gradient is then turned off and the second gradient is turned on, with the same amplitude and different polarity. Spins forced to precess slower than that feeling B_0, in the presence of the first gradient, now are forced to precess faster in the presence of the second gradient and, after some time, the accumulated phase between spins is compensated by inducing a signal echo generated by a gradient: a "gradient echo."

B_0 inhomogeneities are not canceled in this method, because a gradient echo is acquired by manipulating the magnetic field, and the magnetic field felt by spins at the application of the first

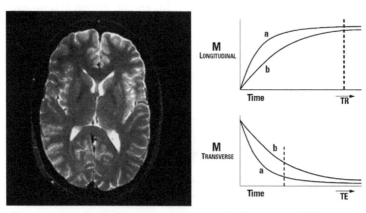

Fig. 10. T2-weighted image acquired using long TR and adequate TE. (*Courtesy of* GE Healthcare, São Paulo, Brazil.)

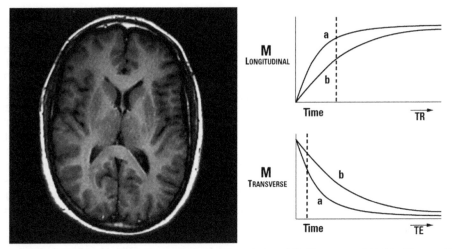

Fig. 11. T1-weighted image acquired using adequate TR and short TE. (*Courtesy of* GE Healthcare, São Paulo, Brazil.)

gradient is not the same in the presence of the second gradient.

Frequency and Phase Encoding

Pulse sequences are not used just to obtain different image contrasts but also to manipulate the spins and form an image. This manipulation is performed by turning gradients on and off, inducing phase and frequency for the spins, and using these properties as spatial information. GRE pulse sequence is used in the following explanation of image formation.

In a GRE pulse sequence, after the emission of excitation pulse, a gradient called "readout gradient" is applied, firstly with a negative polarity (to sample high frequencies of symmetric signal) and afterwards with a positive polarity to place spins in phase and read the echo. When this readout gradient, also known as frequency encoding gradient, is applied, H$^+$ spins precess at different frequencies at the same time the axis gradient was applied (**Fig. 12**).

Although the signal induced in the receiver coil contains all frequencies emitted by the tissues, there is a mathematical tool called Fourier transform (**Fig. 13**) that decomposes this signal in phases and frequencies. With the frequencies contained in the signal and the previous knowledge of the readout gradient amplitude applied, it is possible to correlate signal frequency and spatial location toward an applied gradient.

Unfortunately, it is not possible to apply the same strategy in the other axis, because it would change the spins frequency twice and only the last result would be obtained. To apply another gradient in other direction simultaneously would not be a solution, because magnetic fields would

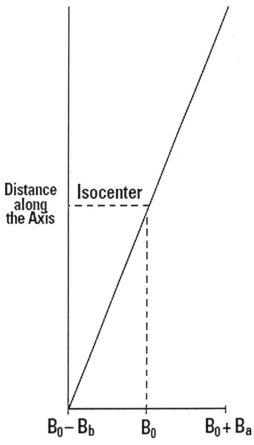

Fig. 12. During the application of a gradient, the magnetic field is modified linearly across the application direction. This change in magnetic field implies a change in precessional frequency, according to the Larmor equation. (*Courtesy of* GE Healthcare, São Paulo, Brazil.)

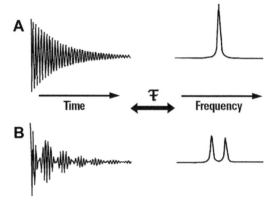

Fig. 13. The Fourier transform indicates the frequencies contained in the signal.

be vector summarized and just one frequency gradient would result. To solve this problem, phase information of spins is used. This information is added by applying a gradient called the "phase-encoding gradient" before the readout gradient and perpendicular to it. The phase-encoding gradient is kept for a short period to modify the magnetic field in the gradient direction, and during this short period spins precess at different frequencies according to equation (1). When the phase-encoding gradient is turned off, spins precess at the same frequency again, but they keep the phase memory acquired in the presence of the gradient (**Fig. 14**). The accumulated phase between spins depends on the gradient amplitude and duration.

In the sampling time, each part of the subject to be imaged will possess a bulk of spins with different phase and frequency information, making possible the image formation. The pulse sequence cycle must be repeated until K-space is filled in a proper way to form the final image.

K-Space and Acquisition Time

After frequency and phase encoding, a continuous signal emitted by the object to be studied is received by the receiver coil and sampled by the equipment, becoming a discrete signal. The signal sampled is converted in voltage and organized in the K-space, which holds the raw data of the image. As the signal is encoded in phase and frequency, both are the coordinates of K-space (**Fig. 15**). The inverse Fourier transform of K-space signal magnitude is the usual magnetic resonance image, thus a good coverage of K-space is needed to guarantee a reasonable image quality.

Pulse sequence controls K-space coverage. The phase-encoding gradient indicates the starting line in K-space to signal sampling, and the frequency-encoding gradient indicates the sampling direction on this line. Refocusing pulses to echo acquisition inverts the sampling direction.

The number of sampled points in K-space must be higher or equal to the number of pixels that compose the final image, thus pulse sequence must be repeated n times, varying the phase-encoding gradient amplitude to the entire coverage of K-space, where n corresponds to the matrix value in the phase direction; this is the first factor that hampers image acquisition time. The frequency encoding does not have a significant impact in acquisition time, because it takes the readout gradient duration (on the order of milliseconds). Nevertheless, the phase encoding to receive one echo depends on the application of one RF pulse, and TR must be taken into account for image contrast. Therefore, TR and phase-encoding steps are primarily the main aspects that affect image acquisition time, and usual methods that optimize acquisition time are multislice acquisition (excitation of multiple slices inside

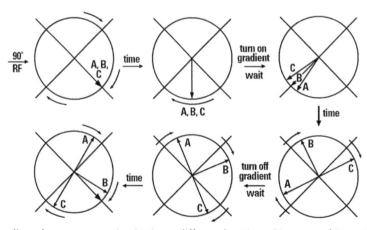

Fig. 14. Phase-encoding scheme representing 3 spins at different locations. (*Courtesy of* GE Healthcare, São Paulo, Brazil.)

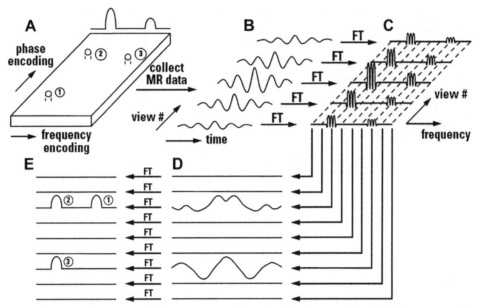

Fig. 15. Image formation by phase and frequency encoding using Fourier transform. (*A*) Slice representation with 3 vials of water. (*B*) Spin echo acquired from the entire slice with different phase encoding. (*C*) Fourier transformation of the signal. (*D*) A new data set is assembled from the columns in (*C*). (*E*) Inverse Fourier transform of (*D*) produces the image. (*Courtesy of* GE Healthcare, São Paulo, Brazil.)

a TR) and acquisition of multiple phase-encoding steps inside a TR, using either RF pulses or readout gradients, between phase-encoding steps.

INTRODUCTION TO DIFFUSION MR IMAGING
Principles and Concepts

Diffusion refers to the transport of gas or liquid molecules through thermal agitation randomly, that is, it is a function of temperature above 0 K. In pure water, collisions between molecules cause a random movement without a preferred direction, called Brownian motion. This movement can be modeled as a "random walk," and its measurement reflects the effective displacement of the molecules allowed to move in a determined period. The random walk is quantified by an Einstein equation: the variance of distance is proportional to $6Dt$, where t is time and D is the proportionality constant called the diffusion coefficient, expressed in SI units of m^2/s.

According to Fick's law, diffusion also occurs from a region of higher concentration to a lower concentration.

In biologic tissue, there is a high probability that water molecules interact with structures such as cell membranes, macromolecules that reduce or impede its motion (**Fig. 16**). Water exchange, between intracellular and extracellular compartments, as well as the shape of extracellular space

and tissue cellularity, affects diffusion. In this case, the term apparent diffusion coefficient (ADC) represents the measured diffusion constants and is commonly reported in cm^2/s or mm^2/s.

Isotropy and anisotropy
Isotropy means uniformity in all directions. A drop of ink placed in the middle of a sphere filled with water spreads over the entire volume, with no directional preference. If the same experiment is repeated in a sphere filled with uniform gel the restriction is increased as compared with free water, but is still isotropic, as the restriction is the same in all directions.

Anisotropy implies that the property changes with the direction. If a bundle of wheat straw with the fibers parallel to each other is placed inside a glass of water, the ink will face severe restriction in the direction perpendicular to the fibers and facilitated along the fibers. This bundle is highly anisotropic (**Fig. 17**).

Diffusion-Weighted Imaging

MR image contrast is based on intrinsic tissue properties and the use of specific pulse sequences and parameter adjustments. The image contrast is based on a combination of tissue properties and is denominated "weighted," as the contribution of different tissue properties are present, but one of them is more expressive than the others.

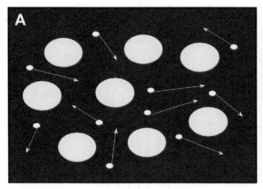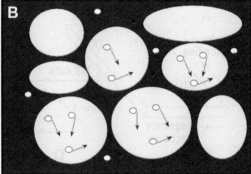

Fig. 16. (*A*) Water molecules travel by "random walk" more freely than (*B*), as the freedom of this movement is reduced by barriers as cell membranes. The diffusion in (*B*) is restricted as compared with (*A*). Finally, ADC (*B*) is less than ADC (*A*). (*Courtesy of* GE Healthcare, São Paulo, Brazil.)

Routine acquisitions have some degree of diffusion influence that is actually quite small. Some strategies have been developed to make diffusion the major contrast contributor, and dedicated diffusion-weighted imaging (DWI) sequences are available nowadays on commercial scanners, as well as several others as investigational sequences that may or not be available in clinical practice.

Diffusion sensitization scheme

Stejskal and Tanner[7] introduced a method to image and quantify DWI with MR imaging in 1960, which was implemented in routine practice by Le Bihan and colleagues[8] in 1986. The sequence was based on a spin echo sequence that has symmetric diffusion sensitizing gradients inserted before and after the 180° refocusing pulse (**Fig. 18**). The idea is as follows.

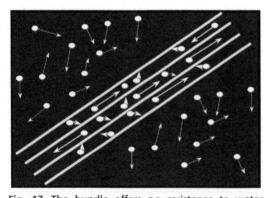

Fig. 17. The bundle offers no resistance to water molecules in the diffusion direction parallel to the fibers but there is a severe restriction if perpendicular. In this case there is preferred water molecule direction due to anisotropy. Outside the bundle, the water molecules are in an isotropic environment and have no preferred direction. (*Courtesy of* GE Healthcare, São Paulo, Brazil.)

Static water spins will experience a precise dephase induced by the first diffusion sensitizing gradient lobe. The 180° pulse will cause a phase compensation for the external field inhomogeneities. The second lobe will rephase the water spins at the same amount they were dephased, as the area is exactly the same and spins were in the same position. Therefore, the signal of the stationary water spins echo is maintained as practically unaltered.

However, moving water spins will be in a different position, so they will not be rephased at the same amount by the second lobe, and the echo will have a reduced signal. The degree of water motion is proportional to the signal attenuation.

The diffusion-sensitizing gradients can be applied to x, y, or z axes, as well as in a combination of them. This direction is called the diffusion-sensitizing direction.

The Stejskal-Tanner scheme can be applied on top of pulse sequences as spin echo, but the most used nowadays is in combination with spin-echo

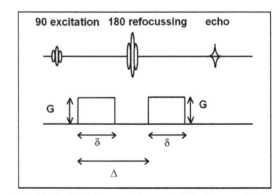

Fig. 18. Stejskal-Tanner Scheme: 2 diffusion-sensitizing gradients inserted before and after 180° RF refocusing pulse using precisely controlled duration and distance. G, amplitude; δ, duration of the sensitizing gradient; Δ, time between the 2 sensitizing gradient lobes.

echo-planar imaging (SE-EPI). A combination with fast spin echo sequence takes longer, but is less sensitive to distortions and susceptibility artifacts than EPI.

Other strategies are also available but are less used in routine practice, as many others are in the research environment and become commercialized eventually.

Diffusion-weighting factor

The sensitivity of the diffusion sequence to water motion can be varied by changing the gradient amplitude, the duration of the sensitizing gradients, and the time between the gradient pair.

The diffusion-weighting factor is named b-value and for the Stejskal and Tanner[8] sequence the value is given in units of s/mm^2 by (2):

$$b = \gamma^2 . G^2 . \delta^2 (\Delta - \delta/3) \qquad (2)$$

where γ is the gyromagnetic ratio, G is the strength of the diffusion-sensitizing gradients; δ is the duration of the gradient pulse, and Δ is the time interval between these gradients. A higher b-value is achieved by increasing the gradient amplitude and duration and by widening the interval between the gradient lobes. In most applications, the gradient amplitude is maximized and the gradient duration and interval changed to control the b-value.

The T2 shine-through phenomena

The signal intensity observed in a diffusion-weighted image can be expressed as:

$$S_{(TE,b)} = PD \left(e^{-TE/T2} \right) \left(e^{-bD} \right) \qquad (3)$$

where S is signal intensity, k is a constant; PD is proton density, TE echo time, D diffusion coefficient, and b the b-value.

As TR (repetition time) is usually long (5000–15,000 ms) and, in case of single shot scans, TR is virtually infinite, T1 contamination is minimal or null. TE is usually kept as low as possible, usually 60 to 100 ms; therefore, the DWI may suffer from T2 contamination if long T2 components are present. This phenomenon is called the "T2 shine-through artifact" and may cause misinterpretation as the signal may be artificially hyperintense or isointense. Parametric ADC maps are used to quantify diffusion, and are insensitive to T2 shine-through artifacts.

Intravoxel incoherent motion

Intravoxel incoherent motion (IVIM) is the random movement of the water inside a voxel, and causes the signal to decay. One example is blood inside tortuous capillary vessels, where the measured diffusion coefficient will be overestimated and fall into the ADC denomination, instead of D. In 1988

Le Bihan and colleagues[9] proposed the name IVIM, instead of diffusion imaging, and D^* as the pseudo-diffusion coefficient dependent on capillary geometry and blood velocity, estimated to be 10 times larger than the diffusion coefficient of water. For high b-values, the perfusion effects are significantly reduced and diffusion information remains. For low b-values, the combined effect of perfusion and diffusion is present. As IVIM measurement involves the acquisition of several small b-values,[10] eddy currents must be well compensated, and motion and single-shot EPI diffusion must be used with high-performance gradients.

Echo-Planar Diffusion-Weighted Sequence

Echo-planar is an ultrafast acquisition, in which all K-space is sampled extremely fast. Although proposed by Peter Mansfield in 1978,[11] it was implemented in routine practice in the 1990s, when high-performance gradients and enhanced analog-to-digital converters, image reconstructors, and support electronics became available. It is fast, robust, and widely available on most scanners today, but it is also sensitive to susceptibility effects that cause artifact and image distortions. The distortion degree depends on several imaging parameters, as well as magnetic susceptibility and field strength.

EPI principles

The EPI strategy to reduce acquisition time is to collect several echoes, with phase and frequency encoding, after the RF excitation pulse, the same way as fast spin echo, but instead of producing an echo train using RF 180° refocusing pulses, EPI uses a series of oscillation gradient reversals that have both positive and negative polarities, to generate "odd" and "even" echoes that take significantly less time to be generated (**Fig. 19**).

EPI can be implemented using different modes such as SE-EPI (spin-echo EPI) or GRE-EPI (gradient-echo EPI), depending on the use of an RF echo or a gradient echo before the EPI echo train. It can collect all echoes needed to acquire an image by using one excitation pulse (single-shot EPI), or splitting into separate shots. SE-EPI is used in conjunction with diffusion-sensitizing gradients, called EPI-DWI, and the single-shot approach is mostly used.

EPI sequences are sensitive to the so-called off-resonance effects of water and fat spins: fat spins accumulate a huge phase shift, proportional to time, in collecting all echoes in a given TR and the frequency distance between water and fat. The effect occurs in the phase direction, and the image of fat can be typically displaced by pixels and is

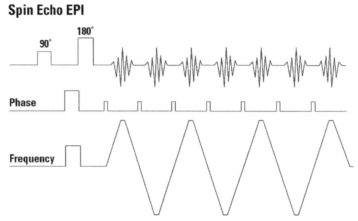

Fig. 19. After a 90° excitation pulse and 180° refocusing pulse is applied, positive-negative gradient oscillations generate frequency-encoded echoes, and the phase encoding is provided by the "blipped" phase encoding gradients. In this case there is an echo train length of 7. (*Courtesy of* GE Healthcare, São Paulo, Brazil.)

increased at higher field strengths. Therefore all EPI sequences, in practice, are fat-suppressed, and different methods can be employed such as spatial-spectral fat suppression, frequency-selective fat suppression, or even short-tau inversion recovery (STIR) in combination with EPI-SE.

The sampling period is typically the "flat-top" part of the readout gradient (**Fig. 20**A). Water spins also accumulate phase shifts in areas near tissue-air or tissue-bone interfaces, which cause disruptions in the local field, and the results are mild to severe distortions depending on the field strength, gradient performance, and sequence parameters (compare **Fig. 20**B with C). The longer the sampling time to collect the echo, the more time water spins accumulate phase shift and the worse is the distortion. The echo spacing is the time from the middle of the echo top to the middle of the next, and is directly related to the degree of the distortions. The shorter the echo spacing, the

less the distortions; this concept is important to optimize sequence parameters and achieve the best results.

High-performance gradients using appropriate acquisition parameters improve EPI image quality significantly (see **Fig. 20**C).

EPI-DWI practical aspects

A common implementation of EPI-DWI acquires 3 separate orthogonal acquisitions with diffusion sensitization in each main gradient direction (X, Y, Z), which are automatically averaged into a final combined image (**Fig. 21**). Usually, 2 b-values are acquired, the first of which is generally b = 0 and is called "T2 image," as no diffusion contribution is present and it is the same as a T2-weighted EPI image. Different implementations allow the acquisition from a single to several b-values in the same scan, at the expense of acquisition time. Respiratory and cardiac compensation can be used to

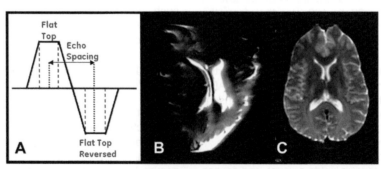

Fig. 20. (*A*) Detail of the oscillating readout gradient echo spacing. Reduction of echo spacing greatly reduces distortion. (*B*) Single-shot EPI with 256 frequency matrix, resulting in severe distortion in the phase-encoding direction on a low-performance gradient of 10 mT/m with 17 T/m/s slew rate. (*C*) Single-shot EPI with 256 frequency matrix, with a gradient of 33 mT/m with 120 T/m/s slew rate. (*Courtesy of* GE Healthcare, São Paulo, Brazil.)

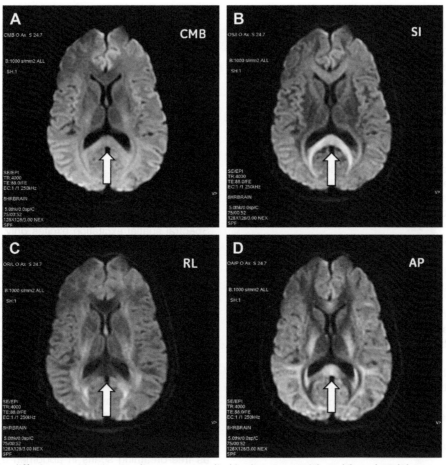

Fig. 21. The diffusion sensitization gradients were applied in directions SI (*B*), RL (*C*), and AP (*D*). Image (*A*) is the average of (*B*), (*C*), (*D*), and is usually denominated combined or "isotropic" image. The white arrow points to splenium of corpus callosum that has restricted diffusion in the SI direction, is facilitated in the RL direction, and has mixed pattern in the AP direction. Combined image (*A*) minimizes the anisotropy effects of the individual images.

minimize motion artifacts, as well as parallel imaging and optimized application of diffusion gradient schemes to improve signal-to-noise ratio and reduce artifacts.

The main sequence parameters are summarized as follows.

Choice of sensitizing directions and combined image The number of sensitizing directions and orientation used depends on the kind of information needed and the isotropic/anisotropic behavior of the structure being studied.

If the goal is to identify areas of altered diffusion in a structure that is normally isotropic, and considering the altered area is also isotropic, one direction would be enough. In this case, the total acquisition time is reduced to a single acquisition per b-value.

A more complex scenario is presented if the object of study and/or the expected altered area of interest are anisotropic. It is important to remember that the diffusion sensitization gradient will affect spins moving along its direction only. Organs such as the brain, kidneys, and muscles have important anisotropy, as others have a more isotropic behavior. This scenario is exemplified in **Fig. 21**: the splenium of the corpus callosum shows restricted diffusion in the SI (superior-inferior) direction (see **Fig. 21**B) and is facilitated in the RL (right-left) direction (see **Fig. 21**C), because of the orientation of the fibers that induces strong directional diffusion dependence. Notice the low-bright pattern in the AP (anterior-posterior) as the inverted "V" disposition of the fibers. In this instance, acquiring diffusion imaging, sensitized in the 3 directions, and averaging them into one combined image is the most used strategy (see **Fig. 21**A).

b-Value The b-value provides diffusion weighting for DWI images as TE provides T2 weighting for T2 images.

The higher the b-value, the more diffusion-weighted the image will be at the cost of signal-to-noise ratio (SNR). As b-value is increased, a structure of lower ADC loses signal faster than structures of higher ADC, and the contrast is increased. If the lower ADC regions have the signal decreased from a certain threshold, the combined image may exhibit increased signal from restricted water motion, due to anisotropy. An example is given in **Fig. 22**.

If the b-value is high enough, only structures with very low ADC will show up and higher ADC structures will fade into the noise floor; this approach can be used as "background suppression" and increase sensitivity. As the minimum TE is increased with the b-value, relatively short T2 tissues such as liver and muscle may be suppressed because of T2 effects rather than diffusion, and this should be taken in account regarding choice of diffusion sequence parameters.

Low b-values have intrinsically high SNR; however, IVIM effects become important and should be taken into consideration. An interesting property is that flow is suppressed, and "black-blood "imaging can be performed (**Fig. 23**).

Receiver bandwidth Receiver bandwidth (rBW) controls the number of frequencies that are detected. The higher the rBW, the shorter the

"flat-top" or readout time, and the fewer the distortions present (**Fig. 24**). Therefore, higher rBW is preferable for EPI-DWI studies.

Frequency direction Echo-planar acquisitions are sensitive to water off-resonance spins in the areas of soft tissue/air/bone interface. With a proper choice of frequency direction, the distortion is more symmetric (**Fig. 25**). Axial plane is the most commonly used acquisition plane with EPI and frequency RL direction.

Fat suppression Due to the large chemical shift, all EPI-DWI acquisitions should be fat-suppressed or fat-saturated. The choice of the method to be employed depends more on the region to be studied. Spectral spatial excitation excites only the water spins on a slice-by-slice basis, instead of the whole volume. Chemical shift selective applies a spectral saturation pulse over the fat spins, but it may be less effective than spectral spatial excitation once the fat saturation pulse is applied over the entire volume. STIR is a good option for a large field of view (FOV), off-center acquisitions, or areas where the other techniques may fail, such as brachial plexus.[12]

Number of measurements The data are acquired several times and averaged into one image, then used to build more SNR, allowing the acquisition of thinner slices and longer b-values at the expense of acquisition time. If motion is present as free-breathing scans in abdomen and chest, some degree of blurring is expected, as the structures are not in the same position in each acquisition and are averaged out. Small structures and

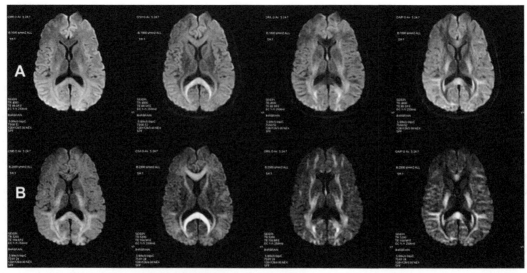

Fig. 22. From right to left the sensitization directions are: combined, SI, RL, and AP. Row (*A*) b = 1000 s/mm², TE = 88 ms; Row (*B*) b = 2500 s/mm², TE = 104 ms.

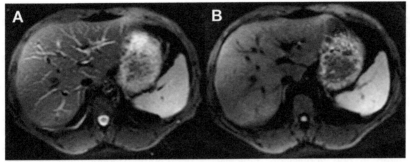

Fig. 23. Diffusion is inherently a black-blood image. Image (*A*) b = 0 s/mm², usually named "T2 image," and Image (*B*), usually named "diffusion image," have b = 90 s/mm².

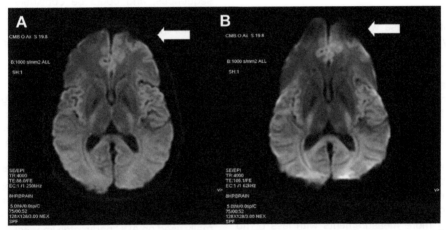

Fig. 24. (*A*) High rBW = ±250 kHz, (*B*) Low rBW = ±62 kHz; both at 3 T field strength. Distortion is reduced using high bandwidth. The unit of the receiver bandwidth can change between vendors, as peak to peak or Hz/pixel, and lead to mistakes if protocol parameters are copied without proper adjustment.

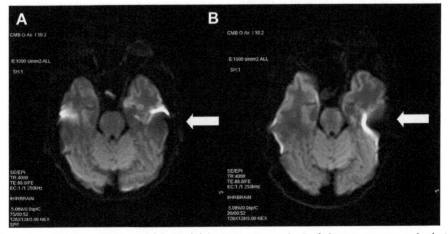

Fig. 25. Frequency direction (*A*) RL and (*B*) AP. (*A*) is more symmetric. Both images were acquired at 3 T field strength.

motion-ghosting artifacts may not show up in the final image as well, due to averaging.

The use of one single acquisition may require adjustment of other parameters, as increased slice thickness or lower acquisition matrix to compensate for the reduced SNR.

Repetition time The number of slices available and acquisition time are proportional to the TR. A TR of 3000 ms is enough to minimize T1 effects and can be as long as needed to accommodate all slices required in one acquisition, typically 5000 ms. Reduced TR acquisition with reduced number of slices can be used to shorten breath-hold time in expiration, but multiple acquisitions are necessary to cover the entire volume, and each group of slices may not be perfectly aligned.

Echo time The TE should be as short as possible and should increase with the b-value. Reduced frequency matrix and the use of parallel imaging decrease the echo spacing, and therefore the minimum TE.

In cases where multiple b-value acquisitions and ADC quantification are needed, it is suggested to use the TE corresponding to the highest used b-value and keep it constant in all other acquisitions of b-values.

Respiratory/cardiac trigger Respiratory trigger synchronizes the acquisition with the respiratory movement, by acquiring data in the expiration phase, reducing movement artifacts, and allowing the use of more measurements with less or no blurring, besides improving lesion detection as compared with breath-hold.[13] It is mostly used for imaging the chest and upper abdomen. Total acquisition time is increased, as only part of the respiration/cardiac cycle is used. The effective TR depends on the respiratory frequency and can be increased using more respiration cycles, to accommodate the number of slices. Cardiac motion is a known source of artifacts (**Fig. 26**)

and can be minimized with cardiac triggering and appropriate trigger delay,[14] but again at the expense of time.

Parallel imaging Parallel imaging plays an important role in EPI-DWI, as the distortion and short T2 blurring are reduced at the expense of SNR. This feat is accomplished by omitting lines of the K-space and increasing the distance between them, just like reduced-phase FOV, but eliminating wrap-around artifacts that use special algorithms and need some K-space reference lines. As such this could be either a separate mask acquisition or a built one, and rely on different coil element sensitivity. Because susceptibility effects are enhanced at higher field strengths, parallel imaging is routinely used at 3 T, in combination with EPI sequences, and could be considered optional, but is recommended at 1.5 T. Other benefits of parallel imaging are increased number of slices for the same TR and reduction of acquisition time.

ADC measurement and ADC maps

The diffusion images have a T2 weighting contamination, and long T2 regions may present an artificial signal enhancement, such as the T2 shine-through artifact. This sign can be removed using exponential images (**Fig. 27**C) that are simply the diffusion image (see **Fig. 27**B) divided by b = 0 image (see **Fig. 27**A), or by using parametric images where the contrast reflects the calculated ADC (see **Fig. 27**D). Gray scale is normally used on ADC parametric images: dark representing low ADC values and bright representing high ADC values. Color scale can be used with low ADC in red and high ADC in blue as a mnemonic for free water, using different colors between the 2 extreme thresholds. However, there is no standard for the use of color scale, and it may be confusing if not properly explained.

In general, ADC (or D depending on the definition) is calculated using b = 0 and another b that

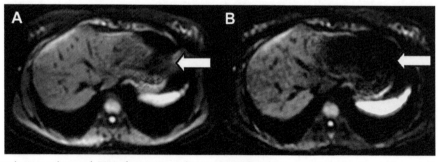

Fig. 26. Respiratory-triggered DWI, but not cardiac triggered. White arrows indicate cardiac motion artifact. (A) b = 150 s/mm^2 and TE = 54 ms; (B) b = 600 s/mm^2 and TE = 68 ms.

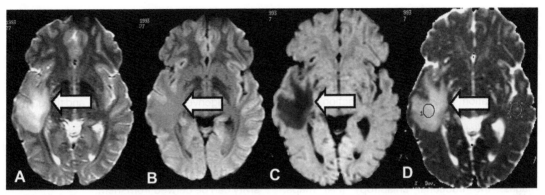

Fig. 27. Example of T2 shine-through effect and correction using exponential and parametric ADC maps: White arrow indicates bright signal on T2 image (*A*), isointense signal on diffusion image (*B*). The exponential map (*C*) has the T2 shine-through artifact removed and the expected low signal of facilitated diffusion is present. The parametric ADC map (*D*) demonstrates high ADC value as a bright region and enables quantification of ADC.

can vary, depending on the organ studied, usually between 600 s/mm^2 and 1000 s/mm^2.

Keeping the TR and TE the same and changing only the b-value, ADC can be calculated using the equation (4):

$$ADC = \ln(S_1/S_0)/(b_1 - b_0) \qquad (4)$$

where S_0 is the signal intensity with the b-value = 0 and S_1, the signal intensity with b-value = b. A monoexponential behavior is assumed.

In the context of research or clinical trial, a more precise estimation can be made using multiple b-values, and in this case, a more complex analysis is necessary because of the microcirculation influence.[9,10,15]

A plot of a multi b-value acquisition in a liver is exemplified in **Fig. 28**: respiratory trigger and b-values of 0 to 1000 s/mm^2. Notice the fast decay in the first part of the curve (b-values 0–100 s/mm^2), due to increased effects of microcirculation and

a slower decay in the second part (b-values 200–1000 s/mm^2), due to increased effects of diffusion.

The low range of b-values from 10 to 200 s/mm^2 may be used to study fast diffusion and is characterized by perfusion parameters D^* (or ADC_{fast}) and f (fraction of volume of water flowing in capillaries). High b-values between 200 and 1000 s/mm^2, or higher, are used to study slow diffusion parameters D (or ADC_{slow}). The term global diffusion is used when b = 0 and b > 200 s/mm^2, and is characterized as ADC_{global}.

The quantification of ADC in moving organs or in the path of its influence is challenging, and the use of free breathing, respiratory triggering, or breath-hold may lead to different results and are under investigation.[16,17]

In summary, diffusion is used as a source of contrast for many different applications in the body, and gives insights on the pathologies by visual inspection. Also, there is a growing number of investigations using quantification; the total process is not completely understood, and a standardization of the acquisition and quantification is yet to be established.

Another aspect of diffusion, the anisotropy, is the study object of diffusion tensor imaging (DTI), which is now discussed.

DIFFUSION TENSOR IMAGING

DTI[18] is based on diffusion-weighted images that investigate the fiber architecture of several regions in the human body as for example of the brain white matter or muscle fibers of the heart. In contrast to DWI, a diffusion tensor $\underline{D}$ (a 3 × 3 matrix) is calculated for each voxel, instead of only one numerical value (such as the ADC), and it enables the possibility to investigate anisotropic

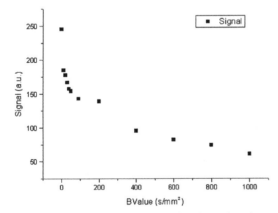

Fig. 28. Signal intensity versus b-value plot from a multi–b-value study on a liver. The signal decays faster between b = 0 and 100 s/mm^2.

diffusion. Anisotropic diffusion means that the water molecules are moving in a specific direction at a specific rate, whereas isotropic diffusion means that the molecules move at equal rates in all directions. This tensor is able to fully describe the molecular mobility along each direction and the correlation between these directions.[18] To achieve this directional information, additional diffusion-weighted images along several gradient directions, using diffusion-sensitized MR imaging pulse sequences, have to be collected. After the postprocessing of the raw diffusion-weighted images, the fractional anisotropy (FA) maps, mean diffusivity (MD), eigenvectors, radial diffusivity, and so forth are calculated, derived from the diffusion tensor.

Physical Basics and Definitions

DWI and DTI use the mathematical model of free diffusion, which is described in physics by the "first Fick's law of diffusion." It can be written as:

$$J = -D\nabla c \qquad (5)$$

where J is the flux density, ∇c the concentration gradient, and D the diffusion coefficient.

When diffusion occurs in the imaged volume, there will be attenuation, A, on the MR signal, which depends on D and on the "b-factor," which characterizes the gradient pulses used in the MR imaging sequence:

$$A = \exp(-bD) \qquad (6)$$

In anisotropic media, the diffusion coefficient depends on the direction of diffusion. Leaving DWI and going to DTI, the diffusion coefficient D has to be substituted through a diffusion tensor $\underline{D}$ (a 3 × 3 matrix).

$$\underline{D} = \begin{pmatrix} D_{xx} & D_{xy} & D_{xz} \\ D_{yx} & D_{yy} & D_{yz} \\ D_{zx} & D_{zy} & D_{zz} \end{pmatrix} \qquad (7)$$

To determine the diffusion tensor one must, as mentioned before, acquire diffusion-weighted images in several gradient directions. In a next step, it is necessary to estimate the entries of the matrix $\underline{D}$ from the set of diffusion-weighted images. As the tensor is symmetric, only 6 different gradient directions are necessary together with one acquisition with no diffusion weighting (b = 0) resulting in a total of 7 acquisition. Using more diffusion directions, it is not necessary, but of advantage, to cover the space more uniformly along many directions, especially for fiber orientation mapping.

Eigenvectors and eigenvalues, mean diffusivity, fractional anisotropy, radial diffusivity, and axial diffusivity

The entries of the tensor reflect average diffusion and degree of anisotropy in each voxel. It is important to determine the main directions of diffusivities, called eigenvectors, in each voxel, and the diffusion values, called eigenvalues, associated with these directions. The eigenvalues represent the diffusion coefficients in the main directions of diffusivities of the medium (**Fig. 29**). Most common parameters, such as MD, FA, radial diffusivity, and axial diffusivity can be derived from them.

The MD gives an overall measure of the diffusion in a voxel or region. It can be calculated from the trace of the diffusion tensor:

$$MD = Tr(\underline{D})/3 = (D_{xx} + D_{yy} + D_{zz})/3 \qquad (8)$$

In the literature, the eigenvalues D_{xx}, D_{yy}, and D_{zz} are often called λ_1, λ_2, and λ_3.

The FA is a measure of the degree of the diffusion anisotropy. The FA values range from 1 (anisotropic diffusion = "directed") to 0 (isotropic diffusion = "not directed").

It can be calculated from:

$$FA = \frac{\sqrt{(D_{xx} - D_{yy})^2 + (D_{yy} - D_{zz})^2 + (D_{zz} - D_{xx})^2}}{\sqrt{2(D_{xx}^2 + D_{yy}^2 + D_{zz}^2)}}$$

$$(9)$$

The diffusivity along the main axis, D_{xx}, is also called axial diffusivity (or parallel diffusivity).

The average diffusivity $(D_{yy} + D_{zz})/2$ of the 2 minor axes is called radial diffusivity.

Visualization of the Tensor Model: the Ellipsoid Model

As the tensor data cannot be simply displayed in one image through gray-scale information or color coding, the diffusion ellipsoid approach has been presented.[19] The ellipsoid is a tridimensional representation of the diffusion distance in space, which the water molecules can reach. In the ellipsoid the x, y, and z axes represent the main diffusion direction in the voxel, corresponding to the direction of the fibers. The eccentricity of the ellipsoid provides information about the degree of anisotropy. This way, an anisotropic diffusion in any direction would be represented as a pole and an isotropic diffusion as a sphere (see **Fig. 29**).

Besides those representations, it is common to visualize FA and MD values in a gray scale or on a direction-coded color map (**Fig. 30**). Their values can be directly measured on these maps with

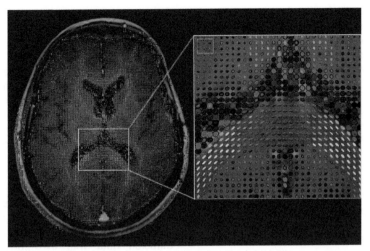

Fig. 29. (*Left*) The ellipsoid model overlaid on a conventional T1 image. (*Right*) The ellipsoid becomes a sphere in areas where no main diffusion directions exist: isotropic diffusion; and the ellipsoid becomes a pole with one main direction where the diffusion is anisotropic.

region of interest (ROI) tools provided by the software manufacturers.

Interpretation

In the brain, the mobility of the water molecules can be limited through obstacles, for example, the cellular membrane. Especially in the nerve fibers, the molecules can only move freely along the length of the axons and can only move short distances perpendicularly across the length. When interpreting diffusion tensor data, the basic

idea is that the direction of the highest diffusion coefficient represents the course of the nerve fiber.

Tractography

The reconstruction of nerve fiber tracts of DTI data is called tractography. This technique is based on connecting voxels in order to build a whole fiber to investigate the fiber architecture in the brain. There are 2 major approaches in tractography: deterministic and probabilistic tractography. With deterministic tractography, the reconstructed fibers

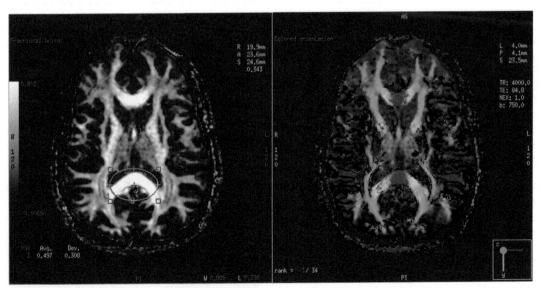

Fig. 30. (*Left*) Gray scale FA map, where the intensity value divided by 1000 corresponds to the FA value. Example: mean intensity value of the ROI of 831 corresponds to an FA of 0.831 in this ROI. (*Right*) FA map where the direction is color-coded.

result from the most likely directions in each voxel, whereas probabilistic fiber-tracking methods use probability distributions to draw several sets of different directions, this way repeating the stream-lining process multiple times.

High Angular Resolution Diffusion Imaging

The diffusion-tensor model describes the behavior of diffusion in a voxel correctly only when the diffusion has one main direction. When nerve fibers cross with others or have ramifications, this model is limited. As a result, over the past few years approaches have been developed that aim to use more gradient directions, in order to gain a better insight into the complex behavior of diffusion. These techniques are called high angular resolution diffusion imaging or HARDI.

Number of diffusion directions

As mentioned before, at least 6 diffusion directions are necessary to determine the elements of the diffusion tensor. But what is the impact of using more directions and the relevance for clinical application? For a robust estimation (using a b-value of 1000 s/mm²) of the FA, which was shown using a Monte Carlo technique, a minimum of 20 unique sampling directions should be used and 30 directions, at least, in the case of MD.[20]

Postprocessing and Evaluation of Diffusion-Weighted Images and Diffusion Tensor Imaging

Evaluation with manufacturers' software

Most MR manufacturers offer their own software to reconstruct the parametric maps for the diffusion parameters, such as ADC (in the case of DWI) and FA, MD, eigenvalues, and trace (in the case of DTI), that are most relevant for the radiologist. The reconstruction is normally performed in an in-line process, whereby the generations of those maps are performed automatically, immediately after running the sequence. In this way a rapid evaluation by the radiologist is possible.

Within the manufacturers' software, in general ROI-based analysis tools are available, enabling the radiologist to draw the ROI directly, such as for example the FA map, providing ROI parameters as the mean value, standard deviation, area, and minimum and maximum value. To obtain a "real" value for the diffusion parameters, sometimes a scaling factor has to be applied.

Region-of-interest based analysis is a common way to analyze, for example, differences in injured tissue with normal tissue (see **Fig. 30**).

Deterministic tractography (streamline tractography)

To reconstruct the trajectories of fibers, first at least one stream particle (seed point) has to be chosen (**Fig. 31**). Then the voxels are connected using pre-chosen calculation criteria for the tract, for example, angular threshold that determines the maximum orientation that a fiber can achieve and FA threshold that determines when the FA value falls below this threshold. Calculation for this tract can then be realized.

Advanced evaluation by third-party software

Instead of or in addition to the use of the software offered by the manufactures, or in addition to it, it is possible to realize advanced evaluation of the diffusion data with third-party software, after transferring the image volume to another workstation.

Especially for the brain, these software programs often offer additional tools that can be useful for analysis, as the image quality potentially can be improved. For instance, it is possible to apply eddy current correction algorithms in the EPI images, which take care of distortion artifacts. Also, distortions of the diffusion-weighted images caused by motion can be corrected. Especially for tractography, when one is interested in quantifying brain connectivity it may be interesting to use such software programs, because they can perform probabilistic tractography instead of more qualitative deterministic tractography offered by most MR manufacturers.

Another interesting option for institutions that are interested in clinical research is the possibility that comes with third-party software, namely the ability to carry out intersubject group analysis. The software includes tools for brain registration

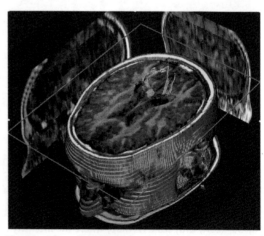

Fig. 31. After choosing a seed point the streaming of the fibers can be realized.

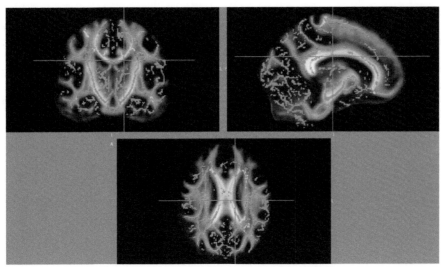

Fig. 32. Tract-based spatial statistical analysis (TBSS; FSL, Oxford, UK). In green: the main tracts (skeleton) where statistical analysis was performed. Overlaid in yellow-red: significant areas of reduction of FA, $P<.05$.

to a pre-chosen target, which may be a mean FA image of the subjects under analysis,[21] to perform voxel-based analysis of the whole brain, using brain atlases as a reference (**Fig. 32**).

REFERENCES

1. Haacke EM, Brown RW, Thompson MR, et al. Magnetic resonance imaging: physical principles and sequence design. Chichester (UK); New York: Wiley-Liss; 1999.
2. Damadian R. Tumor detection by nuclear magnetic resonance. Science 1971;171(976):1151–3.
3. Vlaardingerbroek MT. Magnetic resonance imaging: theory and practice. New York. 3rd edition. Berlin: Springer; 2003.
4. Lauterbur P. Image formation by induced local interactions: examples employing nuclear magnetic resonance. Nature 1973;242:190–1.
5. Mansfield P, Grannell PK. NMR 'diffraction' in solids? J Phys C Solid State Phys 1973;6(22):422–6.
6. Bitar R, Leung G, Perng R, et al. MR pulse sequences: what every radiologist wants to know but is afraid to ask. Radiographics 2006;26(2): 513–37.
7. Stejskal EO, Tanner JE. Spin diffusion measurements: spin echoes in the presence of a time-dependent field gradient. J Chem Phys 1965; 42(1):288–92.
8. Le Bihan D, Breton E, Lallemand D, et al. MR imaging of intravoxel incoherent motions: application to diffusion and perfusion in neurologic disorders. Radiology 1986;161(2):401–7.
9. Le Bihan D, Breton E, Lallemand D, et al. Separation of diffusion and perfusion in intravoxel incoherent motion MR imaging. Radiology 1988;168(2): 497–505.
10. Luciani A, Vignaud A, Cavet M, et al. Liver cirrhosis: intravoxel incoherent motion MR imaging—pilot study. Radiology 2008;249(3):891–9.
11. Mansfield P, Pykett IL. Biological and medical imaging by NMR. J Magn Reson 1978;29: 355–73.
12. Takahara T, Hendrikse J, Yamashita T, et al. Diffusion-weighted MR neurography of the brachial plexus: feasibility study. Radiology 2008;249(2): 653–60.
13. Taouli B, Sandberg A, Stemmer A, et al. Diffusion-weighted imaging of the liver: comparison of navigator triggered and breathhold acquisitions. J Magn Reson Imaging 2009;30(3):561–8.
14. Murtz P, Flacke S, Traber F, et al. Abdomen: diffusion-weighted MR imaging with pulse-triggered single-shot sequences. Radiology 2002; 224(1):258–64.
15. Thoeny HC, Ross BD. Predicting and monitoring cancer treatment response with diffusion-weighted MRI. J Magn Reson Imaging 2010; 32(1):2–16.
16. Nasu K, Kuroki Y, Fujii H, et al. Hepatic pseudo-anisotropy: a specific artifact in hepatic diffusion-weighted images obtained with respiratory triggering. MAGMA 2007;20(4):205–11.
17. Kwee TC, Takahara T, Koh DM, et al. Comparison and reproducibility of ADC measurements in breath-hold, respiratory triggered, and free-breathing

diffusion-weighted MR imaging of the liver. J Magn Reson Imaging 2008;28(5):1141–8.

18. Le Bihan D, Mangin JF, Poupon C, et al. Diffusion tensor imaging: concepts and applications. J Magn Reson Imaging 2001;13(4):534–46.

19. Pierpaoli C, Basser PJ. Toward a quantitative assessment of diffusion anisotropy. Magn Reson Med 1996;36(6):893–906.

20. Jones DK. The effect of gradient sampling schemes on measures derived from diffusion tensor MRI: a Monte Carlo study. Magn Reson Med 2004;51(4): 807–15.

21. Smith SM, Jenkinson M, Johansen-Berg H, et al. Tract-based spatial statistics: voxelwise analysis of multi-subject diffusion data. Neuroimage 2006; 31(4):1487–505.

Diffusion MR Imaging in Central Nervous System

Claudio de Carvalho Rangel, MD[a,b,c,*],
L. Celso Hygino Cruz Jr, MD[a,b,d,e],
Tatiana Chinem Takayassu, MD[a],
Emerson L. Gasparetto, MD, PhD[a,d,e],
Romeu Cortes Domingues, MD[a,d]

KEYWORDS

- Diffusion-weighted imaging • Tractography
- Diffusion tensor • Central nervous system • ADC map

Diffusion describes the spread of particles through random motion, also called Brownian motion. Diffusion sensitization imaging was first introduced in the mid-1960s by Stejskal and Tanner and was first used in the clinical realm in the mid-1980s by Le Bihan and colleagues. In diffusion-weighted imaging (DWI), each voxel has an intensity that reflects the single best measurement of the rate of water diffusion at that location. DWI has been used extensively in clinical practice for the early diagnosis of central nervous system (CNS) conditions that restrict the diffusion of water molecules, as in areas of cytotoxic edema observed in infarction and related conditions. It also provides information about tumor cellularity or abscesses containing viscous fluid. Diffusion tensor imaging (DTI) is actually a mathematical description (ie, the tensor) and is useful when tissue has an internal structure that creates barriers to water motion. For example, the neural axons and myelin sheath allow water molecules to diffuse preferentially along their length. In some cases, DTI can detect brain lesions before any conventional imaging. Tractography gives directional information that can be exploited at a higher structural level to select and follow neural tracts through the brain. This modality is used mainly in planning surgery for tumors and to assess white matter integrity in various other pathologic conditions.

ISCHEMIC CNS LESIONS

Stroke

Stroke involves a rapid onset of neurologic impairment and is the leading cause of adult morbidity and mortality in the developed world. The major cause of stroke is arterial ischemic impairment, followed by intracranial aneurysm rupture and hemorrhage. Stroke is an urgent health issue because the sooner the patients are treated the less brain damage occurs. Imaging studies play a central role in the initial evaluation of patients who have had a stroke.[1]

Nonenhanced computerized tomography (NECT) is an accessible and rapid technique that is usually the first to be performed in suspected

The authors have nothing to disclose.

[a] Clínica de Diagnóstico por Imagem, Avenida das Américas, 4666, sala 325, Barra da Tijuca, Rio de Janeiro, CEP: 22649-900, Brazil
[b] IRM—Ressonância Magnética, Rua Capitão Salomão, 44, Botafogo, Rio de Janeiro, CEP: 22271-040, Brazil
[c] Department of Radiology, Hospital Central da Policia Militar, Rua Estácio Sá, 20 – Estácio, Rio de Janeiro, Brazil
[d] Clínica Multi-Imagem, Rua Saddock de Sá, 266, Ipanema, Rio de Janeiro, Brazil
[e] Department of Radiology, Federal University of Rio de Janeiro, Av. Brigadeiro Trompowisky, S/Nº - Ilha do Fundão, Rio de Janeiro, Brazil
* Corresponding author. Clínica de Diagnóstico por Imagem, Avenida das Américas, 4666, sala 325, Barra da Tijuca, Rio de Janeiro, CEP: 22649-900, Brazil.
E-mail address: cdcrang@gmail.com

Magn Reson Imaging Clin N Am 19 (2011) 23–53
doi:10.1016/j.mric.2010.10.006
1064-9689/11/$ — see front matter © 2011 Published by Elsevier Inc.

cases of acute stroke. NECT detects hemorrhages and other conditions that mimic symptoms of stroke and typically reveals a cortical-subcortical hypodense area within a vascular territory.[2] Conventional MR imaging may depict an acute and subacute infarct as a hypointense area on T1-weighted imaging (WI) and a hyperintense area on T2-WI, but it fails to differentiate between acute stroke and other lesions (**Fig. 1**). However, DWI has the best sensitivity and specificity for the diagnosis of stroke.[3]

Acute stroke causes cytotoxic edema, which decreases water molecule diffusion, leading to a hyperintense area on DWI compared with normal brain tissue. To interpret the diffusion-weighted images, it is important to correlate them with apparent diffusion coefficient (ADC) maps, which should show the region as a dark area when true restriction occurs (**Fig. 2**). Abnormalities can be seen as a reduced ADC as early as 30 minutes after the onset of ischemia, which decreases to a minimum ADC at 3 to 5 days and then increases to baseline levels by 1 to 4 weeks. This evolution is caused by vasogenic edema and further gliosis, leading to increasing extracellular water content.[4] Some areas of moderately low ADC (<15% of normal) escape from infarction, a phenomenon known as DWI reversal.[5]

While DWI is useful to identify irreversibly infarcted tissue, perfusion-weighted MR imaging is capable of identifying areas of reversible ischemia by quantitative and qualitative evaluations of cerebral blood volume, cerebral blood flow, and mean transit time. Cerebral tissue has a vascular autoregulatory mechanism that, in the context of ischemia, causes a hypoperfused peripheral area (ie, decreased blood flow) with no DWI abnormalities, indicating that there is a potential to rescue the affected brain area. The ischemic area surrounds a central core of irreversible ischemia that has both decreased blood volume and restricted diffusion. This mismatch area is called penumbra, and when it occurs, thrombolytic therapy should be considered.[6]

To summarize, DWI is an important tool for diagnosing and evaluating acute ischemic events. Further studies have been developed to determine the ideal selection of patients for thrombolytic treatment based on imaging data rather than on the time of stroke onset alone.

Posterior Reversible Encephalopathy Syndrome

Posterior reversible encephalopathy syndrome (PRES) is a neurotoxic state that occurs in several complex conditions (eg, chemotherapy, autoimmune disease, organ and bone marrow transplants, and preeclampsia/eclampsia). PRES has a unique pattern of brain vasogenic edema, often widespread, but predominating in parietal and occipital regions. On an ADC map, patients with PRES show areas of high signal intensity, indicating vasogenic edema. Such vasogenic edema might be expected to cause decreased signal intensity on DWI relative to the surrounding brain. In reality, however, DWI findings are most often remarkably normal despite obvious abnormalities on conventional MR imaging and ADC maps (**Fig. 3**).[7] These areas of edema usually reverse

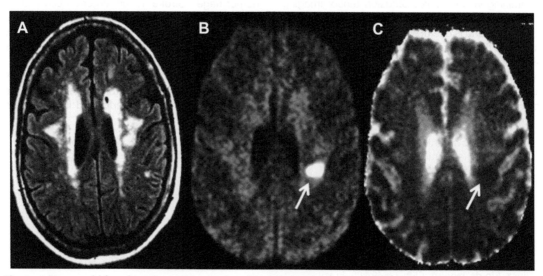

Fig. 1. A 63-year-old female patient with a stroke with right facial palsy for 1 week. FLAIR (*A*) shows hyperintense lesions in the deep white matter. DWI (*B*) and ADC mapping (*C*) show a focal area of restricted diffusion, compatible with ischemic stroke (*arrows*).

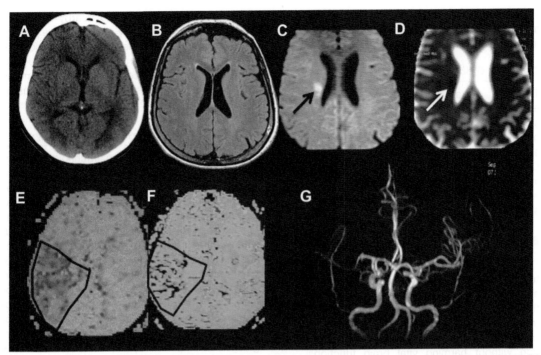

Fig. 2. A 67-year-old female patient with stroke with 2 hours of left hemiparesis. Axial CT (*A*) and axial FLAIR (*B*) show no abnormalities, but a small area of restricted diffusion (*C* and *D arrow*) suggests an infarct. Dynamic susceptibility contrast-MRI (DSC-MRI) maps, time to peak (*E*) and relative cerebral blood volume (*F*) show the penumbra area (*demarcated line*) with potential salvable ischemic tissue. Three dimensional time of flight MR imaging (*G*) reveals reduced flow in the right middle cerebral artery.

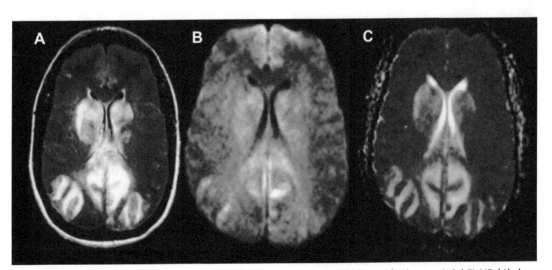

Fig. 3. A 30-year-old pregnant woman with PRES with eclampsia, headache, and seizures. Axial FLAIR (*A*) shows confluent areas of edema and hyperintense signal in the basal ganglia and posterior parieto-occiptal regions. DWI (*B*) and ADC map (*C*) suggest that the major portion of the lesion correspond to vasogenic edema.

completely, following the prompt treatment. Focal areas of restricted diffusion are uncommon and may be associated with an adverse outcome.[8]

Transient Global Amnesia

Transient global amnesia (TGA) is a sudden episode of anterograde memory loss with no other signs of impaired cognitive functioning, lasting no more than 24 hours and having no long-term sequelae. The cause of TGA is unknown, but DWI shows small punctate hyperintense lesions in the lateral aspect of the hippocampus (**Fig. 4**), which are most apparent at 48 hours after the symptom onset.[9]

BRAIN TUMOR

DWI has been used extensively to evaluate brain tumors, including grading, differential diagnosis, and postoperative evaluation. DTI can illustrate the relationship of a tumor with the main fiber tracts nearby.[10] The most desirable approach to brain tumors patients is complete lesion ressection without harming vital brain functions.[11,12] Thus, a preoperative approach that maps the

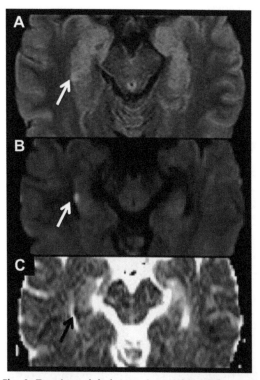

Fig. 4. Transient global amnesia. Axial FLAIR (*A*), DWI (*B*), and ADC map (*C*) show a focal area of hyperintensity with restricted diffusion localized in the lateral aspect of the right hippocampus (*arrows*).

tumor and its relationship to nearby functional structure, even imperfectly, may improve patient outcomes.[13] Although these new applications of DTI have not yet been demonstrated or even widely studied in multicenter clinical trials, many individual practitioners are nonetheless using them.

Epidermoid Tumor Versus Arachnoid Cyst

DWI is used to differentiate an arachnoid cyst from epidermoid tumors (**Fig. 5**).[14] Both lesions present the same signal intensity, characteristic of cerebrospinal fluid (CSF), on conventional T1-WI and T2-WI. On DWI, epidermoid tumors are hyperintense because they are solidly composed, whereas arachnoid cysts are hypointense, demonstrating high diffusivity.[14] The ADC values of epidermoid tumors are similar to those of the brain parenchyma or may be slightly reduced by tumor contents.[15] On the other hand, ADC values of arachnoid cysts are high, similar to those of CSF.[16] DWI can also be used to improve postsurgical follow-up of epidermoid tumor cases because it has been proved to be efficacious in the detection of residual lesions.[17]

Characterization of Intracranial Cystic Masses

DWI can also provide a sensitive and specific method for differentiating a tumor from abscesses because abscesses have a hyperintense signal on DWI and a reduced ADC within the cavity.[18–21] This restricted diffusion is probably related to the high viscosity of the pus, which may lead to reduced water mobility, lower ADC, and high signal intensity on DWI.[22] On the other hand, necrotic and cystic tumors display a low signal intensity on DWI with an increased ADC as well as isointense or hyperintense DWI signal in the lesion margins (**Fig. 6**).[20]

Tumor Grading

In certain settings, diffusion imaging seems to increase both the sensitivity and specificity of MR imaging for evaluating brain tumors by providing information about tumor cellularity, which may, in turn, improve the accuracy of tumor grading.[10,15,23–28] Diffusion of free water molecules is restricted by the increased cellularity present in high-grade lesions.[29,30] The reduction in extracellular space as well as the high nuclear to cytoplasmic ratios of some cancer cells causes a relative reduction in the ADC values.[31] In some studies, however, ADC values from high- and low-grade gliomas have overlapped somewhat.[32] Thus, evaluation of the tumor grade with diffusion

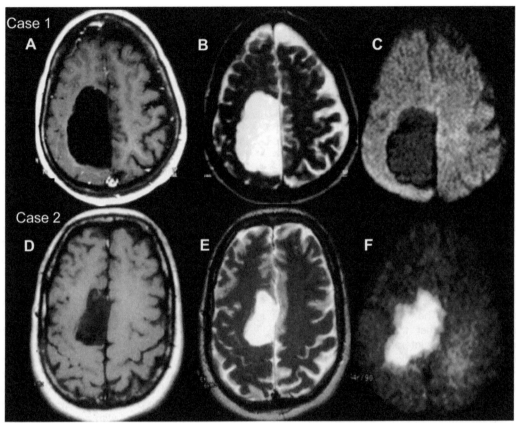

Fig. 5. In case 1, axial contrast-enhanced T1-WI (*A*), T2-WI (*B*) and DWI (*C*) show a large extra-axial cystic lesion with signal intensity similar to the CSF, as well as high diffusion, corresponding to the arachnoid cyst. In case 2, axial T1-WI (*D*), T2-WI (*E*) and DWI (*F*) show an extra-axial lesion with same features of an arachnoid cyst on conventional MRI, but with high signal intensity on DWI, which corresponds to an epidermoid tumor.

imaging remains uncertain and cannot yet be considered reliable.

DWI has also been shown to assist in assessing the high cellularity of other brain neoplasms. In some studies, lymphoma, a highly cellular tumor, has been found to present a hyperintense signal on DWI as well as reduced ADC values.[33]

DWI can play an important role in the differential diagnosis of posterior fossa neoplasms. Medulloblastoma can display a restricted diffusion,

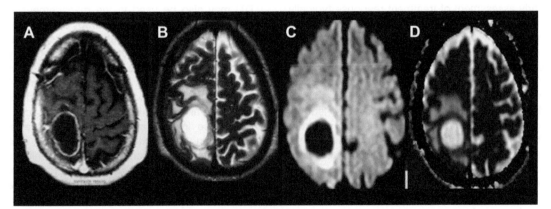

Fig. 6. Glioblastoma multiforme. Axial contrasted-enhanced T1-WI (*A*), coronal T2-WI (*B*), DWI (*C*), and ADC mapping (*D*) demonstrate a large necrotic mass with a central area of facilitated diffusion and a peripheral area of restricted diffusion.

presumably because of the densely packed tumor cells and high nuclear to cytoplasmic ratio.[34,35] The solid enhancing portion of cerebellar hemangioblastomas on postcontrast T1-WI demonstrates hypointensity on DWI and high ADC values because of rich vascular spaces.[36] Pilocytic astrocytoma usually does not present restricted or facilitated diffusion, and its ADC values seem to be similar to those of brain parenchyma.[34]

DTI has also been used as a tool to facilitate grading of brain neoplasms. To date, the additional information provided by DTI has not been shown to correlate with tumor cellularity,[37] perhaps because of the suspected high degree of fiber tract disorganization in the tumor core.[38] Nevertheless, one report has indicated that fractional anisotropy (FA) can distinguish high-grade gliomas from low-grade gliomas.[39] This study found a significant difference between the FA values when analysis was restricted to the solid portion of the lesion, eliminating the necrotic and cystic portions. The FA values in high-grade gliomas were higher than those in low-grade gliomas, which was interpreted to suggest higher symmetry of histologic organization in the former.[39] However, these results are somewhat contradictory to the traditional view of the microstructure of high-grade gliomas, which typically have pleomorphic structures and a regressive organization rather than the increase in parallel histologic organization observed in low-grade gliomas. A separate report found no differences between FA values in the tumor center in low- and high-grade gliomas, which may be consistent with the disorganization of fiber tracts in the center of both types of gliomas, resulting in a loss of structural organization.[38]

Posttreatment Evaluation

Early assessment of treatment response typically relies on imaging with contrast enhancement performed within 24 to 48 hours after the surgical procedure,[40] whereas later assessment uses evaluation of tumor size weeks to months after the conclusion of therapy.[41] The appearance of new enhanced areas often results in changes in the management approach, frequently leading to adjuvant therapy. A recent study reported the benefits of performing DWI in immediate postoperative MR imaging.[40] Areas of restricted diffusion were described adjacent to the tumor resection cavity of low- or high-grade gliomas. Follow-up MR imaging revealed that these areas resolved and showed contrast enhancement, which subsequently regressed to form an area of encephalomalacia. Because conventional MR imaging is done during this enhancement period, this finding can be easily misdiagnosed as tumor recurrence or tumor progression, which leads to an erroneous conclusion of treatment failure and unnecessary initiation of a new adjuvant therapy. Investigators have concluded that a corresponding area of restricted diffusion almost always precedes the delayed contrast enhancement described, which invariably evolves into encephalomalacia or formation of a gliotic cavity on long-term follow-up studies, representing areas of infarct, ischemia, or even venous congestion secondary to acute cellular damage.[31] Such findings are unlikely to represent early recurrence of tumor.

DWI might also serve as a marker for therapeutic response because changes in tumor water diffusion may occur after changes in cell density. In this application, ADC seemed to be a sensitive and an early predictor of therapeutic efficacy[42] when investigators prospectively compared tumor ADC values at 3 weeks after the initiation of therapy with those at pretreatment.[43] If this finding is replicated in multicenter trials, a lack of change in tumor ADC values could become a reliable indication of a failure in therapy. This indication would in turn provide an opportunity to switch to a more beneficial therapy, minimizing the morbidity associated with a prolonged and an inefficient treatment. The logic behind this methodology is that successful treatment results in extensive cell damage, leading to a reduction in cell density. The loss of cellular neoplasm results in an increase in extracellular space that can increase free water molecule diffusion. Because increases in brain tumor ADC correspond to decreases in tumor volume in long-term follow-up studies, DWI may, therefore, be an important surrogate marker for the quantification of treatment response.

DTI may also be used in the management of patients undergoing radiation therapy and chemotherapy. By providing information about the location of white matter tracts, DTI tractography could be successfully used in parallel with functional MR imaging in planning radiosurgery (**Fig. 7**). In theory, this parallel use should reduce necrosis by allowing a lower dose of radioactive tracer to be infused and a smaller volume of normal brain to be irradiated.[44] DTI may also help in the early detection of white matter injuries caused by chemotherapy and radiation therapy. One report in patients with medulloblastoma showed poorer intellectual outcome to be correlated with lower FA values, younger age at treatment, and an increased interval from the beginning of treatment.[45] The possibility of using

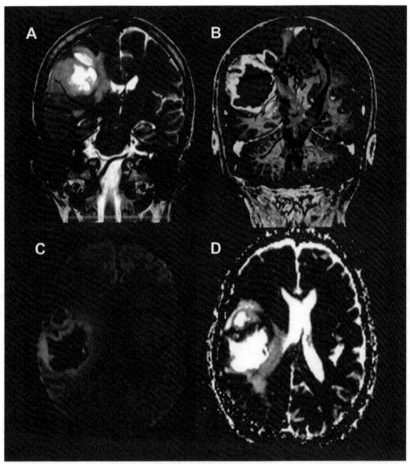

Fig. 7. A 56-year-old male with glioblastoma multiforme. Coronal T2-WI (*A*), tractography (*B*), DWI (*C*) and ADC map (*D*) show a heterogeneous mass located on the right parietal lobe. The peripheral area of the mass shows restricted diffusion, and the central area has a high diffusivity. The lesion seems to dislocate the corticospinal tract contralaterally.

FA or other DTI changes as a biomarker for neurotoxicity is extremely appealing.

INFECTIONS DISEASES
Abscess

An abscess is a pyogenic infection. Most of these infections have a bacterial origin, followed by fungal and parasitic infections. Imaging characteristics depend on the pathologic stage, and the classic appearance is the organized capsulated form. MR imaging with T2-WI may show a hyperintense lesion of liquefied necrosis and inflammatory debris with a hypointense rim of collagen wall surrounded by edema. After intravenous gadolinium administration, MR imaging reveals a nonenhanced central area of necrosis with peripheral enhancement. Daughter abscesses may be seen along the medial wall of the parent abscess.[46]

Conventional images may show similar features in cases of brain abscesses, cystic or necrotic neoplastic lesions, resolving hematomas, demyelination, and subacute infarction. The value of DWI for the diagnosis of various intracranial infections, such as abscesses, is well established, and DWI may help to distinguish infectious abscesses from mimics.[46] The core area of a pyogenic abscess is composed of viscous pus and necrotic material, which reduces water diffusion, explaining the high signal intensity on DWI images and the low signal intensity on ADC maps (**Fig. 8**). Otherwise, the core of most primary and secondary cystic or necrotic brain tumors has unrestricted diffusion and a hyperintense ADC signal. However, restricted diffusion within ring enhancement is found in various other brain diseases and is therefore not pathognomonic for brain abscess.[47] Similar characteristic feature has also been reported in other pyogenic infections,

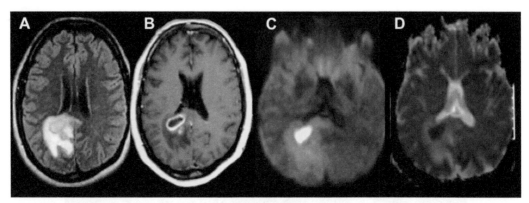

Fig. 8. Pyogenic abscess. Axial FLAIR (*A*), axial contrasted-enhanced T1-WI (*B*), DWI (*C*), and ADC map (*D*) show a round enhancing lesion surrounded by edema with a central area presenting high signal intensity on DWI and low ADC, probably due to the high viscosity of the pus.

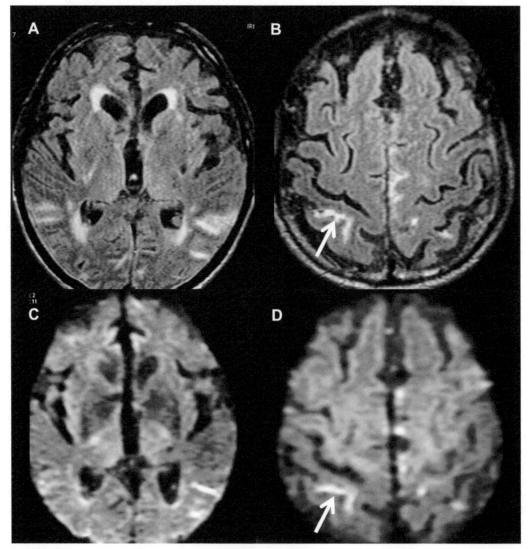

Fig. 9. Meningitis with pyogenic subarachnoid collection. Axial FLAIR (*A, B*) and DWI (*C, D*) demonstrate hyperintense signal on the subarachnoid space, which have restricted diffusion (*arrows* in *B* and *D*).

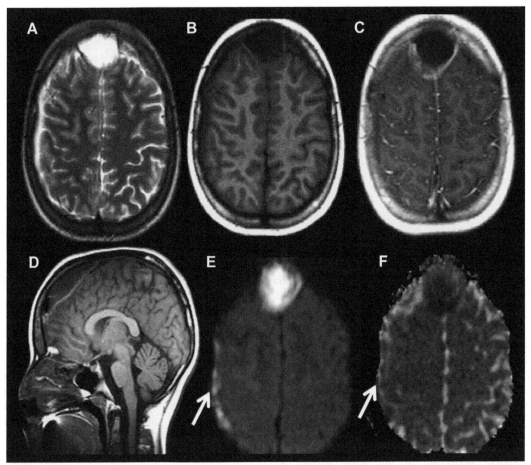

Fig. 10. An 11-year-old female with frontal sinusitis and empyema. Axial T2-WI (*A*), axial T1-WI (*B*), axial and sagittal contrasted-enhanced T1-WI (*C* and *D*), DWI (*E*) and ADC map (*F*) show an extraaxial collection in the frontal region, with restricted diffusion. Note also the small subdural empyema along the right front-parietal region, better visualized by DWI (*arrows*).

such as ventriculitis, pyogenic subarachnoid collection (**Fig. 9**), and subdural empyema (**Fig. 10**).

Septic Embolism

MR imaging shows similar changes in septic embolism and brain abscesses. The main difference in septic embolism is the presence of multiple lesions, usually bilateral with a predominantly subcortical distribution and in terminal zone of vascularization (**Fig. 11**).

Herpes Encephalitis

Herpes encephalitis is the most common cause of viral encephalitis and has a predilection for the temporal lobes. Early treatment is crucial to a positive outcome, and MR imaging may play an important role in the diagnosis.[48]

Conventional MR imaging may show bilateral and asymmetric involvement of temporal lobes with gyriform enhancement. Hemorrhage may be

seen on T1-WI, T2*gradient echo (GRE), or susceptibility weighted imaging. On diffusion-weighted images, herpes encephalitis may show a marked hyperintensity with low ADC. This restricted diffusion is explained by necrosis and cytotoxic edema (**Fig. 12**). Conventional follow-up studies often demonstrate encephalomalacic changes on initially abnormal diffusion-weighted images.

Creutzfeldt-Jakob Disease

Creutzfeldt-Jakob disease (CJD) is an infectious and potentially transmissible disease caused by a prion, characterized by rapidly progressing dementia and eventual death. Conventional MR imaging can demonstrate bilateral and usually symmetric involvement of the basal ganglia and thalami, which usually show no mass effect or contrast enhancement. Likewise, cortical and, less often, white matter involvement has been described. The primary sensorimotor cortex is usually spared, even in advanced illness.[49]

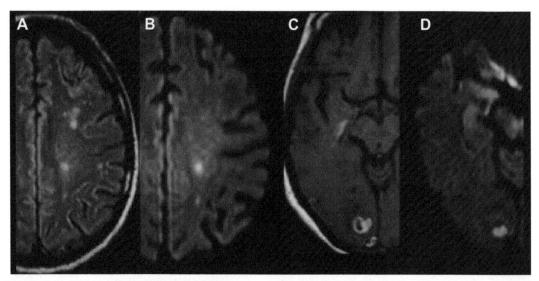

Fig. 11. In septic emboli, axial FLAIR (*A*) and contrasted-enhanced T1-WI (*C*) demonstrate bilateral contrast enhanced lesions with restricted diffusion (*B* and *D*).

A variant of CJD has characteristic MR imaging findings, such as hyperintensity in the pulvinar nucleus of the thalamus, called the pulvinar sign. The "hockey-stick" sign caused by symmetric hyperintensities in both pulvinar and medial dorsal nuclei of the thalamus has also been observed. When lesions are bilateral, the diagnosis of CJD should be highly suspected.

The sensitivity of MR imaging to detect these changes, especially in the early stages, is increased with the use of DWI. Areas of restricted diffusivity in the basal ganglia and cerebral cortex are observed soon after the onset of symptoms, preceding the appearance of changes in T2-WI and fluid-attenuated inversion recovery (FLAIR) sequences by 4 to 6 months (**Fig. 13**).[50–52] The exact mechanism is still unclear, however, it is likely related to deposition of abnormal prion protein, vacuolation, neuronal loss, and gliosis. These restricted DWI areas disappear in the more advanced stages of the disease when atrophy is observed.[50–52]

Influenza Encephalitis

The imaging features of encephalitis caused by influenza include cerebral edema; symmetric involvement of the thalamus, brain stem, and

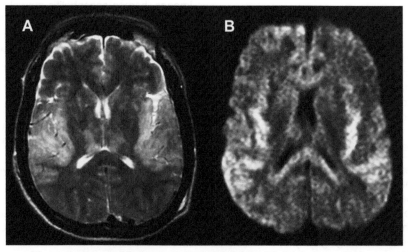

Fig. 12. In a case of herpetic encephalitis, axial T2-WI (*A*) and DWI (*B*) show areas of edema and hyperintense signal as well as restricted diffusion in both temporal lobes.

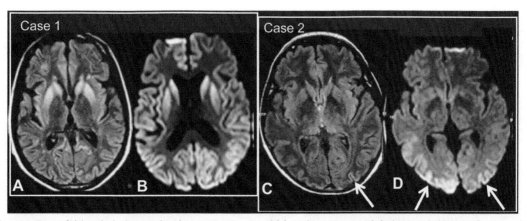

Fig. 13. Creutzfeldt-Jakob disease (CJD). Case 1: 72-year-old female patient with behavioral changes for 2 weeks. Axial FLAIR (*A*) and DWI (*B*) show abnormal areas of hyperintensity with restricted diffusion in the caudate nucleus and putamen, as well as in the cortex of the parieto-occipital lobes, consisting with the classic form of CJD. Case 2: Axial FLAIR (*C*) and DWI (*D*) show abnormal areas of hyperintensity in the cortex of both occipital lobes (*white arrows*), indicating the variant form.

cerebellum (observed as acute necrotizing encephalopathy); and diffuse areas of low signal intensity on T1-WI and mild cerebral atrophy. In addition, a lesion in the splenium of the corpus callosum may be observed as hyperintensity on T2-WI and FLAIR, associated with restricted diffusion but no contrast enhancement. This lesion resolves with improvement of clinical symptoms (**Fig. 14**).[53]

Acute Disseminated Encephalomyelitis

Acute disseminated encephalomyelitis (ADEM) is characterized by multiple lesions of moderate to large size, which are usually asymmetric, have ill-defined limits, and are located in the deep and subcortical white matter of the cerebral hemispheres and brainstem. The lesions generally do not have a mass effect, but when located in the brainstem, they can cause expansion of this structure. Some lesions may show enhancement in the acute phase (30%), presenting as a nodular form, as gyriform, or with irregular or peripheral enhancement.

Although MR imaging is sensitive in detecting these lesions, abnormalities may resolve within 1 month after the onset of symptoms. When present, spinal cord injuries are usually asymmetric and may include hemorrhage and contrast enhancement.[54] Advanced MR imaging sequences have a limited role in evaluating patients with ADEM. In some cases, there is restricted diffusion in acute injuries (**Fig. 15**). Because ADEM involves deep

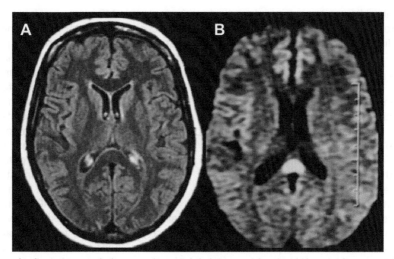

Fig. 14. In a case of influenza encephalitis, axial FLAIR (*A*) shows no abnormal changes but DWI (*B*) reveals a focal area of restricted diffusion on the splenium of the corpus callosum.

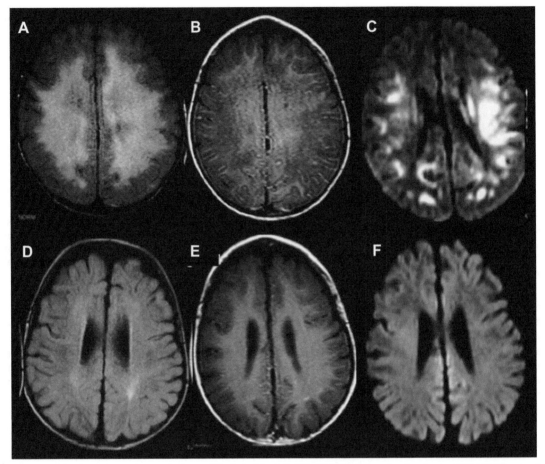

Fig. 15. Acute disseminated encephalomyelitis (ADEM). Axial FLAIR (*A*) and contrast-enhanced T1-WI (*B*) reveals a diffuse hyperintense non-enhancing lesions in the white matter of both hemispheres. DWI (*C*) demonstrates bilateral, diffuse areas of restricted diffusion. In a follow-up MRI performed 3 months later, FLAIR (*D*), contrast-enhanced T1-WI (*E*), and DWI (*F*) show significant improvement, with no areas of restricted diffusion.

and subcortical white matter, cases of cortical lesions with restricted diffusion may be more appropriately diagnosed as vasculitis.[55]

MULTIPLE SCLEROSIS

Diffusion imaging has also been applied to assess multiple sclerosis (MS), specifically the associated plaques and normal-appearing white matter (NAWM). More recently, diffusion imaging has been used to analyze the gray matter, optic nerve, and spinal cord in patients with MS.[56]

Acute plaques may show restricted diffusion, mostly at their margin. This imaging characteristic can also be useful in the differential diagnosis of MS from brain neoplasms, which can present restricted diffusion within the solid portion of the lesion, secondary to high cellularity (**Fig. 16**). Although DWI has been used to differentiate acute

from chronic MS plaques using ADC and FA, the results are discordant. Studies initially indicated that ADC is increased within MS plaques relative to normal white matter[57] and that ADC values were higher in acute than in chronic lesions.[58] The highest diffusion values were found in hypointense lesions, the so-called black holes, compared with enhancing lesions and isointense lesions.[59] More recently, other investigators have been unable to replicate differences in ADC values between the different plaque pathologies. Thus, disease activity cannot be consistently predicted based on ADC maps derived from DWI.[59]

Compared with the contralateral NAWM, MS lesions show decreased FA values on DTI (**Fig. 17**),[60] secondary to disruption of myelin and axonal structures, which leads to disorganization and increased extracellular space.[61] Conflicting results have been reported when FA values are

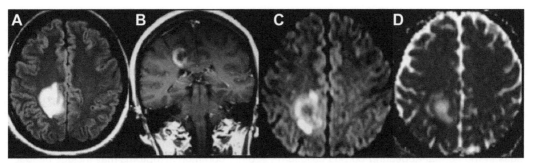

Fig. 16. Acute plaque of multiple sclerosis. Axial FLAIR (*A*), contrasted-enhanced T1-WI (*B*), DWI (*C*), and ADC map (*D*) show a focal hyperintensity, noncontinuous ring contrast enhancement lesion in the right parietal lobe. This peripheral area had restricted diffusion.

used to differentiate acute from chronic plaques. Whereas some investigators have demonstrated greater reduction of FA values in nonenhancing plaques than in enhancing plaques, suggesting that DTI can indicate disease activity,[60] others have not observed any statistically significant difference.[60,62–64]

Statistical correlations with eigenvalues may have some utility for demyelinating disorders.

Recently, demyelination was found to be correlated with a reduction in radial diffusivity values,[65,66] whereas axonal damage was shown to lead to axial diffusivity alterations.[65] Moreover, decreased radial diffusivity was observed during remyelination.[66]

The extension of disease beyond the boundaries of plaques has important ramifications for assessment because disease burden is an

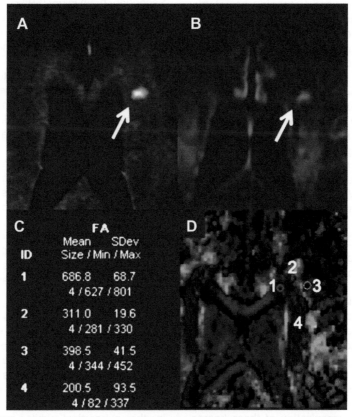

Fig. 17. Multiple sclerosis. Axial contrast-enhanced T1-WI (*A*), DWI (*B*), FA measurement (*C*), and FA color map (*D*) reveal an acute plaque (*arrows*) with enhancement and restricted diffusion in the left frontal lobe. Note the reduced FA in the NAWM surrounding the plaque (**2, 3** and **4**). Normal FA value is seen in (**1**) (*D*).

important surrogate marker of treatment response in trials of therapeutic agents. Several studies have demonstrated diffusion changes in the NAWM of patients with MS, suggesting that histopathologic abnormalities may be widespread. These diffusion abnormalities can be characterized as an increase in mean diffusivity and ADC values as well as a decrease in FA values.[60]

Some reports have also demonstrated the appearance of alterations in diffusion tensor images in the normal-appearing corpus callosum before abnormalities in other NAWM regions, which suggests a preferential occult injury in the corpus callosum.[67] The cumulative effects on the corpus callosum from wallerian degenerative changes secondary to the connecting distal white matter plaques may play an important role in the correlation of corpus callosum diffusion abnormalities and cerebral lesion load.[68]

HEAD TRAUMA

Trauma is a major cause of mortality in children and young adults. Lesions produced after a craniocerebral trauma can be divided into primary effects (eg, epidural hematoma [EDH], subdural hematoma [SDH], and chronic hematoma; subarachnoid hemorrhage [SAH]; cerebral contusion; and diffuse axonal injury [DAI]) and secondary and vascular effects (eg, herniation, cerebral edema and ischemia, brain death, dissection, and fistula).

Computed tomography (CT) is the first imaging examination conducted to evaluate head trauma because it should reveal emergencial neurosurgical lesions and identify lesions that may alter therapy. MR imaging is performed in specific cases to show lesions that are not well visualized by CT and that could explain the clinical status of patients. Both DWI and DTI have gained importance in the evaluation of traumatic brain injury.[58]

Epidural and Subdural Hematoma

EDH involves the collection of blood between the dura mater and the skull, which presents in the acute phase as a spontaneous hyperdense biconvex extra-axial mass that does not usually cross sutures because of the tight attachment of the dura mater to these points. SDH involves a crescent-shaped collection of blood in the subdural space, which may compress and displace the brain, leading to a reversible reduction in cerebral function.

CT density and MR imaging signal intensity vary with age and organization of these hemorrhages. When acute, SDH and EDH are usually hyperdense on CT images, isointense to moderately hypointense on T1-WI, hypointense on T2-WI and T2* GRE, and hyperintense relative to CSF on FLAIR. DWI findings of EDH have not been well described and are nonspecific, but a hypointense signal may facilitate the identification of lesions.

SDH can also have a chronic course, usually in elderly patients, even when a mild traumatic event may precede hemorrhage. Chronic SDH can be an important differential diagnosis for dementia, and other common symptoms may include headache, hemiparesis, and gait disturbance. As surgical treatment is performed, a dramatic and immediate recovery of premorbid function is observed. DTI of the affected descending pyramidal tract can show a significantly reduced FA, which correlates with the severity of motor dysfunction. However, when the hematoma is removed, a significant improvement of the FA ratio and reversal of motor weakness are apparent. These alterations can be explained to be caused by tract compression due to the mass effect and by vasogenic edema rather than by direct damage to the tract.[69]

Ischemia

Secondary brain injury (SBI) occurs after the initial trauma and is defined as damage to neurons because of systemic physiologic responses to the initial injury. The most common cause of SBI is ischemia, which may show delayed symptom onset several hours or days after the trauma. SBI can also result from cerebral herniation, elevation of intracranial pressure, systemic hypoperfusion, cerebral vasospasm from SAH, vascular injury or embolization, or direct vascular compression by mass effects.[70]

When performing a head trauma examination hours or days after symptom onset, the radiologist should consider the cause of ischemia. The most common lesion occurs in the posterior cerebellar artery's vascular distribution, and midsagittal imaging facilitates the evaluation of herniation. A mechanical shift of the brain with herniation across the falx and/or tentorium is present in 80% to 90% of patients with traumatic ischemia.[71]

DAI

DAI is characterized by the disorganization of axonal membranes and cytoskeletal network, which occurs in the first few hours after a traumatic brain injury.[72] These lesions are caused by a shear-strain mechanism that leads to multifocal petechial and nonhemorrhagic lesions, especially in the subcortical white matter, the corpus callosum, and the dorsolateral aspect of the upper brain stem.[73]

CT is the initial examination modality for head trauma, although MR imaging is more sensitive for detecting DAI lesions. Petechial lesions vary in signal intensity depending on the sequence used and the type of blood products involved. Sequences that are sensitive to paramagnetic properties of iron-containing products may detect a greater number of lesions and show a strong correlation with Glasgow Coma Scale (GCS) scores.[74]

DWI may be more sensitive than conventional MR imaging for the detection of DAI. Because the lesions present with cytotoxic edema there is restricted diffusion.[75] However, these lesions evolve into vasogenic edema, which presents as unrestricted diffusion. DTI is also more sensitive than conventional MR imaging, demonstrating diminished mean FA histograms compared with controls. The FA parameters are also correlated with the GCS scores and posttraumatic amnesia (**Fig. 18**).[76]

DEGENERATIVE DISEASES
Alzheimer Disease

Alzheimer disease (AD) is an incurable, degenerative, and terminal disease and the most common cause of dementia.[77] AD pathologic changes begin in the parahippocampal gyrus and hippocampus, moving to frontal, temporal, and parietal lobes, explaining the appearance of memory deficits before the loss of other cognitive functions. The diagnosis of AD is commonly confirmed with behavioral assessments, cognitive tests, and brain imaging. The current role of imaging in AD is to exclude treatable causes of dementia and to identify early stages of the disease for potential early intervention therapies.[78]

CT and MR imaging are important tools for the detection of cortical atrophy, which is commonly observed in AD. The images show temporal and parietal atrophy associated with a disproportionate loss of hippocampal volume and enlargement of the parahippocampal fissures.[79] Coronal MR imaging may help to identify early atrophy of the hippocampus and entorhinal cortex. MR imaging volumetric analysis of the hippocampus, parahippocampus, and amygdala is a promising method of visualizing hippocampal volume loss.[80]

DWI is not yet a common imaging method for AD in clinical practice, but it can be considered a tool to explore the pathogenesis and to confirm a suspected clinical diagnosis.[81] The destruction of cell membranes and later loss of myelin and axons

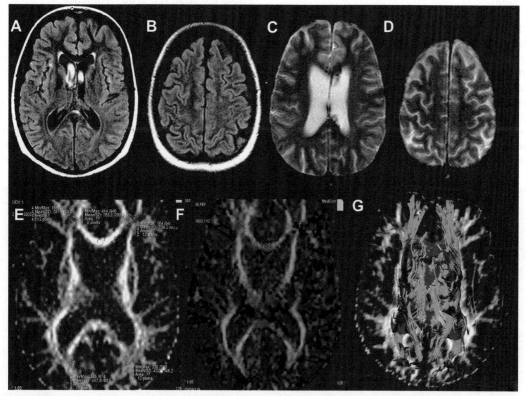

Fig. 18. Diffuse axonal injury. Multiple small hypointense lesions of the subcortical white matter and corpus callosum are better visualized by T2 GRE (*C, D*) than by FLAIR (*A, B*) images. DTI shows reduced FA values within the lesion and in the surrounding NAWM (*E, F*). Tractography (*G*) demonstrated reduced fiber density, mainly in the corpus callosum.

because of wallerian degeneration may reduce the restriction of water diffusion in the hippocampus and afferent white matter tracts. Therefore, DWI of patients with AD compared with that of controls can show differences in mean diffusion, especially in the hippocampus and in the temporal, parietal, and cingulate lobes.

DTI can depict subtle changes even when imaging the NAWM (Fig. 19). Therefore, researchers are using this technique to study the initial white matter involvement in AD. The suggested microstructural degradation of white matter in AD may result in decreased FA that follows a regional gradient, with the greatest changes seen in the temporal lobe, followed by the parietal and frontal lobes; no changes are observed in the occipital lobe.[82]

Amyotrophic Lateral Sclerosis

Degeneration of motor neurons of the corticospinal tract (CST) leads to a progressive and fatal neurodegenerative disease known as amyotrophic lateral sclerosis (ALS). This disease is characterized by muscle weakness, atrophy, and fasciculation without any alteration in cognitive function.[83]

For patients with ALS, CT is less sensitive than MR imaging and may show progressive atrophy. The most specific findings on MR imaging are symmetric, bilateral, hyperintense areas on T2-WI along the CST, extending from the corona radiata, internal capsule, cerebral peduncles, and anterolateral column of the spinal cord.[84] ALS leads to axonal loss, reflected as increases of extracellular water volume and high ADC. DTI is more sensitive than conventional MR imaging for ALS and may detect lesions before pyramidal

symptoms appear, revealing a reduction in FA that is most likely caused by axonal degeneration. DTI detects alterations in early disease stages, whereas DWI can reveal chronic axonal loss.[85]

HYPOXIC-ISCHEMIC ENCEPHALOPATHY

Despite technological improvements in obstetric and perinatal care, ischemic brain injury remains a major cause of infant morbidity and mortality. Most hypoxic-ischemic brain injuries in neonates are a result of cerebral hypoperfusion, secondary to the complex mechanisms of asphyxia. Episodes of ischemic insults to newborn brains can be mild, moderate, or severe; can be isolated, repetitive, or ongoing; and can occur antenatally, perinatally, or postnatally. Sequelae of perinatal brain ischemia include developmental delays, seizures, spasticity, behavioral disturbances, and focal deficits. The early use of pharmacologic agents and induced cerebral hypothermia may help to ameliorate the deleterious effects of brain ischemia.

Periventricular leukomalacia, or cerebral white matter injury, is the major form of brain injury observed in premature infants. Border vascular zones are observed in periventricular white matter as well as optic and acoustic radiations. In unpublished data, authors analyzed 34 extremely premature infants (birth weights <1500 g) who underwent MR imaging at term equivalent (37–42 weeks) and demonstrated that the most common findings were diffuse and excessive high signal intensity (DEHSI) in the white matter (79.5%, n = 27), ventricular dilation (52.9%, n = 18), and enlargement of the extracerebral spinal fluid spaces (35.3%, n = 12), indicating periventricular white matter lesions evolving to white

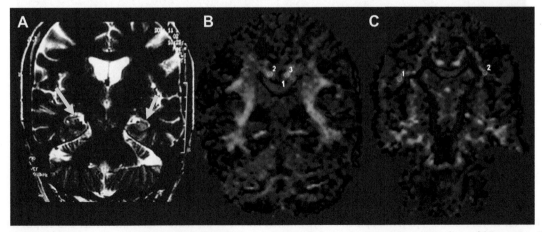

Fig. 19. Alzheimer's disease. Coronal T2-WI (A) demonstrates slight and symmetric volume loss of hippocampi (arrows). A coronal FA color map shows reduced FA values on the splenium of the corpus callosum (B, 1), bilaterally on the posterior cingulate gyrus (B, 2 and 3), and on the superior longitudinal fasciculus (C, 1 and 2).

matter loss in many of these premature infants. Using DWI, Counsell and colleagues[86] found objective evidence that DEHSI represents diffuse white matter lesion. Conventional MR imaging results are often normal within the first hours after ischemic insult, an early period that overlaps with the narrow, finite therapeutic window during which neuroprotective interventions will most likely be effective. DWI can show areas of infarction in perinatal brain ischemia before abnormalities are apparent by conventional MR imaging.[87]

Some reports have addressed changes in the patterns of injury that occur during the first few days of life.[88] Although anatomic images were normal or nearly normal on the first 2 days after birth in most patients, abnormalities were detected on DTI, both visually and by quantitative interrogation of FA maps (Fig. 20). These DTI parameters tend to worsen until about day 5 and then gradually normalize. Of interest, as areas of abnormal FA pseudonormalized within one region of the brain, they develop in other areas. Pseudonormalization indicates that although diffusivity may normalize, other DTI parameters remain abnormal for life.[89] Based on these changing areas of diffusivity, the pattern of injury appeared different when imaging was performed at different times. Knowledge of these evolving patterns is essential for studies performed during this critical period of life.

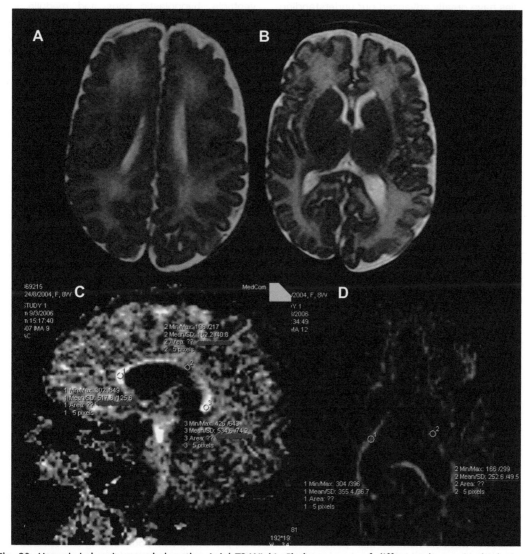

Fig. 20. Hypoxic-ischemic encephalopathy. Axial T2-WI (*A, B*) shows areas of diffuse and excessive high signal intensity (DEHSI) in white matter of a premature asphyxiated newborn. FA map (*C, D*) shows areas of reduced anisotropy in posterior portions of the corpus callosum and left posterior limb of the internal capsule secondary to Wallerian degeneration of axons.

Neonatal Infarction

Neonatal focal infarctions are most often caused by arterial occlusions in the left middle cerebral artery territory.[90] The imaging characteristics of focal infarctions differ from those of hypoxia-ischemia. Earlier and more consistent changes have been reported on both diffusion and conventional MR imagings in focal infarctions compared with hypoxia-ischemia (**Fig. 21**).[91,92]

BRAIN MALFORMATIONS

DTI and tractography provide information about white matter organization and architecture that is not available using conventional MR imaging. DTI studies have greatly advanced our understanding of the anatomy underlying some congenital brain malformations (**Fig. 22**). For example, DTI has been used to demonstrate that the size of CSTs and middle cerebellar peduncles correlates strongly with both the holoprosencephaly type

and neurodevelopmental score.[93,94] Furthermore, in molar tooth malformation (ie, Joubert syndrome), patients lack superior cerebellar peduncle decussations, which are visualized using tractography (**Fig. 23**).

Horizontal Gaze Palsy with Progressive Scoliosis

Horizontal gaze palsy with progressive scoliosis is a congenital malformation caused by a rare autosomal recessive condition. Symptoms are limited to the hindbrain and spine and include congenital absence of normal horizontal gaze and scoliosis. Both structural and diffusion imaging commonly show a depression in the floor of the fourth ventricle, hypoplastic pons and medulla with a butterfly medulla sign from an anterior median fissure, and a deep midline pontine cleft.[95] DTI studies have shown an absence of normal decussating fibers in the pons, including superior cerebellar peduncles and pontocerebellar fibers.[96]

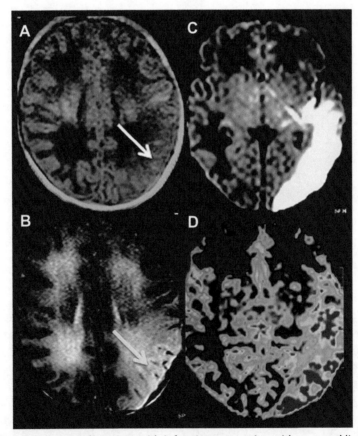

Fig. 21. A 40-week-old newborn male patient with infarction, presenting with poor suckling and seizures. MRI obtained 72 hours after birth shows barely visible areas of hypointensity on T1-WI (*A*) and hyperintensity on T2-WI (*B*), corresponding to the "missing cortical sign" (*arrows*). DWI (*C*) shows a core area of reduced diffusion in the parieto-occipital cortex, with high relative cerebral blood volume (*D*), representing arterial infarction associated with reperfusion.

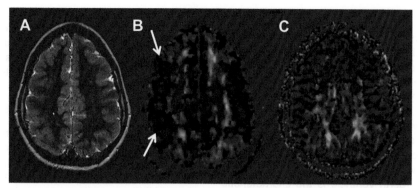

Fig. 22. A 5-year-old female patient with congenital cytomegalovirus infection and polymicrogyria. Axial T2-WI (*A*) shows polymicrogyria and some foci of heterotopia. FA color map (*B*) at the same level shows a horizontally oriented pattern of subcortical white matter fibers (*arrows*). A normal control FA color map (*C*) is shown for comparison.

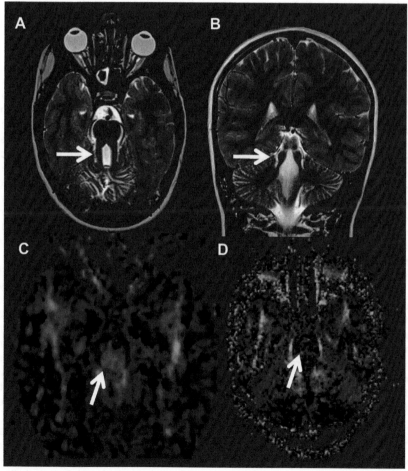

Fig. 23. A 6-year-old male patient with Joubert syndrome. Axial and coronal T2-WI (*A, B*) show the molar tooth malformation with increased width of the superior cerebellar peduncle (*arrows*). The absence of the superior cerebellar peduncle decussation (*arrow*) was apparent in the FA color map (*C*). A control patient with normal superior cerebellar decussation at the pons (*arrow*) is shown for comparison (*D*).

Pontine Tegmental Cap Dysplasia

The mechanisms underlying pontine tegmental cap dysplasia are less clear than those of other brain malformations. Clinical findings are varied and include multiple cranial neuropathies (ie, acoustic nerve palsy in all patients with variable involvement of facial and trigeminal nerves), impaired swallowing, and cerebellar and pyramidal motor symptoms. Conventional MR imaging has revealed several hindbrain abnormalities. A hypoplastic ventral pons with a dorsal cap projecting into the fourth ventricle is the characteristic finding, although other cerebellar and supratentorial abnormalities also occur. Tractography studies have revealed the absence of the superior and middle cerebellar peduncle decussations as well as an ectopic fiber tract that crosses the midline in the dorsal aspect of the pons, forming the characteristic tegmental cap.[97,98]

Dysgenesis of the Corpus Callosum

Dysgenesis of the corpus callosum (AgCC) is characterized by the partial or complete absence of callosal fibers, accompanied by various neuropsychological deficits, including many that are within the autistic spectrum.[99] A large amount of imaging research in AgCC has focused on identifying and characterizing other possible anatomic features that contribute to the phenotype. Studies using conventional MR imaging have found polymicrogyria and cortical and subcortical heterotopias. Diffusion imaging and tractography studies have focused on several anatomic features of AgCC, such as the presence of Probst bundles.[100] Early DTI studies confirmed the anteroposterior direction of the Probst bundles, established that fibers within the bundles are at least partially topographically organized,[101] and showed that a significant number of these fibers project to subcortical regions, including the thalamus and brainstem,[102] rather than to other cortical areas (**Fig. 24**). In the case of partial agenesis, callosal fragments of similar size and position were found to have vastly different connectivity patterns, and these variations could correlate with behavioral and cognitive performances.[103] Another study examined the microstructural organization of the cingulum bundle in patients with AgCC.[104]

Future Directions

Diffusion imaging has been applied to more common pediatric conditions that typically do not show atypical features on conventional neuroimaging, such as autism. White matter alterations in these neurodevelopmental disorders have been found to be more widespread. Because diffusion imaging provides uniquely detailed quantitative information about white matter microstructural organization and connectivity, its applications to pediatric neuroradiology are likely to proliferate.

TOXIC AND METABOLIC DISEASES

MR imaging of patients with toxic and metabolic diseases is useful in diagnosis, but may show nonspecific features. DWI can add information to facilitate the early diagnosis and treatment of some of these conditions.

Krabbe Disease

DTI with quantitative tractography has been used to detect significant differences in the CST of asymptomatic neonates who had early-onset Krabbe disease.[105] Umbilical cord blood transplantation is the only available treatment and is effective only in presymptomatic infants. Other inborn errors of metabolism can also be evaluated using DWI.

Mitochondriopathies

Mitochondrial diseases are a group of inherited disorders caused by a disturbance of mitochondrial respiration because of enzyme deficiency, which primarily affect the CNS and skeletal muscles. The genetic defects are easily detected in blood cells as well as muscles.[106,107] Some well-defined disorders in this category include Leigh syndrome (LS), mitochondrial encephalopathy with lactic acidosis (MELAS), Kearns-Sayre syndrome, and myoclonus epilepsy with ragged red fibers.

MR spectroscopy detects abnormal accumulation of lactate in brain parenchyma and CSF in association with multiple mitochondrial disorders, such as LS.[108] LS is characterized by a heterogeneous combination of developmental delay, ataxia, hypotonia, optic atrophy, and lactic acidosis. Neuroimaging studies in patients with LS have demonstrated a focal, bilaterally symmetric subacute necrosis of the basal ganglia, thalamus, or brain stem.[109] DWI and DTI have been shown to help in the early diagnosis and management of acute LS (**Fig. 25**).[110] DWI and ADC mapping are of particular interest during the acute stages of a strokelike episode in MELAS (**Fig. 26**). Results reported to date are conflicting because some lesions in the acute phase show clearly restricted diffusion, whereas others do not. Lesions in the acute phase may show normal or even elevated ADC values in MELAS, indicating vasogenic edema.[111] There is evidence that most of these findings are reversible,

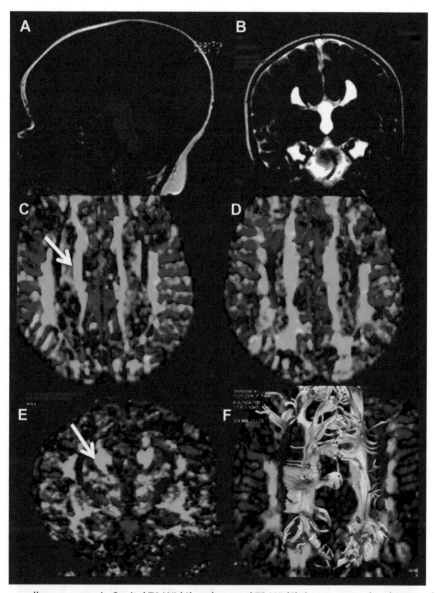

Fig. 24. Corpus callosum agenesis. Sagital T1-WI (*A*) and coronal T2-WI (*B*) demonstrate the absence of the corpus callosum and the characteristic ventricle shape. Axial (*C, D*) and coronal (*E*) FA color maps depict Probst bundles (*C, E, arrows*) as green bundles lying in an anteroposterior orientation. Tractography superimposed on the FA color map (*F*) shows that these fibers do not cross the midline.

disappearing after a couple of weeks, whereas others persist or result in focal atrophy.[112]

Chemotherapy-Induced Leukoencephalopathy

Intrathecal or intravenous methotrexate (MTX), with or without radiation therapy, can cause diffuse white matter changes.[113] Subacute MTX neurotoxicity is manifested by abrupt onset of focal cerebral dysfunction occurring days to weeks after MTX administration, usually in children. High-dose chemotherapy, including

carmustine, cyclophosphamide, cisplatin, 5-fluo-rouracil and carmofur can also cause diffuse white matter disease.[114] MR imaging shows diffuse or multifocal white matter lesions that are hyperintense on FLAIR and T2-WI. DWI shows these white matter changes as diffuse hyperintensity with decreased ADC in the white matter, even before conventional MR imaging can detect the lesions. Pathologically, these lesions represent intra-myelinic and axonal swelling. Chemotherapy-associated leukoencephalopathy can be fatal. Thus, early diagnosis and discontinuation of therapy can be lifesaving.

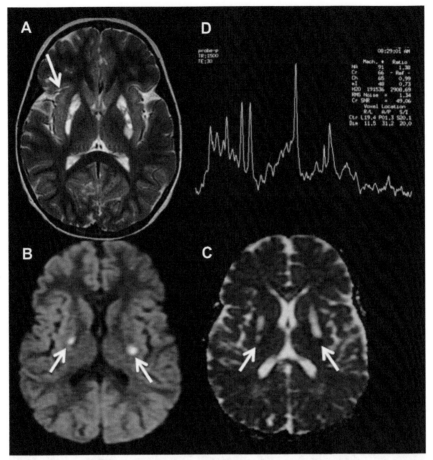

Fig. 25. Leigh syndrome. High signal areas on the putamen are visualized by T2-WI (*A, arrow*), whereas foci of high DWI signal intensity (*B, arrows*) and low ADC values (*C, arrows*) demonstrate an acute exacerbation of Leigh encephalopathy. Spectroscopy (*D*) shows metabolic peaks of lactate probably secondary to anaerobic glycolysis.

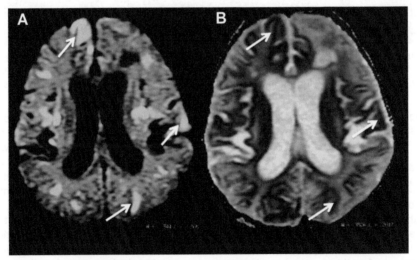

Fig. 26. Mitochondrial encephalopathy with lactic acidosis (MELAS). DWI (*A*) shows hyperintense cortical and subcortical signals with low ADC values (*B, arrows*), corresponding to acute exacerbation of mitochondriopathy and atrophic changes.

Central Pontine Myelinolysis and Extrapontine Myelinolysis

Central pontine myelinolysis (CPM) and extrapontine myelinolysis (EPM) represent destruction of myelin sheaths in characteristic regions within the brain stem and cerebrum, with the central part of the basis pontis as the most common site. The most prevalent osmotic insult is a rapid correction of hyponatremia[115]; however, CPM and EPM can also occur in normonatremic or hypernatremic states in patients with chronic alcoholism, postliver transplantation, malnutrition and AIDS. MR imaging has a fundamental role in diagnosis, demonstrating hyperintense lesions on T2-WI with or without enhancement on gadolinium-enhanced T1-WI. In the early phase, DWI can be useful in visualizing lesions as hyperintense areas with decreased ADC, which indicates cytotoxic edema (**Fig. 27**).[116]

Wernicke Encephalopathy

Thiamine (vitamin B_1) deficiency can cause Wernicke encephalopathy, characterized by confusion, ataxia, and abnormal eye movements. Pathologic findings include decreased myelination, edema, astrocytic swelling, and necrosis in the mammillary bodies, thalamic and hypothalamic nuclei, periaqueductal gray matter, walls of the third ventricle and floor of the fourth ventricle, and less commonly, in the caudate, frontal, and parietal cortex. MR imaging shows hyperintense lesions in these areas on T2-WI (**Fig. 28**) and may or may not show enhancement on T1-WI after injection of a contrast agent.[117] DWI shows these lesions as

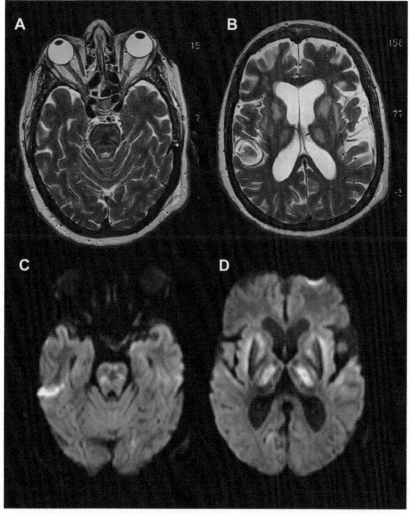

Fig. 27. In pontine myelinolysis and extrapontine myeinolysis, T2-WI shows foci of hyperintense signal on the pons (*A*) and bilateral and symmetric areas of high signal intensity on the putamen and thalami (*B*). DWI shows areas of restricted diffusion on the pons (*C*), putamen, and thalami (*D*).

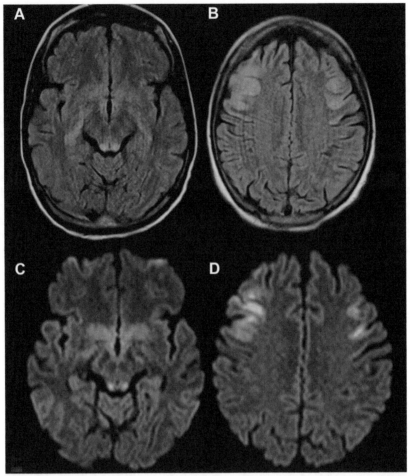

Fig. 28. Wernicke's encephalopathy. Areas of high signal intensity on FLAIR images (*A, B*) and restricted diffusion on DWI (*C, D*) are demonstrated bilaterally on the mammillary bodies, periaqueductal gray matter, and in the frontal cortex bilaterally.

hyperintense with decreased ADC, indicating cytotoxic edema, or increased ADC, indicating vasogenic edema. Both types of lesions are reversible.[118]

Marchiafava-Bignami Disease

Marchiafava-Bignami disease is a rare form of toxic demyelination that is most frequently observed in long-term alcoholics, but may also occur in nondrinkers who are poorly nourished. Clinical signs are nonspecific and include seizures, impairment of consciousness, and interhemispheric disconnection. The genu of the corpus callosum is most frequently involved. However, degeneration can extend throughout the corpus callosum, and other cerebral structures may also be involved.[119] The corpus callosum appears hyperintense on T2-WI and FLAIR images, which is essential to confirm the diagnosis. These lesions can be

partially reversed with treatment. DWI shows lesions in the early phase as hyperintense with decreased ADC, indicating cytotoxic edema. In the subacute phase, the lesions are hyperintense on DWI with increased ADC, indicating demyelination or necrosis.

Heroin-Induced Spongiform Leukoencephalopathy

Heroin can lead to toxic leukoencephalopathy, characterized by spongiform degeneration of the white matter as a result of fluid accumulation within the myelin sheaths. CT and MR imaging show abnormalities in the cerebral and cerebellar white matter, cerebral peduncles, CST, lemniscus medialis, and solitary tracts. On DWI, these areas may be hyperintense with decreased ADC. In cases of less severe heroin-induced leukoencephalopathy, the changes in the DWI signal intensity may be reversed on follow-up MR imaging.[120]

Cocaine, Amphetamines, and Related Catecholaminergics

Catecholaminergic drugs can cause hemorrhage or infarction because of vasculitis, vasculopathy, or acute hypertensive effects. DWI can be useful

for the detection of these lesions in the acute phase.[121]

SPINAL CORD

Even though the role of DWI, DTI, and tractography is well defined for many neurologic lesions that affect the brain, its clinical application in spinal cord diseases is increasing. The imaging evaluation

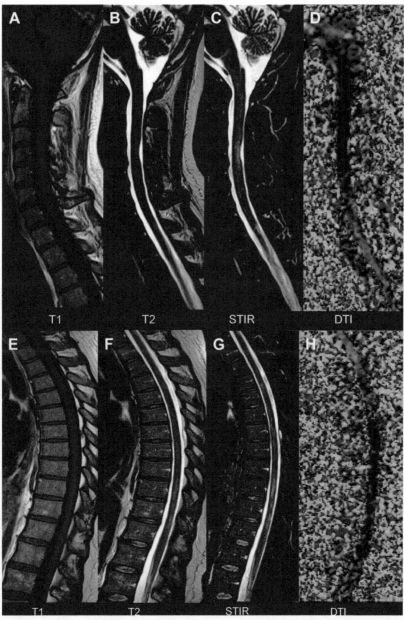

Fig. 29. Multiple sclerosis. Demyelinating plaques can be detected as diffuse hyperintense lesions on both T2-WI (*B, F*) and STIR (*C, G*) images. Contrast-enhanced T1-WI (*A, E*) does not demonstrate any abnormal enhancement. Sagittal DTI (*D, H*) shows reduced FA values within the lesion and in the surrounding normal-appearing spinal cord, suggesting a more extensive abnormality. STIR, short *tau* inversion recovery.

of demyelinating diseases, tumors, vascular malformations, infection, ischemia, and traumatic injuries affecting the spinal cord can benefit from diffusion imaging information. Several challenges have to be considered when obtaining spinal cord DWI and DTI, but recent advances in MR image acquisition offer several helpful options.[122,123]

Although technical details regarding diffusion imaging acquisition and postprocessing is beyond the scope of this article, a couple of points should be considered. First, because of its small size, the spinal cord requires the use of small voxel sizes. Macroscopic motion, field inhomogeneities, and routine echo planar sequences are drawbacks that can be partially solved with the use of faster alternative techniques, such as multishot echo planar imaging, diffusion-weighted PROPELLER, spin echo navigator spiral DTI, and parallel imaging methods. Cardiac pulse gating is also useful, but it lengthens the acquisition time and increases the likelihood of swallowing and respiratory artifact.[122]

Many potential clinical applications of DWI and DTI in spinal cord lesions have been suggested. In patients with MS, these applications have demonstrated significant changes in DTI metrics in the cervical spinal cord, even in the absence of spinal cord signal abnormality at conventional MR examination (**Fig. 29**).[123] Tractography has been used to differentiate astrocytomas from ependymomas because the former shows a pattern of infiltration of the fibers, whereas the latter has a pattern of fiber displacement (**Fig. 30**).[124] The same pattern of fiber displacement can also be seen in spinal cord vascular malformations such as cavernomas (**Fig. 31**) and arteriovenous malformations. In patients with cervical spondylotic myelopathy, there are studies suggesting increased sensitivity of DTI for early detection of myelopathic changes. DWI and DTI have also been used to demonstrate acute and chronic spinal cord abnormalities after traumatic injury. It seems that diffusion imaging is more sensitive than conventional MR imaging for detecting the exact extension of the spinal cord injury.[125] Finally, the diagnosis of spinal cord ischemia is difficult in some cases when using only conventional MR imaging. However, diffusion imaging can add valuable information, showing the ischemic areas with high signal intensity on

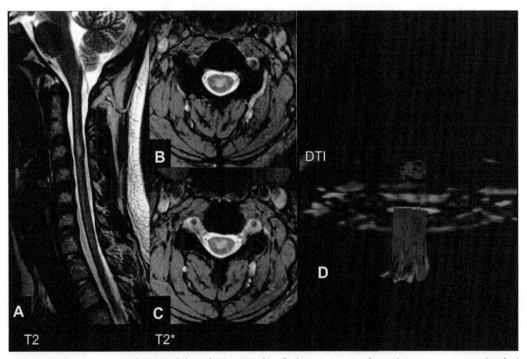

Fig. 30. Ependimoma. Sagital T2-WI (*A*) and T2* GRE (*B, C*) demonstrate a hyperintense on expansive lesion located at the middle portio of the cervical spine, which does not cause disruption, but only a mild dislocation of the main fibers, demonstrated on tractography (*D*).

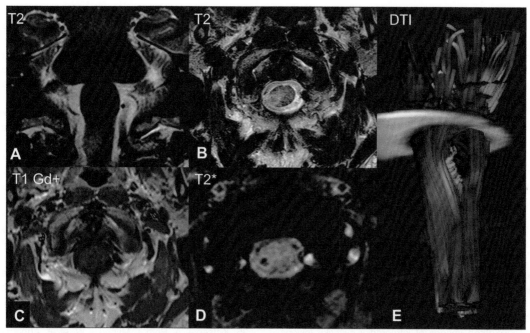

Fig. 31. Cavernoma. Coronal (*A*) and axial T2-WI (*B*), and T2* GRE (*B*), show hyperintense expansive lesion on the posterior and right lateral aspects of the cervical spinal cord at C1-C2 level, which does not enhances after intravenous contrast administration on contrast-enhanced T1-WI (*C*). Axial T2* GRE (*D*) demonstrates a foci of hypointense signal intensity within the lateral aspect of the lesion. There is no disruption of the main fibers demonstrated on tractography (*E*). Gd, gadolinium.

DWI and low signal intensity on ADC maps (restricted diffusion).

REFERENCES

1. Srinivasan A, Goyal M, Al Azri F, et al. State-of-the-art imaging of acute stroke. Radiographics 2006; 26(Suppl 1):S75–95.
2. de Lucas EM, Sanchez E, Gutierrez A, et al. CT protocol for acute stroke: tips and tricks for general radiologists. Radiographics 2008;28(6):1673–87.
3. Beauchamp NJ Jr, Ulug AM, Passe TJ, et al. MR diffusion imaging in stroke: review and controversies. Radiographics 1998;18(5):1269–83 [discussion: 1283–65].
4. Saini M, Butcher K. Advanced imaging in acute stroke management-part II: magnetic resonance imaging. Neurol India 2009;57(5):550–8.
5. Kidwell CS, Saver JL, Mattiello J, et al. Thrombolytic reversal of acute human cerebral ischemic injury shown by diffusion/perfusion magnetic resonance imaging. Ann Neurol 2000;47(4):462–9.
6. Kidwell CS, Alger JR, Saver JL. Beyond mismatch: evolving paradigms in imaging the ischemic penumbra with multimodal magnetic resonance imaging. Stroke 2003;34(11):2729–35.
7. Casey S. "T2 washout": an explanation for normal diffusion-weighted images despite abnormal apparent diffusion coefficient maps. AJNR Am J Neuroradiol 2001;22(8):1450.
8. Provenzale JM, Petrella JR, Cruz LC Jr, et al. Quantitative assessment of diffusion abnormalities in posterior reversible encephalopathy syndrome. AJNR Am J Neuroradiol 2001;22:1455–61.
9. Weon Y, Kim J, Lee J, et al. Optimal diffusion-weighted imaging protocol for lesion detection in transient global amnesia. AJNR Am J Neuroradiol 2008;29(7):1324.
10. Brunberg JA, Chenevert TL, McKeever PE, et al. In vivo MR determination of water diffusion coefficients and diffusion anisotropy: correlation with structural alteration in gliomas of the cerebral hemispheres. AJNR Am J Neuroradiol 1995;16(2): 361–71.
11. Laundre BJ, Jellison BJ, Badie B, et al. Diffusion tensor imaging of the corticospinal tract before and after mass resection as correlated with clinical motor findings: preliminary data. AJNR Am J Neuroradiol 2005;26(4):791–6.
12. Maldjian JA, Schulder M, Liu WC, et al. Intraoperative functional MRI using a real-time neurosurgical navigation system. J Comput Assist Tomogr 1997; 21(6):910–2.
13. Schulder M, Maldjian JA, Liu WC, et al. Functional image-guided surgery of intracranial tumors located in or near the sensorimotor cortex. J Neurosurg 1998;89(3):412–8.

14. Tsuruda JS, Chew WM, Moseley ME, et al. Diffusion-weighted MR imaging of the brain: value of differentiating between extraaxial cysts and epidermoid tumors. AJR Am J Roentgenol 1990;155(5): 1059–65 [discussion: 1066–58].

15. Tsuruda J, Chew W, Moseley M, et al. Diffusion-weighted MR imaging of extraaxial tumors. Magn Reson Med 1991;19(2):316–20.

16. Chen S, Ikawa F, Kurisu K, et al. Quantitative MR evaluation of intracranial epidermoid tumors by fast fluid-attenuated inversion recovery imaging and echo-planar diffusion-weighted imaging. AJNR Am J Neuroradiol 2001;22(6):1089.

17. Laing AD, Mitchell PJ, Wallace D. Diffusion-weighted magnetic resonance imaging of intracranial epidermoid tumours. Australas Radiol 1999; 43(1):16–9.

18. Guo AC, Provenzale JM, Cruz LC Jr, et al. Cerebral abscesses: investigation using apparent diffusion coefficient maps. Neuroradiology 2001;43(5): 370–4.

19. Bergui M, Zhong J, Bradac G, et al. Diffusion-weighted images of intracranial cyst-like lesions. Neuroradiology 2001;43(10):824–9.

20. Chang SC, Lai PH, Chen WL, et al. Diffusion-weighted MRI features of brain abscess and cystic or necrotic brain tumors: comparison with conventional MRI. Clin Imaging 2002;26(4):227–36.

21. Chan J, Tsui E, Chau L, et al. Discrimination of an infected brain tumor from a cerebral abscess by combined MR perfusion and diffusion imaging. Comput Med Imaging Graph 2002;26(1):19–23.

22. Ebisu T, Tanaka C, Umeda M, et al. Discrimination of brain abscess from necrotic or cystic tumors by diffusion-weighted echo planar imaging. Magn Reson Imaging 1996;14(9):1113–6.

23. Tien RD, Felsberg GJ, Friedman H, et al. MR imaging of high-grade cerebral gliomas: value of diffusion-weighted echoplanar pulse sequences. AJR Am J Roentgenol 1994;162(3):671–7.

24. Eis M, Els T, Hoehn-Berlage M, et al. Quantitative diffusion MR imaging of cerebral tumor and edema. Acta Neurochir Suppl (Wien) 1994;60:344–6.

25. Krabbe K, Gideon P, Wagn P, et al. MR diffusion imaging of human intracranial tumours. Neuroradiology 1997;39(7):483–9.

26. Le Bihan D, Douek P, Argyropoulou M, et al. Diffusion and perfusion magnetic resonance imaging in brain tumors. Top Magn Reson Imaging 1993;5(1): 25–31.

27. Yanaka K, Shirai S, Kimura H, et al. Clinical application of diffusion-weighted magnetic resonance imaging to intracranial disorders. Neurol Med Chir (Tokyo) 1995;35(9):648–54.

28. Cruz Junior LC, Sorensen AG. Diffusion tensor magnetic resonance imaging of brain tumors. Neurosurg Clin N Am 2005;16(1):115–34.

29. Pierpaoli C, Jezzard P, Basser PJ, et al. Diffusion tensor MR imaging of the human brain. Radiology 1996;201(3):637–48.

30. Sugahara T, Korogi Y, Kochi M, et al. Usefulness of diffusion-weighted MRI with echo-planar technique in the evaluation of cellularity in gliomas. J Magn Reson Imaging 1999;9(1):53–60.

31. Cha S. Update on brain tumor imaging: from anatomy to physiology. AJNR Am J Neuroradiol 2006;27(3):475–87.

32. Kono K, Inoue Y, Nakayama K, et al. The role of diffusion-weighted imaging in patients with brain tumors. AJNR Am J Neuroradiol 2001;22(6): 1081–8.

33. Guo AC, Cummings TJ, Dash RC, et al. Lymphomas and high-grade astrocytomas: comparison of water diffusibility and histologic characteristics. Radiology 2002;224(1):177–83.

34. Gauvain KM, McKinstry RC, Mukherjee P, et al. Evaluating pediatric brain tumor cellularity with diffusion-tensor imaging. AJR Am J Roentgenol 2001;177(2):449–54.

35. Kotsenas A, Roth T, Manness W, et al. Abnormal diffusion-weighted MRI in medulloblastoma: does it reflect small cell histology? Pediatr Radiol 1999; 29(7):524–6.

36. Quadery F, Okamoto K. Diffusion-weighted MRI of haemangioblastomas and other cerebellar tumours. Neuroradiology 2003;45(4):212–9.

37. Witwer BP, Moftakhar R, Hasan KM, et al. Diffusion-tensor imaging of white matter tracts in patients with cerebral neoplasm. J Neurosurg 2002;97(3): 568–75.

38. Goebell E, Paustenbach S, Vaeterlein O, et al. Low-grade and anaplastic gliomas: differences in architecture evaluated with diffusion-tensor MR imaging. Radiology 2006;239(1):217–22.

39. Inoue T, Ogasawara K, Beppu T, et al. Diffusion tensor imaging for preoperative evaluation of tumor grade in gliomas. Clin Neurol Neurosurg 2005; 107(3):174–80.

40. Smith JS, Cha S, Mayo MC, et al. Serial diffusion-weighted magnetic resonance imaging in cases of glioma: distinguishing tumor recurrence from post-resection injury. J Neurosurg 2005;103(3):428–38.

41. Sandler A, Gray R, Perry M, et al. Paclitaxel-carboplatin alone or with bevacizumab for non-small-cell lung cancer. N Engl J Med 2006;355(24):2542.

42. Chenevert T, Stegman L, Taylor J, et al. Diffusion magnetic resonance imaging: an early surrogate marker of therapeutic efficacy in brain tumors. J Natl Cancer Inst 2000;92(24):2029–36.

43. Moffat BA, Chenevert TL, Lawrence TS, et al. Functional diffusion map: a noninvasive MRI biomarker for early stratification of clinical brain tumor response. Proc Natl Acad Sci U S A 2005; 102(15):5524–9.

44. Price SJ, Burnet NG, Donovan T, et al. Diffusion tensor imaging of brain tumours at 3T: a potential tool for assessing white matter tract invasion? Clin Radiol 2003;58(6):455–62.

45. Khong PL, Kwong DL, Chan GC, et al. Diffusion-tensor imaging for the detection and quantification of treatment-induced white matter injury in children with medulloblastoma: a pilot study. AJNR Am J Neuroradiol 2003;24(4):734–40.

46. Luthra G, Parihar A, Nath K, et al. Comparative evaluation of fungal, tubercular, and pyogenic brain abscesses with conventional and diffusion MR imaging and proton MR spectroscopy. AJNR Am J Neuroradiol 2007;28(7):1332–8.

47. Hartmann M, Jansen O, Heiland S, et al. Restricted diffusion within ring enhancement is not pathogno-monic for brain abscess. AJNR Am J Neuroradiol 2001;22(9):1738–42.

48. Schaefer PW, Grant PE, Gonzalez RG. Diffusion-weighted MR imaging of the brain. Radiology 2000;217(2):331–45.

49. Prusiner SB. Shattuck lecture–neurodegenerative diseases and prions. N Engl J Med 2001;344(20):1516–26.

50. Murata T, Shiga Y, Higano S, et al. Conspicuity and evolution of lesions in Creutzfeldt-Jakob disease at diffusion-weighted imaging. AJNR Am J Neurora-diol 2002;23(7):1164–72.

51. Ukisu R, Kushihashi T, Kitanosono T, et al. Serial diffusion-weighted MRI of Creutzfeldt-Jakob disease. AJR Am J Roentgenol 2005;184(2):560–6.

52. Demaerel P, Sciot R, Robberecht W, et al. Accuracy of diffusion-weighted MR imaging in the diagnosis of sporadic Creutzfeldt-Jakob disease. J Neurol 2003;250(2):222–5.

53. Bulakbasi N, Kocaoglu M, Tayfun C, et al. Transient splenial lesion of the corpus callosum in clinically mild influenza-associated encephalitis/encepha-lopathy. AJNR Am J Neuroradiol 2006;27(9):1983.

54. Honkaniemi J, Dastidar P, Kahara V, et al. Delayed MR imaging changes in acute disseminated encephalomyelitis. AJNR Am J Neuroradiol 2001;22(6):1117.

55. Albayram S, Bilgi Z, Selcuk H, et al. Diffusion-weighted MR imaging findings of acute necrotizing encephalopathy. AJNR Am J Neuroradiol 2004;25(5):792–7.

56. Rovaris M, Gass A, Bammer R, et al. Diffusion MRI in multiple sclerosis. Neurology 2005;65(10):1526–32.

57. Horsfield MA, Larsson HB, Jones DK, et al. Diffusion magnetic resonance imaging in multiple sclerosis. J Neurol Neurosurg Psychiatr 1998;64(Suppl 1):S80–4.

58. Larsson H, Thomsen C, Frederiksen J, et al. In vivo magnetic resonance diffusion measurement in the brain of patients with multiple sclerosis. Magn Re-son Imaging 1992;10(1):7–12.

59. Roychowdhury S, Maldjian JA, Grossman RI. Multiple sclerosis: comparison of trace apparent diffusion coefficients with MR enhancement pattern of lesions. AJNR Am J Neuroradiol 2000;21(5):869–74.

60. Filippi M, Inglese M. Overview of diffusion-weighted magnetic resonance studies in multiple sclerosis. J Neurol Sci 2001;186(Suppl 1):S37–43.

61. Ge Y. Multiple sclerosis: the role of MR imaging. AJNR Am J Neuroradiol 2006;27(6):1165–76.

62. Bammer R, Augustin M, Strasser-Fuchs S, et al. Magnetic resonance diffusion tensor imaging for characterizing diffuse and focal white matter abnormalities in multiple sclerosis. Magn Reson Med 2000;44(4):583–91.

63. Filippi M, Iannucci G, Cercignani M, et al. A quantitative study of water diffusion in multiple sclerosis lesions and normal-appearing white matter using echo-planar imaging. Arch Neurol 2000;57(7):1017–21.

64. Castriota-Scanderbeg A, Sabatini U, Fasano F, et al. Diffusion of water in large demyelinating lesions: a follow-up study. Neuroradiology 2002;44(9):764–7.

65. Song SK, Sun SW, Ramsbottom MJ, et al. Dysmye-lination revealed through MRI as increased radial (but unchanged axial) diffusion of water. Neuro-image 2002;17(3):1429–36.

66. Song SK, Yoshino J, Le TQ, et al. Demyelination increases radial diffusivity in corpus callosum of mouse brain. Neuroimage 2005;26(1):132–40.

67. Rueda F, Hygino LC Jr, Domingues RC, et al. Diffu-sion tensor MR imaging evaluation of the corpus callosum of patients with multiple sclerosis. Arq Neuropsiquiatr 2008;66(3A):449–53.

68. Ciccarelli O, Werring DJ, Barker GJ, et al. A study of the mechanisms of normal-appearing white matter damage in multiple sclerosis using diffusion tensor imaging–evidence of wallerian degenera-tion. J Neurol 2003;250(3):287–92.

69. Yokoyama K, Matsuki M, Shimano H, et al. Diffusion tensor imaging in chronic subdural hematoma: correlation between clinical signs and fractional anisotropy in the pyramidal tract. AJNR Am J Neu-roradiol 2008;29(6):1159–63.

70. Klufas RA, Hsu L, Patel MR, et al. Unusual manifes-tations of head trauma. AJR Am J Roentgenol 1996;166(3):675–81.

71. Osborn AG, Hedlund GL, Blaser SI, et al. Traumatic cerebral ischemia. In: Diagnostic imaging brain. Salt Lake City: Amirsys; 2004. p. I2.51–53.

72. Arfanakis K, Haughton VM, Carew JD, et al. Diffusion tensor MR imaging in diffuse axonal injury. AJNR Am J Neuroradiol 2002;23(5):794–802.

73. Li XY, Feng DF. Diffuse axonal injury: novel insights into detection and treatment. J Clin Neurosci 2009;16(5):614–9.

74. Yanagawa Y, Tsushima Y, Tokumaru A, et al. A quantitative analysis of head injury using T2*-weighted gradient-echo imaging. J Trauma 2000;49(2):272–7.

75. Kinoshita T, Moritani T, Hiwatashi A, et al. Conspicuity of diffuse axonal injury lesions on diffusion-weighted MR imaging. Eur J Radiol 2005;56(1):5–11.

76. Benson RR, Meda SA, Vasudevan S, et al. Global white matter analysis of diffusion tensor images is predictive of injury severity in traumatic brain injury. J Neurotrauma 2007;24(3):446–59.

77. Berchtold NC, Cotman CW. Evolution in the conceptualization of dementia and Alzheimer's disease: Greco-Roman period to the 1960s. Neurobiol Aging 1998;19(3):173–89.

78. Fox NC, Cousens S, Scahill R, et al. Using serial registered brain magnetic resonance imaging to measure disease progression in Alzheimer disease: power calculations and estimates of sample size to detect treatment effects. Arch Neurol 2000;57(3):339–44.

79. de Leon MJ, Golomb J, George AE, et al. The radiologic prediction of Alzheimer disease: the atrophic hippocampal formation. AJNR Am J Neuroradiol 1993;14(4):897–906.

80. Norfray JF, Provenzale JM. Alzheimer's disease: neuropathologic findings and recent advances in imaging. AJR Am J Roentgenol 2004;182(1):3–13.

81. Ito S. Brain diffusion changes in patients diagnosed with Alzheimer's disease. Curr Med Imaging Rev 2008;4(4):226–30.

82. Parente DB, Gasparetto EL, da Cruz LC Jr, et al. Potential role of diffusion tensor MRI in the differential diagnosis of mild cognitive impairment and Alzheimer's disease. AJR Am J Roentgenol 2008;190(5):1369–74.

83. Rowland LP. Diagnosis of amyotrophic lateral sclerosis. J Neurol Sci 1998;160(Suppl 1):S6–24.

84. Cheung G, Gawel MJ, Cooper PW, et al. Amyotrophic lateral sclerosis: correlation of clinical and MR imaging findings. Radiology 1995;194(1):263–70.

85. Ulug AM, Grunewald T, Lin MT, et al. Diffusion tensor imaging in the diagnosis of primary lateral sclerosis. J Magn Reson Imaging 2004;19(1):34–9.

86. Counsell SJ, Allsop JM, Harrison MC, et al. Diffusion-weighted imaging of the brain in preterm infants with focal and diffuse white matter abnormality. Pediatrics 2003;112(1 Pt 1):1–7.

87. Rutherford MA, Pennock JM, Schwieso JE, et al. Hypoxic ischaemic encephalopathy: early magnetic resonance imaging findings and their evolution. Neuropediatrics 1995;26(4):183–91.

88. Johnson AJ, Lee BC, Lin W. Echoplanar diffusion-weighted imaging in neonates and infants with suspected hypoxic-ischemic injury: correlation with patient outcome. AJR Am J Roentgenol 1999;172(1):219–26.

89. Huppi P, Murphy B, Maier S, et al. Microstructural brain development after perinatal cerebral white matter injury assessed by diffusion tensor magnetic resonance imaging. Pediatrics 2001;107(3):455.

90. Volpe JJ. Neurology of the newborn. São Paulo (Brazil): Elsevier; 2008.

91. Robertson RL, Ben-Sira L, Barnes PD, et al. MR line-scan diffusion-weighted imaging of term neonates with perinatal brain ischemia. AJNR Am J Neuroradiol 1999;20(9):1658–70.

92. Rumpel H, Ferrini B, Martin E. Lasting cytotoxic edema as an indicator of irreversible brain damage: a case of neonatal stroke. AJNR Am J Neuroradiol 1998;19(9):1636–8.

93. Albayram S, Melhem ER, Mori S, et al. Holoprosencephaly in children: diffusion tensor MR imaging of white matter tracts of the brainstem—initial experience. Radiology 2002;223(3):645–51.

94. Rollins N. Semilobar holoprosencephaly seen with diffusion tensor imaging and fiber tracking. AJNR Am J Neuroradiol 2005;26(8):2148–52.

95. Rossi A, Catala M, Biancheri R, et al. MR imaging of brain-stem hypoplasia in horizontal gaze palsy with progressive scoliosis. AJNR Am J Neuroradiol 2004;25(6):1046.

96. Sicotte NL, Salamon G, Shattuck DW, et al. Diffusion tensor MRI shows abnormal brainstem crossing fibers associated with ROBO3 mutations. Neurology 2006;67(3):519–21.

97. Barth PG, Majoie CB, Caan MW, et al. Pontine tegmental cap dysplasia: a novel brain malformation with a defect in axonal guidance. Brain 2007;130(Pt 9):2258–66.

98. Jissendi-Tchofo P, Doherty D, McGillivray G, et al. Pontine tegmental cap dysplasia: MR imaging and diffusion tensor imaging features of impaired axonal navigation. AJNR Am J Neuroradiol 2009;30(1):113–9.

99. Badaruddin DH, Andrews GL, Bolte S, et al. Social and behavioral problems of children with agenesis of the corpus callosum. Child Psychiatry Hum Dev 2007;38(4):287–302.

100. Hetts SW, Sherr EH, Chao S, et al. Anomalies of the corpus callosum: an MR analysis of the phenotypic spectrum of associated malformations. AJR Am J Roentgenol 2006;187(5):1343–8.

101. Lee SK, Mori S, Kim DJ, et al. Diffusion tensor MR imaging visualizes the altered hemispheric fiber connection in callosal dysgenesis. AJNR Am J Neuroradiol 2004;25(1):25–8.

102. Paul LK, Brown WS, Adolphs R, et al. Agenesis of the corpus callosum: genetic, developmental and functional aspects of connectivity. Nat Rev Neurosci 2007;8(4):287–99.

103. Wahl M, Strominger Z, Jeremy RJ, et al. Variability of homotopic and heterotopic callosal connectivity in partial agenesis of the corpus callosum: a 3T diffusion tensor imaging and Q-ball tractography study. AJNR Am J Neuroradiol 2009;30(2):282–9.

104. Nakata Y, Barkovich AJ, Wahl M, et al. Diffusion abnormalities and reduced volume of the ventral cingulum bundle in agenesis of the corpus callosum: a 3T imaging study. AJNR Am J Neuroradiol 2009; 30(6):1142–8.

105. Escolar ML, Poe MD, Smith JK, et al. Diffusion tensor imaging detects abnormalities in the corticospinal tracts of neonates with infantile Krabbe disease. AJNR Am J Neuroradiol 2009;30(5):1017–21.

106. Hammans S, Sweeney M, Brockington M, et al. Mitochondrial encephalopathies: molecular genetic diagnosis from blood samples. Lancet 1991;337(8753):1311–3.

107. Holt IJ, Harding AE, Morgan-Hughes JA. Deletions of muscle mitochondrial DNA in patients with mitochondrial myopathies. Nature 1988;331(6158):717–9.

108. Lin D, Crawford T, Barker P. Proton MR spectroscopy in the diagnostic evaluation of suspected mitochondrial disease. AJNR Am J Neuroradiol 2003;24(1):33.

109. Munoz A, Mateos F, Simon R, et al. Mitochondrial diseases in children: neuroradiological and clinical features in 17 patients. Neuroradiology 1999; 41(12):920–8.

110. Sakai Y, Kira R, Torisu H, et al. Persistent diffusion abnormalities in the brain stem of three children with mitochondrial diseases. AJNR Am J Neuroradiol 2006;27(9):1924–6.

111. Yoneda M, Maeda M, Kimura H, et al. Vasogenic edema on MELAS: a serial study with diffusion-weighted MR imaging. Neurology 1999;53(9):2182–4.

112. Wray SH, Provenzale JM, Johns DR, et al. MR of the brain in mitochondrial myopathy. AJNR Am J Neuroradiol 1995;16(5):1167–73.

113. Eichler AF, Batchelor TT, Henson JW. Diffusion and perfusion imaging in subacute neurotoxicity following high-dose intravenous methotrexate. Neuro Oncol 2007;9(3):373–7.

114. Brown MS, Stemmer SM, Simon JH, et al. White matter disease induced by high-dose chemotherapy:

longitudinal study with MR imaging and proton spectroscopy. AJNR Am J Neuroradiol 1998;19(2): 217–21.

115. Sterns RH, Riggs JE, Schochet SS Jr. Osmotic demyelination syndrome following correction of hyponatremia. N Engl J Med 1986;314(24): 1535–42.

116. Cramer SC, Stegbauer KC, Schneider A, et al. Decreased diffusion in central pontine myelinolysis. AJNR Am J Neuroradiol 2001;22(8):1476–9.

117. Antunez E, Estruch R, Cardenal C, et al. Usefulness of CT and MR imaging in the diagnosis of acute Wernicke's encephalopathy. AJR Am J Roentgenol 1998;171(4):1131–7.

118. Halavaara J, Brander A, Lyytinen J, et al. Wernicke's encephalopathy: is diffusion-weighted MRI useful? Neuroradiology 2003;45(8):519–23.

119. Johkura K, Naito M, Naka T. Cortical involvement in Marchiafava-Bignami disease. AJNR Am J Neuroradiol 2005;26(3):670–3.

120. Wolters EC, van Wijngaarden GK, Stam FC, et al. Leucoencephalopathy after inhaling "heroin" pyrolysate. Lancet 1982;2(8310):1233–7.

121. Maschke M, Fehlings T, Kastrup O, et al. Toxic leukoencephalopathy after intravenous consumption of heroin and cocaine with unexpected clinical recovery. J Neurol 1999;246(9):850–1.

122. Thurnher MM, Law M. Diffusion-weighted imaging, diffusion-tensor imaging, and fiber tractography of the spinal cord. Magn Reson Imaging Clin N Am 2009;17:225–44.

123. Cruz LC Jr, Domingues RC, Gasparetto EL. Diffusion tensor imaging of the cervical spinal cord of patients with relapsing-remising multiple sclerosis: a study of 41 cases. Arq Neuropsiquiatr 2009;67: 391–5.

124. Setzer M, Murtagh RD, Murtagh FR, et al. Diffusion tensor imaging tractography in patients with intramedullary tumors: comparison with intraoperative findings and value for prediction of tumor resectability. J Neurosurg Spine 2010;13:371–80.

125. Shanmuganathan K, Gullapalli RP, Zhuo J, et al. Diffusion tensor MR imaging in cervical spine trauma. AJNR Am J Neuroradiol 2008;29:655–9.

Diffusion Magnetic Resonance Imaging in the Head and Neck

James Schafer, MD, Ashok Srinivasan, MD*,
Suresh Mukherji, MD

KEYWORDS

- Diffusion weighting • Head and neck imaging
- Apparent diffusion coefficient • ADC histogram

Diffusion weighting (DW) represents a magnetic resonance (MR) imaging contrast distinct from T1 and T2 in terms of imaging physics and its relationship to underlying physiology and pathophysiology. Researchers have long been aware of DW imaging and although it is conceptually no more daunting than traditional MR imaging,[1] it became practical only with the advent of higher performance field gradients. However, since its widespread deployment in the late 1990s, it has become a sine qua non of neuroimaging because of its exquisite sensitivity to the molecular motion of water that is altered in multiple pathologic conditions, including the classic example of impeded water motion in acute brain ischemia.[2] More recently, because of the improvement in the spatial resolution and the postprocessing analytic tools of DW imaging, its utility as more than just a tool to evaluate for acute stroke has become apparent.

Continuous improvements in computed tomography (CT) and MR imaging have made the anatomic challenges of head and neck imaging less daunting. Now, the tumor size and extent can be reliably described, the macroscopic invasion of adjacent structures can be assessed, and the gross morphologic derangement of nodal architecture, including that of nodes in clinically inaccessible areas such as the retropharyngeal space, can be identified. Distinguishing normal physiology from more subtly disrupted diseased tissue and robustly characterizing the latter remain difficult. Often the radiologist is still forced to surrender the field to

the surgeon and the pathologist, particularly in the posttreatment neck. Thus, there is an ongoing drive to develop more sophisticated, noninvasive biologic imaging techniques that evaluate tissue functional status (eg, cellularity, metabolic response to chemotherapy) to differentiate the areas of posttherapeutic ambiguous soft tissue that can be left alone (because they are nonneoplastic granulation tissue and are no-touch lesions) from those that need excision (because there is residual or recurrent neoplasm). This article reviews the physical principles of DW imaging in the head and neck and describes how it can help to solve this and several other related problems. Many excellent articles review the physical principles of DW imaging in greater detail.[3–6]

PRINCIPLES

DW imaging measures the random motion of water protons by increasing the magnetic fields applied in opposite directions along a given axis. For example, consider a proton within a given voxel exposed to gradients such that if it moved along the x-axis in one direction from that voxel, it would experience increasingly positive field strength. Similarly, if it moved along the x-axis in the opposite direction, it would experience increasingly negative field strength. These gradients are symmetric such that the positive magnitude at a given distance in the x direction is equal to the negative magnitude at the same distance in the anti-x direction. In freely

Division of Neuroradiology, Department of Radiology, University of Michigan Health System, 1500 East Medical Center Drive, Ann Arbor, MI 48109, USA
* Corresponding author.
E-mail address: ashoks@med.umich.edu

Magn Reson Imaging Clin N Am 19 (2011) 55–67
doi:10.1016/j.mric.2010.10.002

moving water, that is, water in which there are no impediments to diffusion, the same number of water protons (in a given voxel) move in the x and anti-x directions and for the same distance such that the positive and negative magnetic fields cancel each other out. Likewise, if there was a reason why water molecules within a voxel preferentially move in the x direction rather than the anti-x, then there would be a net positive magnetization from the increased number of protons moving along the x direction. Thus, DW is not based on inherent magnetization characteristics like T1 or T2 relaxation times but on a modification of local field strength by externally applied gradients. Therefore, the practical acquisition of DW images requires an underlying sequence (usually a T2-weighted echo planar sequence because of its speed) which is in turn modified by gradients applied not just in the x and anti-x directions but also in the y- and z-axes to assess for disruptions of free water flow in those directions as well. The need to piggyback the DW onto a spin echo sequence creates a problem in that the pure DW signal must then be extracted from the inherent T2 tissue contrast. The variety of methods of this disambiguation results, directly and indirectly, in the proliferation of DW images (DW imaging, apparent diffusion coefficient [ADC], exponential ADC, and so forth), which causes such consternation for radiology residents and neurologists.

The signal intensity (S) measured in a DW voxel is calculated by the following formula:

$$S = S_0 \times \exp(-b \times D)$$

where D is the diffusion coefficient, S_0 is the pure T2-weighted signal, and b is the diffusion sensitivity factor defined by the formula:

$$b = \gamma^2 G^2 \delta^2 (\Delta - \delta/3)$$

in which γ is the gyromagnetic ratio, G is the strength of the gradients applied along the given axes to assess for diffusion, δ is the width of those gradients, and Δ is their time.[3] The true diffusion coefficient D cannot be controlled or measured directly by MR. Instead, an approximation, the ADC, must be calculated by measuring S with multiple b values and solving for the ADC algebraically.[5]

In contrast to DW imaging, diffusion tensor imaging (DTI) not only generates the degree of freedom of diffusion (or diffusivity, a conceptualization akin to ADC) but also provides directionality to the diffusion characteristics within a voxel. It thus becomes possible to ascertain the direction of the diffusion vector in each voxel. Applying this principle, fiber tracts of a nerve or neural pathway can be delineated because the primary diffusion vector in a nerve or nerve bundle is oriented along the direction of its axon.[4,7–9]

An alternative method, diffusion spectrum imaging (DSI), can evaluate multiple fiber orientations within a single voxel.[10] Although DSI has promising applications within the complex white matter of the central nervous system, DTI is probably sufficient to identify the large peripheral nerves of the head and neck.[11]

PROTOCOLS

Table 1 provides a sample neck diffusion protocol that is used at the authors' institution at 3 T. This protocol is almost identical to that used for DW imaging of the brain and is based on a single-shot, spin echo, echo planar sequence with eddy current correction that can be performed rapidly, adding less than 2 minutes to the overall scan time. Images are acquired using the same 16-channel head and neck coil as for the rest of the scan, with the ADC images generated using the terminal hardware before transmission to the reading workstation.

An additional consideration is that in organs with an intrinsically high ADC (eg, prostate), higher b-values are needed to give good contrast with lesions. In general, the b-value should be kept as low as possible because there is a signal-to-noise ratio penalty for higher b-values. However, with the use of low b-values (<300 s/mm^2), the perfusion component of the tissue hampers the pure diffusion measurement. Therefore, many researchers have used 2 b-values (such as 500 and 1000 s/mm^2) to calculate ADCs of head and neck lesions.[12]

USING DW IMAGING TO EVALUATE TISSUES

DW imaging addresses 2 questions related to head and neck imaging. The first relates to lesion

Table 1 Sample neck diffusion protocol		
Slice Orientation	**Axial**	**Sagittal**
Extent	Skull base to thoracic inlet	Skull base to thoracic inlet
Field of view (mm)	240	260
Slice thickness (mm)	4	4
Echo time (ms)	45	49
Repetition time (ms)	2454	2468
Flip angle (°)	90	90
b values (s/mm^2)	0 and 800	0 and 1000

characterization in de novo imaging. For example, if a patient presents with a palpable neck mass, it is imperative to determine whether the mass is benign or malignant; or perhaps a new but morphologically indeterminate node may be identified in a patient with a history of malignancy. The second relates to the ongoing evaluation of a previously identified and characterized lesion. This lesion might be indeterminate on prior imaging, a surgical bed being followed for local recurrence, or a tumor being irradiated. Providing the correct answer to these clinical problems has a dramatic effect on patient care and outcomes.

METHODS OF EXPRESSING ADC
Mean ADC Values

Using diffusion to assess the newly identified lesions is comparatively straightforward because only instantaneous findings need comment, not how those findings have changed over time. The metric with the best validation is the mean ADC. Measured in square millimeters per second (reflecting the average diffusion of a proton in a given area per unit time), the mean ADC value is just that, an assessment of the average magnitude of diffusion of water molecules in a volume of tissue. A region of interest (ROI) is drawn around the lesion or its components (eg, necrotic core, enhancing periphery), and the average ADC value of that volume is computed (**Fig. 1**). This average ADC value is compared with the published values for benign and malignant lesions and used in conjunction with other imaging to characterize the tissue.

Mean ADC values are also used to quickly approximate changes in lesions over time and with treatment. It is comparatively simple to draw an

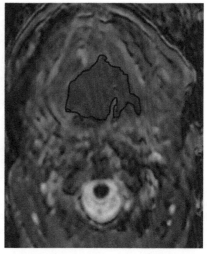

Fig. 1. A freehand ROI drawn around the lesion (squamous cell carcinoma of the oral tongue) on the ADC map, used to generate the mean ADC of the lesion (which measured 0.8×10^{-3} mm^2/s in this lesion).

ROI around the same lesion in multiple scans and assess how the mean ADC has changed. Even if the lesion has changed significantly in size or shape, a comparison can be made with the mean ADC.

However, measurements and comparisons made with the mean ADC values do have limitations. The obscuration of lesion heterogeneity with a single average value is a primary limitation. For example, a completely homogeneous lesion may yield the same ADC as a lesion composed of an equal combination of densely cellular and necrotic elements (**Fig. 2**). Such obscuration continues with comparisons. A tissue volume in which most voxels are stable with only a few changing dramatically

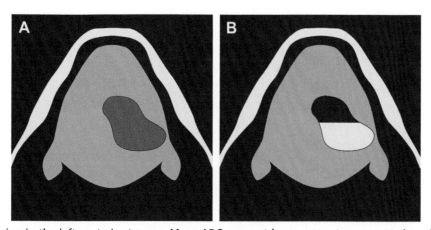

Fig. 2. A lesion in the left posterior tongue. Mean ADC may not be an accurate representation of the lesion because a homogeneous lesion demonstrating intermediate ADC values (*gray*) (*A*) can have the same mean as a heterogeneous lesion that contains areas of increased ADC values (*white*) and decreased ADC values (*black*) (*B*).

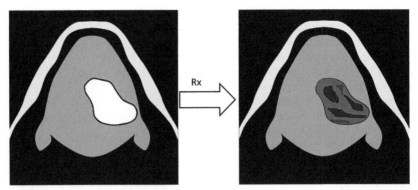

Fig. 3. The parametric response map principle comparing pre- and posttherapy ADC maps. A user-defined color coding is used to visually represent the change in ADC that occurs on a voxel-to-voxel basis between the 2 scans. In this example, voxels showing an increase in ADC are red, those showing a decrease are blue, and those that show no change are gray. This visual technique is a quick way of comparing tumors that show different responses to therapy.

may have the same mean ADC as a volume in which most of the voxels change only slightly. This limitation of ADC has led to the development of alternative ADC measures described below.

Parametric ADC Maps

Although measuring the average ADC values of a given ROI is the most common option for a de novo scan, there are alternatives to the mean ADC approach when making comparisons. A parametric ADC map, as shown in **Fig. 3**, is a graphical representation of changes in the ADC on a voxel-to-voxel basis.[13] Specifically, such a map displays those voxels that have increased in ADC, decreased in ADC, or show no change in ADC in different colors to enable instantaneous visual representation of the changes within the lesion. Such a map makes it easy to assess the overall

change in diffusion within a lesion and to identify particular areas that may deviate from the overall trend.

Although more complex and more informative than the mean ADC strategy, there are significant hurdles to the application of this technique. The most significant are the difficulties in spatial registration necessitated by voxel-to-voxel comparisons. Under ideal circumstances, these difficulties merely involve altered partial volume effects. However, if the lesion has significantly changed in size or orientation, comparisons are likely to be grossly inaccurate, if they are possible at all (**Fig. 4**).

ADC Histogram

An alternative to the mean ADC approach, which also takes into account the potential heterogeneity of a lesion, is the ADC histogram. In this approach,

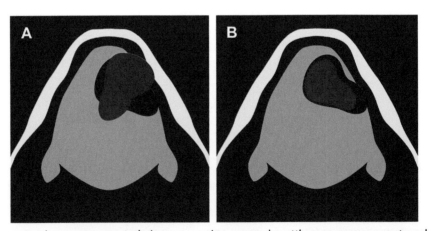

Fig. 4. The parametric response map technique comparing pre- and posttherapy scans may not work well if the tumor has changed in its axis (*A*) or changed substantially in size (*B*) because the voxel-to-voxel correlation is then lost for a large number of voxels, rendering the technique less effective in demonstrating changes.

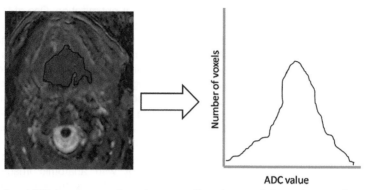

Fig. 5. (*Left*) A freehand ROI drawn around a squamous cell carcinoma of the tongue on the ADC map. (*Right*) A histogram is then generated for this lesion, where the x-axis represents the ADC values and the y-axis represents the number of voxels within the lesion for a particular ADC value.

the ROI of a lesion is identified in multiple scans and a plot of the number of voxels at each ADC value is depicted as a histogram (**Fig. 5**). Such histograms have several advantages over other methods. First, because they do not require one-to-one correlation of voxels, they are not dependent on precise concordance of ROI and thus are applicable even if a lesion has changed significantly in size or shape. Second, they provide an easy qualitative comparison of diffusion contrast that accounts for heterogeneity. Consider 2 lesions: one with uniform mid-range ADC values and the other with an equal number of very high and very low ADC values. Although these lesions are identical according to the mean ADC approach, their graphic representation in an ADC histogram is markedly distinct (**Fig. 6**). Third, this comparison can be made quantitatively with the simple addition of a numerical threshold determining the fraction of voxels above or below a certain value.

CLINICAL APPLICATIONS

From a clinical perspective, the underlying physics of an imaging modality or contrast are only relevant insofar as they allow that modality to be used quickly, easily, and reliably to answer a particular question. Although speed, ease of use, and reproducibility have been well documented for DW imaging in the head and neck, their clinical utility is only now becoming apparent. This article briefly reviews the evidence that DW can be used as a contrast to discriminate between normal and pathologic tissue.

Evaluation of Primary Malignancy

The most common and most critical clinical question in head and neck imaging is whether a mass represents a malignant cancer, a benign mass, or normal tissue. Although the diffusion characteristics of more

obscure lesions are not well known, those of squamous cell cancer, by far the most common head and neck malignancy, have been extensively studied. Pathophysiologically, such cancers have disordered and hypercellular growth, which impedes diffusion more (ie, has a lower ADC) than normal tissues or benign masses, which have lower cell densities and less disrupted extracellular matrices. There is some uncertainty about the optimal ADC cutoff to use to help differentiate benign and malignant lesions. In 3-T systems, for example, lesions with a mean ADC greater than 1.3×10^{-3} mm^2/s

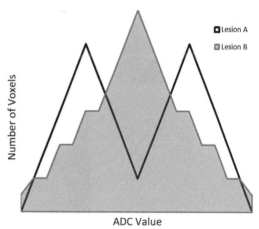

Fig. 6. ADC histograms provide another way of comparing lesions that otherwise have the same mean ADC value. In this example, the histograms show a different spread of voxels within 2 lesions that have the same mean ADC value. Lesion B shows a normal distribution centered at a single value; lesion A, despite having the same mean ADC, shows a bimodal distribution with 2 peaks that represent 2 parts of the same mass with very different physiologies. Therefore, ADC histograms are a more accurate way of characterizing a lesion.

are more likely to be benign and those with a mean ADC less than 1.3×10^{-3} mm²/s are more likely to be malignant.[14] Although this value will likely remain in flux for some time as sample sizes increase, the difference in ADC values between benign and malignant lesions has been consistent in multiple studies.[15,16] In the case of major salivary gland lesions, some studies have shown these differences but others have not, suggesting that more research in this area is required to establish the utility of DW in major salivary gland lesions.[17–19] To summarize, malignant head and neck lesions tend to demonstrate lower ADC values compared with normal tissue or benign lesions (**Figs. 7** and **8**).

Evaluation of Lymph Nodes

After determination of malignancy, whether by imaging or pathology, staging becomes critical for treatment optimization. One of the most important elements of this staging is the identification of pathologic lymph nodes. Although nodes are grossly abnormal or classically benign, many are indeterminate with borderline size and no obvious fatty hila. Although positron emission tomography (PET)-CT has become the gold standard in imaging for determining nodal abnormalities in head and neck cancer,[20] the same principles described earlier for a primary mass may also be used in nodal tissues (**Fig. 9**). Long before the architectural changes are apparent with anatomic imaging, nodes, even normal-sized ones, show metastatic foci that manifest as decreased ADC and can be measured on DW imaging. In a patient with known primary malignancy in the head and neck, the lower the ADC in a normal-sized lymph node in the neck, the greater the chances of it being metastatic. Various studies have tried to evaluate the threshold value below

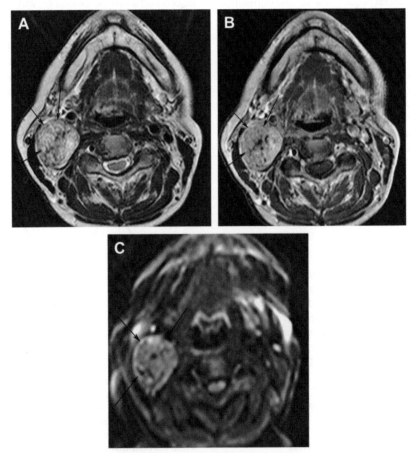

Fig. 7. T2-weighted, postcontrast T1-weighted, b1000 DW images of a 47-year-old patient demonstrate a large T2 hyperintense lesion (*A*) in the right carotid sheath that shows moderate heterogeneous enhancement (*B*) and mild increased diffusion signal (*C*). The ADC in the lesion measured 1.6×10^{-3} mm²/s, and pathology confirmed the lesion to be a schwannoma. The high ADC in the lesion is consistent with a benign process that tends to show increased ADC values.

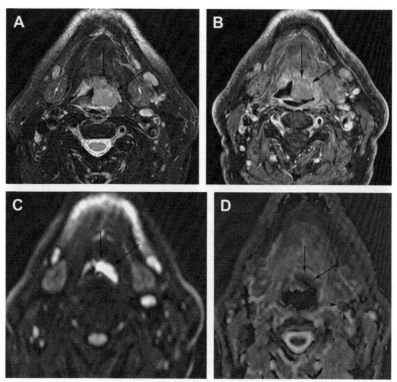

Fig. 8. T2-weighted, postcontrast T1-weighted, b1000 DW images and an ADC map of a 65-year-old patient demonstrate a T2 hyperintense (*A*), intensely enhancing (*B*) lesion along the posterior tongue base. The lesion shows bright diffusion signal (*C*) and decreased ADC (*D*), with the ADC measuring 0.7×10^{-3} mm²/s. Pathology confirmed the presence of a squamous cell carcinoma. The low ADC in the lesion is likely because of the hyper-cellularity seen within malignant neoplasms.

which the node is highly likely to be metastatic, with the results ranging from an ADC of 0.9 to 1.0 mm²/s.[21–23]

Monitoring Response to Nonsurgical Treatment

The traditional imaging metric of treatment response is based on tumor size, which is necessarily a late finding after a substantial volume of tumor mass has died and contracted. In addition, it is confounded by proliferative reactive changes that result in stable or increased tumor size despite a decrease in the volume of malignant cells. A far superior biologic imaging modality would directly measure the death of malignant cells or, more ominously, their proliferation. DW imaging shows promise in monitoring tumors during the course of chemoradiotherapy because it measures the changes in free water diffusion (which result when the tumor cells become necrotic).

Examination of tumor treatment response with DW imaging in a mouse model, in which histologic changes can be more systematically characterized,

showed that mice whose tumors responded better (and who thus survived longer) also had a more pronounced increase in tumor ADC value, as would be expected with more tumor necrosis.[24] Such results have been replicated in humans receiving treatment of head and neck cancer; however, the best method of correlating changes in proton diffusivity with tumor response remains uncertain. Whereas some studies have shown that changes in the mean ADC of the ROI of a tumor are adequate markers,[25] others suggest that more sophisticated means of mapping diffusivity changes, such as parametric ADC maps, correlate with tumor response and patient survival; the mean ADC is too coarse a measure and its association is not statistically significant.[26] One study has shown that changes in parametric color-coded ADC maps and percentage change in tumor volumes between baseline DW imaging and mid-therapy DW imaging at 3 weeks showed correlation with outcomes, as opposed to percentage change in mean ADC that did not correlate with tumor control at 6 months, implying that this technique could be better than mean ADC measurements alone.[26]

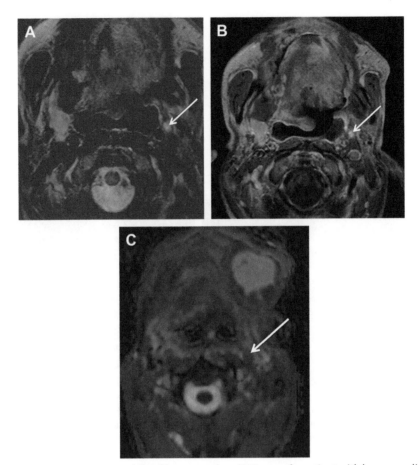

Fig. 9. T2-weighted, postcontrast T1-weighted images and an ADC map of a patient with known malignancy in the head and neck show a small, mildly T2 hyperintense lymph node at left level II, adjacent to the carotid artery (*A*). The lymph node shows only mild enhancement (*B*) and measured 1.0×0.8 cm, which is below the size for suspicion of metastasis. However, the lymph node was dark on the ADC map (*C*) and showed an ADC of 0.8×10^{-3} mm^2/s, suggesting that there may be metastatic deposits. This lymph node was removed at surgery and confirmed to be metastatic. Hence, in patients with known head and neck malignancies, the presence of decreased ADC within normal-sized lymph nodes should be viewed with suspicion in the appropriate clinical setting.

Prediction of Response to Nonsurgical Treatment

The increasing complexity of potential oncologic treatments makes it imperative to know as much as possible about a patient's malignancy. Such critical information includes gross anatomic considerations, histology, and, increasingly, tumor genetics. If the pretherapy probability of success of a therapy (eg, chemoradiotherapy) can be predicted, appropriate modification of the treatment protocol can be made if the chances of success are poor or, in some instances, the treatment plan can be changed altogether to a more aggressive approach (eg, salvage surgery). This approach can minimize the cohort of patients who undergo extensive chemoradiotherapy only to respond poorly but who thus are precluded from salvage surgery because of significant radiation-induced tissue architectural changes that make surgery more complicated and risky. In this context, DW imaging provides additional information about a tumor's composition, particularly about its cellularity, which has been correlated with response to therapy and survival. One group demonstrated a strong correlation between low ADC (high cellularity) and tumor regression after therapy.[27] An even better predictor of tumor response is based on early changes in response to therapy.[25] In both studies, patients with lower ADCs in the baseline scan were more likely to be complete responders to chemoradiotherapy, possibly attributed to better response in hypercellular lesions (the more cellular a lesion, the less hypoxic it is, which is a major impediment to the success of radiotherapy).[28]

Posttherapeutic Changes Versus Disease Recurrence

Although the initial therapeutic approach is the most critical branch point in terms of clinical decision making and patient survival, determining it is often less frustrating from a clinical perspective and less disquieting to patients than the follow-up decision. Tissue planes may be completely disrupted after surgery; radiotherapy may provoke extensive fibrosis with distortion, and healing granulation tissue may enhance avidly.[29] Distinguishing persistent or recurrent disease from normal tissue in the posttreatment neck is challenging at best and impossible at worst. Although unnecessary additional treatment is likely to increase morbidity, delay in salvage treatment decreases the likelihood of a positive outcome.[30]

Every treated neck is a unique entity, and every decision to intervene or cautiously wait is undertaken after scraping together every available piece of information. Under such circumstances, DW imaging should be seen as one part of a much larger puzzle. However, many studies suggest that ADC measurements are an increasingly useful part of that puzzle. In particular, preliminary work has used the increased free water in necrotic tissue and the decreased ADC values in areas of increased cellularity to discriminate viable or recurrent tumor from adjacent normal tissues.[31–35] Posttherapy masses that demonstrate a decreased ADC value have been shown to be more likely to be tumor recurrences than those that show increased ADC values (**Figs. 10** and **11**).

CHALLENGES AND FUTURE DIRECTIONS

Diffusion imaging has passed out of its infancy and childhood into its adolescence. Although many

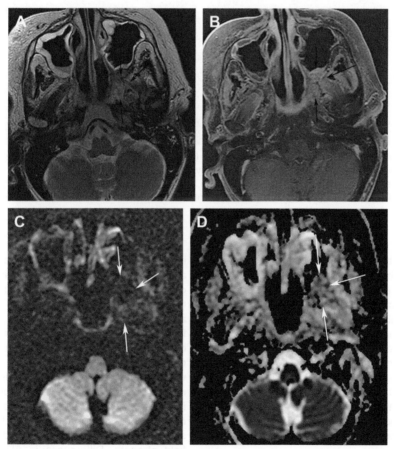

Fig. 10. T2-weighted, postcontrast T1-weighted, b1000 DW images and an ADC map of a patient treated with malignancy in the left masticator space demonstrate a T2 hyperintense, enhancing region along the medial left pterygoid (*A*, *B*). However, this region is not increased in diffusion signal (*C*) and shows an ADC values (*D*) that is brighter than the brain on the same image. The ADC measured 1.3×10^{-3} mm²/s, and there was no evidence of recurrent neoplasm on surgical pathology.

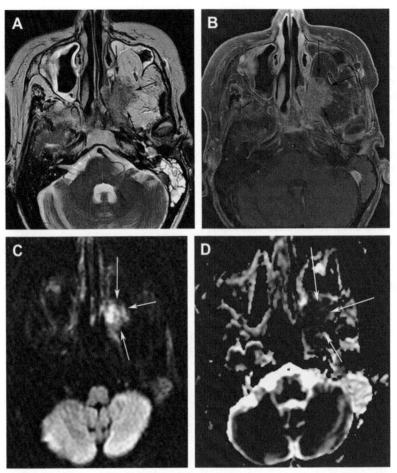

Fig. 11. T2-weighted, postcontrast T1-weighted, b1000 DW images and an ADC map of the same patient as in Fig. 10 (performed 10 months later) demonstrate a T2 hypointense, enhancing region along the medial left pterygoid (*A, B*) This region now shows increased diffusion signal (*C*) and decreased ADC values (*D*). The ADC now measured 0.6×10^{-3} mm^2/s, suggesting the possibility of neoplastic recurrence, which was confirmed on pathology.

technical problems remain, the fundamental technologies that will resolve those problems are already in place and merely need refinement. The potential applications of DW imaging are numerous and increasing. There is no question that some of these will never come to fruition, nor is there any doubt that other modalities may surpass diffusion imaging in many areas. However, DW represents an entirely different type of MR contrast; and just as we are continuing to find new ways to extract clinical information from T2 signal and patterns of contrast enhancement, diffusion is likely to provide a wealth of information in the years to come.

Field Strength

As with MR imaging in other modalities, increase in magnetic field strength represents an obvious gain

in signal-to-noise ratio that must be weighed against additional imaging complications. Some of these are well known and simply represent technical hurdles to be overcome. Field inhomogeneity at tissue interfaces, for example, increases with field strength. Although this problem is not significant in the homogeneous intracranial space, it is much more problematic within the head and neck where airspaces abound. Nevertheless, the awareness of such problems calls forth solutions such as improved shimming algorithms. More problematic are the less easily appreciated (and thus corrected) subtle differences in imaging introduced at higher field strength. Differences in ADC values, and more importantly in ADC variance, have been described as field strength increases,[36] making it impossible from a theoretic perspective to confidently extrapolate findings from 1.5 to 3 T. Because the drive to higher field strength is unlikely to abate, the need to empirically determine differences is necessary. However, it is reassuring that early studies in this regard suggest that the association between malignancy and low ADC persists from 1.5 to 3 T.[14,37]

Diffusion Tractography

Although diffusion tractography, accomplished with DTI or DSI, is likely to become increasingly important for central nervous system imaging, its role in head and neck imaging is more specific, but no less important. In particular, because of their propensity for perineural spread, a critical question related to malignancies of the neck is whether they have invaded nearby nerves. Nerves are often difficult to visualize on even the highest resolution anatomic scan. Tractography, with its dedicated evaluation of fiber paths through anisotropy evaluation, is an ideal means of determining the location of peripheral nerves.[11] Although the technical challenges described above (eg, tissue-air interfaces) make tractography more challenging in the head and neck, the peripheral nerves are larger and more isolated than those being studied within the brain and spine.

Diffusion Kurtosis

The mathematics described above with respect to the calculation of the various diffusion values assumes an ideal Gaussian movement of water. This assumption is numerically straightforward, and its utility is borne out by the well-demonstrated effectiveness of DW imaging in a variety of circumstances. It is, however, an approximation: real neural tissues, whether healthy or diseased, deviate from this ideal. Techniques are being developed to quantify the deviation of the actual diffusivity from the Gaussian model.[38] Although now essentially experimental, diffusion kurtosis has the potential to become yet another type of MR imaging contrast. In its current formulation, it, like DTI, has more obvious applications to fiber-rich brain tissues; however, as more data are collected, diffusion kurtosis imaging may show applicability to the head and neck as well.

SUMMARY
Diffusion Imaging as Part of a Neck Imaging Protocol

Because it is based on rapid echo planar sequences, DW imaging can be added to a neck protocol without a significant effect on patient throughput, and because these sequences are used extensively in brain imaging, any contemporary MR system should be able to accommodate them without difficulty. However, MR examinations must balance clinical information against scan time and image volume. Already, a combination brain and neck scan runs to more than a dozen sequences with more than a thousand images and an hour or more of scanning time. To add another sequence (or to displace one already present), DW imaging must justify its inclusion. There may come a time when DW images of the neck will be considered as critical as a T2-weighted or postcontrast sequence for basic assessment of pathology and anatomy. However, at the moment, DW imaging would best be described as a problem-solving sequence. It has significant utility in terms of malignancy workup and can provide information about tissue necrosis as seen with abscesses. Neoplasms and infections are the major reasons why clinicians are interested in neck imaging; however, if, for some reason, these elements were not of clinical concern, then DW imaging might not have anything to offer and could probably be safely excluded.

Diffusion Imaging as a Window onto Physiology

It is hard to imagine that in the not-too-distant past, clinical assessment was entirely dependent on physical examination. Imaging has revolutionized the care of patients with disease of the head and neck. From diagnosis to surgical planning and posttherapy surveillance, anatomic changes can be followed up at incredible resolution. The next step is to expand on this anatomic knowledge with insights into physiology and cell biology. This step will be a multifactorial process with input from PET-CT, MR spectroscopy, and other assorted modalities, some of which have not even been invented yet. However, DW imaging is a technique currently available on clinical scanners and it is already used every day to assess the cell biology of brain matter, looking for the cytotoxic edema that heralds ischemia. This article reviews the cutting edge applications of readily available DW sequences to the assessment of neck physiology. At the moment, these applications are limited to broad categorizations of neck lesions based on cellularity and necrosis as proxies for malignancy and treatment response, but as experience grows, so too will the certainty of diagnoses using diffusion. Over the next few years, diffusion imaging may become the next best thing to cutting out tissue and making histologic stains.

ACKNOWLEDGMENTS

The authors acknowledge Priya Rajdev for the illustrations in this article.

REFERENCES

1. Stejskal E, Tanner J. Spin diffusion measurements: spin echoes in the presence of time-dependent field gradient. J Chem Phys 1965;42:288–92.

2. Warach S, Chien D, Li W, et al. Fast magnetic resonance diffusion-weighted imaging of acute human stroke. Neurology 1992;42(9):1717–23.

3. Schafer PW, Grant PE, Gonzalez RG. Diffusion-weighted MR imaging of the brain. Radiology 2000;217:331–45.

4. Mukherjee P, Berman JI, Chung SW, et al. Diffusion tensor MR imaging and fiber tractography: theoretic underpinnings. AJNR Am J Neuroradiol 2008;29: 632–41.

5. Neil JJ. Measurement of water motion (apparent diffusion) in biological systems. Concepts Magn Reson 1997;9(6):385–401.

6. Hagman P, Jonasson L, Maeder P, et al. Understanding diffusion MR imaging techniques: from scalar diffusion-weighted imaging to diffusion tensor imaging and beyond. Radiographics 2006;26: S205–33.

7. Ito R, Mori S, Melhem ER. Diffusion tensor brain imaging and tractography. Neuroimaging Clin N Am 2002;12(1):1–20.

8. Alexander AL, Lee JE, Lazar M, et al. Diffusion tensor imaging of the brain. Neurotherapeutics 2007;4(3):616–29.

9. Le Bihan D, Mangin JF, Poupon C, et al. Diffusion tensor imaging: concepts and applications. J Magn Reson Imaging 2001;13(4):534–46.

10. Wedeen VJ, Wang RP, Schmahmann JD, et al. Diffusion spectrum magnetic resonance imaging (DSI) tractography of crossing fibers. Neuroimage 2008; 41(4):1267–77.

11. Akter M, Hirai T, Minoda R, et al. Diffusion tensor tractography in the head-and-neck region using a clinical 3-T MR scanner. Acad Radiol 2009;16:858–65.

12. Theony HC, De Keyzer F, Boesch C, et al. Diffusion-weighted imaging of the parotid gland: influence of the choice of b-values on the apparent diffusion coefficient value. J Magn Reson Imaging 2004; 20(5):786–90.

13. Galban CJ, Chenevert TL, Meyer CR, et al. The parametric response map is an imaging biomarker for early cancer treatment outcome. Nat Med 2009; 15(5):572–6.

14. Srinivasan A, Dvorak R, Perni K, et al. Differentiation of benign and malignant pathology in the head and neck using 3T apparent diffusion coefficient values: early experience. AJNR Am J Neuroradiol 2008; 29(1):40–4.

15. Wang J, Takashima S, Takayama F, et al. Head and neck lesions: characterization with diffusion-weighted echo-planar MR imaging. Radiology 2001;220:621–30.

16. Maeda M, Kato H, Sakuma H, et al. Usefulness of the apparent diffusion coefficient in line scan diffusion-weighted imaging for distinguishing between squamous cell carcinomas and malignant lymphomas of the head and neck. AJNR Am J Neuroradiol 2005;26:1186–92.

17. Eida S, Sumi M, Sakihama N, et al. Apparent diffusion coefficient mapping of salivary gland tumors: prediction of the benignancy and malignancy. AJNR Am J Neuroradiol 2007;28(1):116–21.

18. Habermann CR, Gossrau P, Graessner J. Diffusion-weighted echo-planar MRI: a valuable tool for differentiating primary parotid gland tumors? Rofo 2005; 177(7):940–5.

19. Habermann CR, Arndt C, Graessner J, et al. Diffusion-weighted echo-planar MR imaging of primary parotid gland tumors: is a prediction of different histologic subtypes possible? AJNR Am J Neuroradiol 2009;30(3):591–6.

20. Ng SH, Yen TC, Liao CT, et al. 18F-FDG PET and CT/MRI in oral cavity squamous cell carcinoma: a prospective study of 124 patients with histologic correlation. J Nucl Med 2005;46:1136–43.

21. de Bondt RBJ, Hoeberigs MC, Nelemans PJ, et al. Diagnostic accuracy and additional value of diffusion-weighted imaging for discrimination of malignant cervical lymph nodes in head and neck squamous cell carcinoma. Neuroradiology 2009; 51:183–92.

22. Holzapfel K, Duetsch S, Fauser C, et al. Value of diffusion-weighted MR imaging in the differentiation between benign and malignant cervical lymph nodes. Eur J Radiol 2009;72(3):381–7.

23. Vandercaveye V, De Keyzer F, Vanderpoorten V, et al. Head and neck squamous cell carcinoma: value of diffusion-weighted MR imaging for nodal staging. Radiology 2009;251(1):134–46.

24. Hamstra DA, Lee KC, Moffat BA, et al. Diffusion magnetic resonance imaging: an imaging treatment response biomarker to chemoradiotherapy in a mouse model of squamous cell cancer of the head and neck. Transl Oncol 2008;1(4): 187–94.

25. Kim S, Loevner L, Quon H, et al. Magnetic resonance imaging for predicting and detecting early response to chemoradiation therapy of squamous cell carcinomas of the head and neck. Clin Cancer Res 2009;15(3):986–94.

26. Galban CJ, Mukherji SK, Chenevert TL, et al. A feasibility study of parametric response map analysis of diffusion-weighted magnetic resonance imaging scans of head and neck cancer patients for providing early detection of therapeutic efficacy. Transl Oncol 2009;2(3):184–90.

27. Kato H, Kanematsu M, Tanaka O, et al. Head and neck squamous cell carcinoma: usefulness of diffusion-weighted MR imaging in the prediction of

a neoadjuvant therapeutic effect. Eur Radiol 2009; 19(1):103–9.

28. Buck A, Krause BJ, Scheidhauer K, et al. Clinical applications of FDG PET and PET/CT in head and neck cancer. J Oncol 2009;2009:ID208725.

29. Hermans R. Post-treatment imaging in head and neck cancer. Eur J Radiol 2008;66(3):501–11.

30. de Bree R, van der Putten L, Brouwer J, et al. Detection of locoregional recurrent head and neck cancer after (chemo)radiotherapy using modern imaging. Oral Oncol 2009;45(4):386–93.

31. Razek AA, Sadek AG, Kombar OR, et al. Role of apparent diffusion coefficient values in differentiation between malignant and benign solitary thyroid nodules. AJNR Am J Neuroradiol 2008;29(3):563–8.

32. Razek AA, Megahed AS, Denewer A, et al. Role of diffusion-weighted magnetic resonance imaging in differentiation between the viable and necrotic parts of head and neck tumors. Acta Radiol 2008;49(3): 364–70.

33. Vandecaveye V, de Keyzer F, Vanderpoorten V, et al. Evaluation of the larynx for tumour recurrence by diffusion-weighted MRI after radiotherapy: initial experience in four cases. Br J Radiol 2006;79:681–7.

34. Vandecaveye V, De Keyzer F, Nuyts S, et al. Detection of head and neck squamous cell carcinoma with diffusion weighted MRI after (chemo)radiotherapy: correlation between radiologic and histopathologic findings. Int J Radiat Oncol Biol Phys 2007;67(4): 960–71.

35. Abdel Razek AA, Kandeel AY, Soliman N, et al. Role of diffusion-weighted echo-planar MR imaging in differentiation of residual or recurrent head and neck tumors and post-treatment changes. AJNR Am J Neuroradiol 2007;28:1146–52.

36. Huisman TA, Loenneker T, Barta G, et al. Quantitative diffusion tensor MR imaging of the brain: field strength related variance of apparent diffusion coefficient and fractional anisotropy scalars. Eur Radiol 2006;16:1651–8.

37. Srinivasan A, Dvorak R, Rohrer S, et al. Initial experience of 3-tesla apparent diffusion coefficient values in characterizing squamous cell carcinomas of the head and neck. Acta Radiol 2008;49(9): 1079–84.

38. Jensen JH, Helpern JA, Ramani A, et al. Diffusional kurtosis imaging: the quantification of non-gaussian water diffusion by means of magnetic resonance imaging. Magn Reson Med 2005;53:1432–40.

Diffusion-Weighted Imaging of the Chest

Antonio Luna, MD[a],*, Javier Sánchez-Gonzalez, PhD[b],
Pilar Caro, MD[c]

KEYWORDS

- Pulmonary nodule • Diffusion-weighted imaging
- Lung cancer • Diffusion tensor imaging
- Intra-voxel incoherent motion • Heart fiber
- Hyperpolarized gases

MR imaging of the chest has been traditionally challenging and difficult. Shortcomings for thoracic MR imaging are motion artifacts related to breathing and heart and vascular pulsation, susceptibility artifacts associated to air–tissue interfaces, and low proton density in both lungs creating low signal in all pulse sequences.[1] Improvements in MR imaging systems, including more powerful gradients and phased-array coils, development of fast imaging techniques, such as echo-planar sequences (EPI), and application of parallel imaging, have made it possible to increase the clinical applications of thoracic MR imaging, although it is still far from being a first-line imaging test in pulmonary and mediastinal pathology. In a similar manner, cardiovascular MR imaging has developed in the last few years, with more clinical impact than pulmonary MR imaging.

In the era of functional imaging, diffusion-weighted imaging (DWI) has been proposed as a cancer biomarker.[2] DWI allows the analysis of tissue characteristics based on the diffusivity of water molecules within the tissues. Although it was first used to detect acute cerebral ischemia, the use of DWI outside the brain has been possible in the last few years because of the previously mentioned technologic developments. Despite these advances, its use in the chest is still very challenging because of the high sensitivity of DWI to artifacts. Because of this, almost all the clinical studies of DWI in the chest have been performed in 1.5-T magnets. In addition, different methods of acquisition and quantification of DWI have been used. All of these facts have limited the clinical use of DWI in the thorax, with scarce clinical experience, mostly limited to detection and characterization of pulmonary nodules and mediastinal lymph nodes. Ongoing research with DWI in such areas as cardiac imaging and pulmonary ventilation makes DWI a potential clinical imaging tool in different areas and systems of the chest, which should be fully developed in the coming years.

This article clarifies which are the most appropriate sequences and technical adjustments for the different chest applications of DWI, including its use in 3-T magnets. Current realistic and potential clinical applications of DWI in the lungs, mediastinum, pleura, and heart are also analyzed.

TECHNICAL CONSIDERATIONS

DWI is an MR imaging technique sensitive to the Brownian molecular motion of spins.[3] The molecular motion (diffusion) is related to the thermal kinetic energy of the molecules, which is proportional to the temperature. In 1950, Hahn[4] described that the presence of a magnetic field gradient during an MR imaging spin-echo (SE) experiment results in a signal attenuation because of the molecular diffusion of the spins. In 1965, Stejskal and Tanner[5] proposed an MR imaging

Javier Sánchez is an employee of Philips Healthcare as a MR clinical scientist in Spain. The other authors have no disclosures to declare.

[a] MR Unit, SERCOSA, Health Time Group, Clinica las Nieves, Carmelo Torres 2, 23007 Jaén, Spain
[b] Philips Healthcare, Maria de Portugal 1, 28050, Madrid, Spain
[c] MR Unit, DADISA, Health Time Group, Avenida Consejo de Europa, 11011 Cadiz, Spain
* Corresponding author.
E-mail address: aluna70@sercosa.com

sequence to quantify the diffusion coefficient (D) in an MR imaging experiment. In their experiment, a pair of additional gradient pulses was inserted into a pulse sequence, the so-called "Stejskal–Tanner diffusion gradients." This pulse sequence is still in use today in most DWI experiments, although some modifications have been proposed for moving organs, such as the heart.[6–8] A new parameter (b, measured in seconds per square millimeter), is derived from the Stejskal–Tanner experiment, to control the image contrast in diffusion. This parameter is mainly controlled by the area under the two gradient lobes and the separation between them is used to weight diffusion. When higher b values are applied, the signal from the molecules that suffer a higher displacement is lost, with only the signal from those molecules with less displacement remaining.

The early DWI experiments were performed in stimulated-echo and SE pulse sequences.[9–11] However, these pulse sequences required very long acquisition times of several minutes to acquire a single multislice data set, because they filled the required raw-data line by line. Therefore, these slow sequences were very prone to motion artifacts, which limited their usefulness in clinical applications, mainly in moving organs, such as the chest. Nowadays, the most extended pulse sequence for DWI is the single-shot (SS) SE EPI sequence.[12] This sequence is relatively insensitive to macroscopic patient motion because of its very fast readout of the complete image data, within about 100 ms. It has become the standard technique for DWI and diffusion tensor imaging (DTI) not only for the brain but also for body applications.

Unfortunately, EPI images frequently suffer from gross geometric distortion in the presence of B0 inhomogeneities because of the accumulation of phase error during the long echo train length (ETL).[13] This error is accumulated in phase acquisition direction, limiting the achievable resolution to maintain the geometric distortion under control. These distortions are particularly important in regions prone to magnetic susceptibility, such as bone–soft tissue interfaces or those structures in contact with air-filled spaces, as occurs in the chest.

To avoid the artifacts associated to SS EPI acquisitions, different strategies have been proposed. The most sensible one is to segment the ETL of the EPI acquisition in different shots, reducing the phase error accumulated during different readouts. Although this approach has fewer geometric artifacts, the acquisition time increases proportionally to the number of EPI shots. Besides, these sequences are more prone to motion artifacts, making it necessary to apply motion correction techniques, such as navigation echoes.[14] A special application of the multishot EPI readout is the "periodically rotated overlapping parallel lines with enhanced reconstruction" acquisition.[15,16] This sequence organizes the segmented (PROPELLER) acquisition in a radial way around the center of k-space. This approach has the advantage that the results are less sensible to motion artifacts. A different strategy to reduce the ETL without increasing the acquisition time is to apply parallel imaging, where the phase encoding lines that are not acquired are recovered using the sensitivity profile of phased array coils.[17,18]

Recent innovations in hardware and acquisition techniques have substantially improved the suitability of EPI for chest DWI. Improved gradient systems with reduced eddy-current effects have allowed faster EPI readout, which can decrease geometric distortions. Moreover, new gradient technology, reaching gradient strength of 80 mT/m, makes it feasible to acquire DWI with a b value up to 1000 s/mm^2 and an echo time (TE) under 45 milliseconds, with an acquisition matrix of 128 × 128.

Another important aspect related to the combination of EPI readout with DWI is the intensity of fat signal for very high b values. Fat signal has a very low diffusion coefficient, which makes it very relevant for high b values. However, the difference in precession frequency between the water and the fat produces a water-fat shift of several voxels in the phase encoding direction of the EPI readout. Because of both factors, the fat signal usually overlaps on the studied anatomy making it mandatory to apply fat suppression techniques for more accurate apparent diffusion coefficient (ADC) estimation. When studying the chest, the short tau inversion recovery (STIR) approach has been most commonly used as a fat suppression technique in such sequences as DWI with background suppression (DWIBS). The main problem of sequences using STIR is the low signal to noise ratio (SNR) caused by water signal reduction after the inversion pulse. To overcome this problem, different spectral fat suppression techniques, such us spectral presaturation inversion recovery (SPIR) and spectral selection attenuated inversion recovery, have been proposed, because of their superior SNR to acquisitions using STIR (Fig. 1).

To solve the lack of spatial resolution of DWI sequences, the use of higher field magnets as 3 T has been proposed for body applications. For example, a signal improvement of 50% has been reported in kidney studies when comparing 3 T

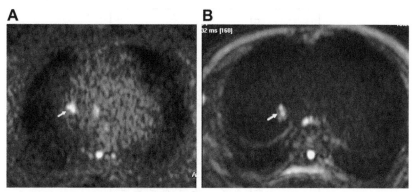

Fig. 1. Differences in DWI using STIR and SPIR acquisition on a 3-T magnet. Two DWI images were acquired in the same patient affected by an epidermoid carcinoma (*arrows*) using the same b value (1000 s/mm²). (*A*) DWI with STIR (DWIBS) and (*B*) DWI with spectral fat suppression. Spectral fat suppression DWI has a higher signal-to-noise ratio compared with the DWIBS sequence.

with 1.5 T within the same acquisition time.[19] The increase of signal of 3-T magnets may be used to obtain higher resolution or to reduce scan time. The acquisition problems inherent to DWI increase in 3-T magnets, because of higher magnetic field variation and susceptibility artifacts, which produce image distortion, and SAR limitations, which make fat suppression diffcult.[20] These limitations can be overcome using appropriately higher strength of the gradient systems of 3-T scanners in combination with parallel imaging and advanced fat suppression sequences.[21] In our experience, all these tools make it feasible to acquire thoracic DWI studies in 3-T systems (**Fig. 2**). Moreover, Gill and colleagues[22] recently reported the first clinical series of DWI performed on a 3-T magnet, with satisfactory evaluation of 57 patients with malignant pleural mesothelioma (MPM), although ADC quantification could not be obtained in seven patients because of image distortion.

The authors' standard sequences for DWI of the chest at 1.5- and 3-T magnets are detailed in **Table 1**; their sequence recommendation when possible is as follows:

- SS SE EPI
- Phased array surface coil
- b-values: several values between 0 and 100 s/mm² until 1000 s/mm²
- Field of view: 320–400
- Parallel Imaging acceleration factor of 2
- Pixel resolution 2.5 × 2.5 × 7 mm³
- Spectral fat suppression
- Number of slices, 24
- TR: 5000 ms
- TE: 53 milliseconds (shortest)
- Respiratory triggered
- Three orthogonal motion probing gradients.

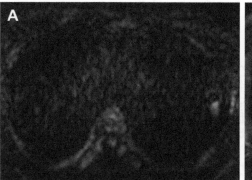
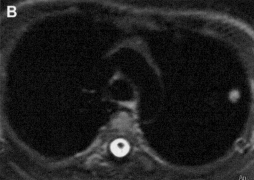

Fig. 2. Pulmonary metastasis of renal carcinoma at 3-T magnet. (*A*) Respiratory-triggered SS EPI DWI sequence with spectral fat suppression and a b value of 900 s/mm² nicely depicts a metastasis in the upper lobe of left lung. (*B*) Black-blood STIR TSE shows the lesion similarly to DWI.

Table 1
DWI sequences performed at our centers at 1.5- and 3-T magnets

	Sequence Type/Parallel Acceleration Factor	B values (s/mm²)	TR/TE (ms)	Resolution (mm³)	Synchronization	Fat Suppression Technique	Image Evaluation
IVIM 3-T	SS EPI/factor 2	0, 10, 20, 30, 50, 100, 150, 300, 450, 600, 750, 1000	5000/55	2.5 × 2.5 × 7	Respiratory triggered	Spectral fat suppression	IVIM model
DWIBS 3-T	SS EPI/factor 2	0–1000	5000/55	2.5 × 2.5 × 7	Respiratory triggered	STIR (inversion time 260 ms)	ADC
IVIM 1.5-T	SS EPI/factor 2	0, 50, 100, 150, 400, 600, 1000	1400/100	3 × 3 × 7	Respiratory triggered	Spectral fat suppression	IVIM model
DWIBS 1.5-T	SS EPI/factor 2	0–1000	632/60	3 × 3 × 7	Respiratory triggered	STIR (inversion time 160 ms)	ADC

Abbreviations: TE, echo time; TR, repetition time.

ADC Quantification

From the Stejskal and Tanner[5] acquisition sequence, it can be derived that the signal attenuation caused by DWI has an exponential behavior, modulated by the control sequence parameter, b value, and the diffusion properties of the tissue. In the presence of single water compartment the diffusion signal can be expressed as:

$$S(b) = S_0 e^{-bD},$$

where S(b) represents the acquired signal, S_0 is the signal taking into account the T1 and T2 relaxation effects. When more than a single DWI is acquired the diffusion coefficient D can be estimated as

$$D = \frac{1}{b_{max} - b_{min}} \ln\left(S(b_{min})/S(b_{max}) \right).$$

There are many parameters that can affect the in vivo measured diffusion coefficient, such as the presence of cell membranes and organelles or blood flow along the vessels. For these reasons, the diffusion coefficient is referred to as ADC.

To isolate the effect of the blood flow from the estimation of the diffusion coefficient, Le Bihan and colleagues[11] proposed the Intra Voxel Incoherent Motion (IVIM) model of the diffusion signal. This model separates the diffusion signal decay in two different diffusion compartments. For low b values, between 0 and 100 s/mm², the diffusion signal experiments a fast decay because of the blood flow along the microvasculature, whereas for higher b values, over 100 s/mm², the signal decay corresponds to the conventional diffusion of the tissue, following this equation:

$$\frac{S(b)}{S_0} = (1 - f)e^{-bD} + fe^{-b(D+D^*)},$$

where f represents the perfusion fraction, D is the perfusion free diffusion coefficient, and D* is the perfusion diffusion coefficient.

This model has been successfully evaluated in several pathologic conditions, such as brain tumors[11] and liver cirrhosis. To differentiate patients with and without cirrhosis, Luciani and colleagues[23] compared the diffusion coefficient (D), estimated from an IVIM DWI sequence with 10 different b values (0, 10, 20, 30, 50, 80, 100, 200, 400, and 800 s/mm²), with the ADC value obtained from a separate DWI measurement with four b values (0, 200, 400, and 800 s/mm²). In this series, ADC values were significantly higher than D in both cirrhotic and noncirrhotic patients. This difference between ADC and D values is probably secondary to the perfusion effect in the diffusion signal decay. Therefore, the IVIM approach allows one to avoid the perfusion effects (**Fig. 3**).

Synchronization of DWI

Another problem involving the diffusion signal is the macroscopic movement produced by the respiratory motion and heartbeat, which are critical in thoracic acquisitions. To avoid this movement, different strategies have been proposed, which have been carefully studied in the liver.[24–26] Kwee and colleagues[24] reported good agreement in the estimation of ADC value comparing breath-hold and free-breathing sequences, whereas respiratory-triggered acquisitions systematically showed an overestimation in the ADC values. In

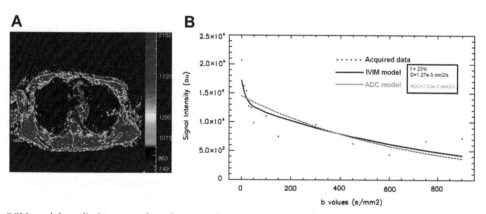

Fig. 3. IVIM model applied to a renal carcinoma pulmonary metastasis (same case as **Fig. 2**). (*A*) Parametric D map shows a nodule in the upper left lobe with restricted diffusion. (*B*) Comparison of diffusion signal decay within the lesion using either the IVIM model estimation (*solid line*) or the conventional ADC estimation from the monoexponential model (*dotted line*). The effect of the perfusion contribution to the ADC estimation can be appreciated as fast signal decay in the lower b values caused by perfusion effect. The results of both models show a clear difference between the conventional ADC and the D measurements.

contrast, Kandpal and colleagues[25] found good agreement in the ADC values acquired with respiratory-triggered and breathhold strategies for normal liver and focal lesions, although respiratory-triggered acquisitions showed higher SNR in normal liver and higher contrast-to-noise ratio between normal liver and focal lesion than with breathhold sequences. Finally, in another report, Kwee and colleagues[26] also studied the effect of the heart motion on DWI of the liver, showing a strong degradation of those images acquired during the heart systole because of the effect of the heart movement. Although the effect of cardiac movement in the ADC estimation was not studied in this paper, the authors suggest that the signal loss in DWI images should affect the ADC estimation. Similar approaches have been applied in DWI of the chest with current lack of consensus. Most of the time the use of respiratory trigger improves the quality of DWI sequences compared with those using breath-holding, according to our experience. A cardiac trigger is also useful to avoid pulsation artifacts, but it is not always necessary except in the case of lesions located immediately around the heart or in dedicated cardiac acquisitions, because it is time consuming (**Fig. 4**).

Region of Interest Analysis

As in other organs, there is a lack of standardization in region of interest analysis, which is prone to errors because it is operator-dependent. The number and size of region of interest varies from series to series. There is also no consensus as to whether or not it is more appropriate to use the mean or minimal ADC value. Areas of necrosis and those with susceptibility artifacts should be avoided. Misregistration of the trace images may cause variations of the ADCs, which may be partially solved using coregistration software.

CLINICAL APPLICATIONS
Detection of Pulmonary Nodules

Pulmonary MR imaging with conventional sequences, including STIR, has demonstrated good results in the detection of pulmonary nodules.[27-29] CT with breathholding at end inspiration is considered the best imaging technique for nodule detection.[30] In comparison with multidetector CT (MDCT), STIR sequences have achieved better results with sensitivities superior to 90% for nodules measuring 3 mm in size or larger.[29]

There are scarce reports of the capability of DWI to detect pulmonary nodules, which are most commonly included in whole-body acquisitions for tumor staging or detection. In most of the series comparing the detection of pulmonary metastasis in either positron emission tomography (PET) or integrated PET-CT cameras with whole-body (WB) DWI MR imaging, the accuracy and sensitivity of both methods are similar, with similar rates of false-positive lesions.[30-32] However, in a recent series by Chen and colleagues,[33] WB-DWI MR imaging missed three of five pulmonary metastasis of non–small cell lung cancer (NSCLC), with a size of less than 10 mm. Koyama and colleagues[34] recently showed that the detection rate of pulmonary adenocarcinomas was significantly lower for a dedicated chest DWI sequence than that of STIR. In another series, small metastases and non-solid adenocarcinomas showed low signal intensity on DWI sequence with high b value (1000 s/mm^2), which makes them very difficult to be detected (**Fig. 5**).[35] Furthermore, in the same series, a bronchioalveolar carcinoma (BAC) of 2 cm was missed on DWI. Similar results were presented by Liu and colleagues,[36] where seven metastasis and two moderately differentiated adenocarcinomas demonstrated only moderate hyperintensity on DWI with a b value of 500 s/mm^2.

In most of the reports evaluating pulmonary nodules with a dedicated chest DWI sequence, the size of the studied nodules is usually superior to 1 cm, which supposes a limitation to find out the real potential of DWI in the detection of lung lesions, making further research with smaller nodules necessary. Therefore, with the available data, DWI may be inferior to STIR in the detection of pulmonary nodules, and similar to PET and PET-CT. Larger series are necessary to define the behavior of well-differentiated adenocarcinomas and lung metastasis.

Pulmonary Nodules and Lung Cancer Characterization

The characterization of pulmonary nodules is still a common clinical dilemma. The probability of malignancy increases with the nodule's size. Only 20% of nodules larger than 20 mm are benign. For instance, the prevalence of malignancy for nodules larger than 20 mm ranges from 64% to 82%.[37] To avoid unnecessary surgical resection of benign nodules, it is important to get as precise as possible noninvasive characterization. CT is the most used test in pulmonary nodule evaluation, but still is based on morphologic criteria, showing obvious limitations, mainly in areas of altered pulmonary anatomy. Dynamic enhanced CT shows an excellent sensitivity but a limited specificity, because there is some overlap in enhancing nodules between active granulomas, hypervascular benign nodules, and

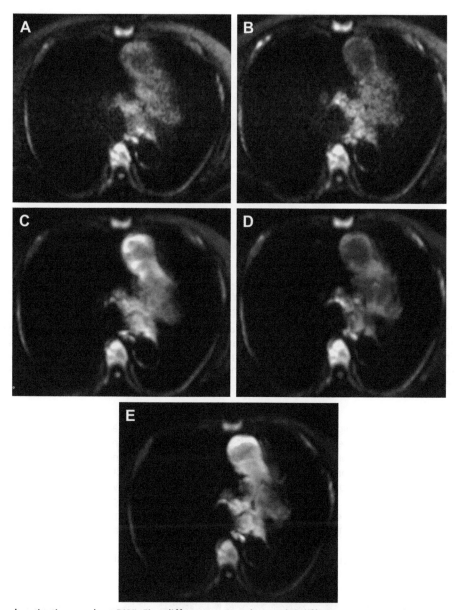

Fig. 4. Synchronization on chest DWI. Five different approaches under different strategies of motion compensation of the same DWI sequence are shown, using the same b value (800 s/mm²) at a 3-T magnet, in a patient with small cell lung cancer (SCLC). (*A*) Free-breathing. (*B*) Breathhold. (*C*) Breathhold and cardiac trigger. (*D*) Respiratory trigger. (*E*) Respiratory and cardiac trigger. Higher signal of the mediastinal mass is shown in acquisitions with cardiac and respiratory control (*C, E*), caused by reduction of the signal loss on DWI related to respiratory and cardiac movement. On the contrary, in acquisitions without cardiac synchronization (*A, B,* and *D*), a loss of signal within the tumor is evident because of the cardiac movement effect over the DWI signal.

malignant nodules.[37,38] PET has demonstrated usefulness in this task, but it is also limited in the detection of adenocarcinomas and shows an important false-positive rate caused by inflammation.[39]

Conventional MR imaging has been proposed for the evaluation of solitary pulmonary nodules according to their relaxation times with significant overlap between benign and malignant tumors.[40] More recently, dynamic enhanced MR imaging

has shown better specificity and accuracy than multidetector CT and coregistered PET-CT in the differentiation between benign and malignant nodules,[41] although an overlap is still present in the patterns of enhancement between malignant and inflammatory lesions.[42]

Based on the concept that malignant lesions demonstrate increased cellularity, higher tissue disorganization, and increased extracellular space

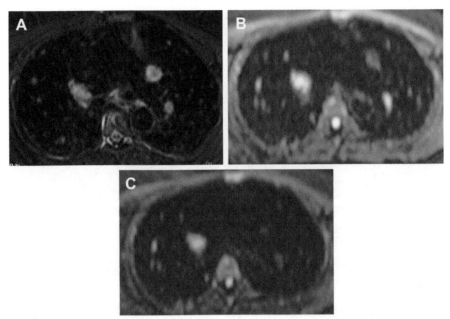

Fig. 5. Pulmonary metastases of papillary thyroid carcinoma. (*A*) Axial black-blood STIR image shows several bilateral millimetric pulmonary metastases and enlarged prevascular and bilateral hilar lymphadenopathies, probably representing lymph node metastases. Respiratory-triggered SS EPI DWI sequence with SPIR on a 1.5-T magnet with b values of 150 s/mm² (*B*) and 500 s/mm² (*C*) demonstrate a lesser number of pulmonary metastases than STIR. The enlarged lymph nodes are also less evident.

tortuosity compared with benign lesions, diffusion of interstitial water should be restricted in cases of lung cancer (**Fig. 6**). Several series have been published in the last 5 years exploring the capabilities of DWI in the characterization of pulmonary lesions (**Table 2**).

Using a visual assessment of a DWI sequence with a maximum b value of 1000 s/mm², Satoh and colleagues[35] evaluated 54 nodules larger than 5 mm. They could accurately differentiate

benign from malignant nodules, with an area under the curve of 0.80. Small metastasis and some non-solid adenocarcinomas were predominantly hypo-intense on DWI with high b value. Granulomas, active inflammatory, and fibrous nodules occasionally showed high signal intensity in a similar fashion to malignant lesions (**Fig. 7**).

In contrast, Liu and colleagues[36] analyzed 66 pulmonary lesions and did not find significant differences in the signal intensity between benign

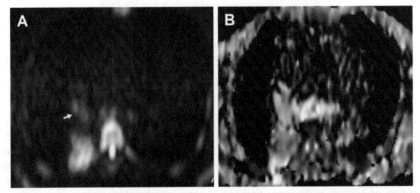

Fig. 6. Poorly differentiated adenocarcinoma. (*A*) Free breathe SS EPI DWI sequence with SPIR and a b value of 800 s/mm² performed in a 1-T magnet shows restricted diffusion of the lesion, which is confirmed in the ADC map (*B*). The mass demonstrated an ADC value of 1.2×10^{-3} mm²/s. Notice the presence in *A* of a metastatic right hilar lymphadenopathy, which is detectable on the DWI sequence (*arrow*), which was not evident on T2 weighted (not shown).

Table 2
Resume of technical parameters of DWI sequences used in the published series evaluating pulmonary nodulesx

	Sec Type/Parallel Acceleration Factor	B values (s/mm²)	TR/TE (ms)	Resolution (mm³)	Synchronization	Fat Suppression	Image Evaluation
Koyama et al[34]	SS EPI/factor 2	0–1000	5000/70	3.3 × 3.3 × 5	Free breathing	STIR	ADC + comparison with muscle SI
Satoh et al[35]	SS EPI/factor 2	0–1000	4650–9059/50–70	3.3 × 3.3 × 4	Free breathing	STIR	Visual inspection
Liu et al[36]	SS EPI/factor 2	0–500	4000/48.9	2.8 × 2.8 × 6	Free breathing	Not available	Qualitative + ADC
Uto et al[43]	SS EPI/factor 2	0–1000	4100–5100/50	2.08 × 2.08 × 5	Breathhold	Spectral	ADC + comparison with spinal cord SI
Matoba et al[45]	SS FSE	68.46–577.05	Not available/65	Not available	Breathhold and cardiac triggered	No fat suppression	ADC
Tanaka et al[46]	SS EPI/factor 2	1000	2900–3900/60–70	3.5 × 3.5 × 8	Respiratory triggered	Spectral	Visual inspection
Baysal et al[70]	SS EPI	0–1000	5000/100	2.3 × 1.56 × 7	Breathhold	Not available	ADC
Qi et al[54]	SS EPI/factor 2	0–500	2450/57.6	3.6 × 3.6 × 8	Breathhold	Not available	Visual inspection
Kanauchi et al[47]	SS EPI/not available	1000	Not available/52	3.3 × 1.4 × 5	Free breathing	STIR	Comparison with spinal cord SI
Okuma et al[55]	SS EPI/not available	0–500–1000	5700/81	3 × 3 × 6	Breathhold	Spectral	ADC
Mori et al[44]	SSEPI/not available	0–1000	5900/60–90	3.6 × 4 × 6	Breathhold	Not available	ADC

Abbreviations: Sec type, sequence type; SI, signal intensity; TE, echo time; TR, repetition time.

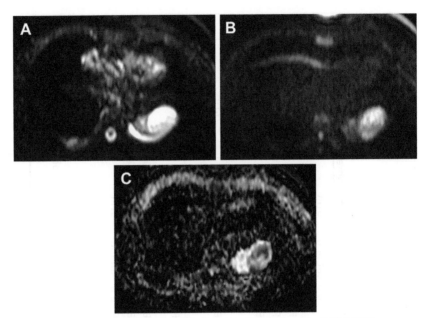

Fig. 7. Pulmonary abscess and exudative pleural effusion. (*A, B*) Free breathe SS EPI DWI sequence with SPIR on a 1-T magnet with b values of 0 s/mm^2 (*A*) and 800 s/mm^2 (*B*) show a hyperintense mass located in the left lung along with an exudative pleural effusion. (*C*) The ADC map confirms the restriction of the mass, because it shows a minimal ADC value of 1×10^{-3} mm^2/s.

and malignant nodules using a DWI sequence with a maximum b value of 500 s/mm^2. However, in this report, a threshold ADC value of 1.4×10^{-3} mm^2/s allowed the distinction between benign and malignant lesions with a sensitivity of 83% and a specificity of 74%. Furthermore, small cell lung cancer (SCLC) demonstrated statistically significant lower ADC values than NSCLC.

Different results were obtained in a series by Uto and colleagues.[43] They evaluated 28 pulmonary lesions larger than 1 cm with a DWI sequence with a maximum b value of 1000 s/mm^2. They compared a semiquantitative approach, measuring the signal intensity of the lesions and the spinal cord, with the ADC values to differentiate between benign and malignant nodules. In the receiver operating characteristic curve analysis, the semiquantitative approach had a higher area under the curve compared with ADC values (0.911 vs 0.600).[43]

Mori and colleagues[44] achieved better results in the distinction of benign from malignant pulmonary nodules with DWI with a b value of 1000 s/mm^2 compared with PET. Using a cut-off ADC value of 1.1×10^{-3} mm^2/s, they obtained a sensitivity of 70% and specificity of 97%, compared with the 72% and 79% obtained by PET, respectively. DWI also reduced the rate of false-positive lesions compared with PET.

DWI has been defined as an in vivo biomarker of tumoral grade and differentiation in oncologic lesions in other organs, because more aggressive lesions are more hypercellular than well-differentiated lesions.[2] In this sense, Matoba and colleagues[45] performed a split acquisition of fast SE signals for diffusion imaging with two b values (68.46 and 577.05 s/mm^2) in 30 patients with lung carcinoma, demonstrating an adequate correlation between the ADC values of lung cancer and tumor cellularity. Although there was an overlap between the ADC values of the different types of lung carcinoma, they demonstrated that well-differentiated adenocarcinomas showed higher ADC values than those of more aggressive adenocarcinomas and epidermoid carcinomas in a significant manner, because well-differentiated adenocarcinomas showed lesser tumor cellularity and cellular differentiation than the other types of pulmonary carcinoma.

In another series, Tanaka and colleagues[46] studied 46 peripheral adenocarcinomas lesser than 3 cm, with DWI with a higher b value of 1000 s/mm^2. Adenocarcinomas were histologically classified as BAC, advanced-BAC, mixed subtype, and non-BAC. The first one shows a favorable prognosis and the last two subtypes are invasive cancers. They did not use ADC quantification, if not a visual assessment of the signal intensity on DWI of the nodules compared with spinal cord. They were able to significantly differentiate invasive adenocarcinomas from BAC, because invasive adenocarcinomas usually showed higher signal intensity (see **Fig. 6; Fig. 8**).

Following the same histologic classification for lung adenocarcinoma, Koyama and colleagues[34] evaluated 33 adenocarcinomas with DWI and a higher b value of 1000 s/mm^2. The ADC values were not useful to differentiate the subtypes of adenocarcinoma.

Kanauchi and colleagues[47] studied 41 patients with clinical stage IA NSCLC who had undergone curative resection with DWI and PET-CT. Using a visual qualitative analysis, DWI was found to be an independent predictive factor to detect patients with invasive cancer with a sensitivity of 90%, a specificity of 81%, a positive predictive value of 60%, and a negative predictive value of 96%. In another report, DWI was equivalent to PET in distinguishing NSCLC from benign pulmonary nodules. PET was able to predict tumoral aggressiveness, showing significant differences between pathologic stages IA versus IB or more advanced stages and between well-differentiated and moderately or poorly differentiated adenocarcinomas. However, DWI using ADC quantification was of no value in the prediction of tumoral invasion.[48]

It is difficult to compare results from the previously referred series because of the different DWI sequences performed, and different qualitative and quantitative assessment methods. As a general rule, DWI of pulmonary nodules achieves good results in the differentiation between benign and malignant nodules (**Fig. 9**). Limitations of the technique are the presence of a significant number of false-positives related mainly to benign inflammatory lesions and potential false-negatives of low-grade adenocarcinomas and metastasis. In the limited series available comparing DWI with PET, both perform equivalently in pulmonary lesion characterization, with similar limitations, although DWI tends to have fewer false-positives.

The selection of b values is another topic of discussion. Conversely to the opinion of Matoba and colleagues,[45] the authors' experience indicates that with current state-of-the-art magnets, a b value of 1000 s/mm^2 can be performed perfectly without significant image quality loss or increase of susceptibility artifacts, allowing a better differentiation between benign and malignant lesions. With regard to the most appropriate assessment of pulmonary DWI, Uto and colleagues[43] correctly stated that ADC calculations of pulmonary lesions were significantly affected by perfusion phenomena. They proposed to increase the higher b value over 1000 s/mm^2 to prevent perfusion effects, because DWI sequences obtained with higher b values are more sensitive to diffusion. Additionally, ADC measurements obtained with higher b values are generally smaller than those obtained using lower b values. In addition, the IVIM model of diffusion signal decay has demonstrated that microvascular perfusion is detected at low b values (under 100 s/mm^2), allowing one to calculate the perfusion-free diffusion parameter (D) in several organs, such as brain, abdominal organs, or muscle.[11,23,49–51] ADC values are usually significantly higher than D values, as demonstrated in abdominal organs.[49] If an IVIM sequence may not be performed, another approach to avoid perfusion contamination, proposed in other organs,[52] is to avoid b values under 100 in the ADC quantification, to partially avoid perfusion effects. In the authors' experience, the IVIM model is feasible in the thorax, allowing differentiation of the diffusion and perfusion in pulmonary nodules, although it remains to be proved whether this approach improves lesional detection and characterization (see **Figs. 3** and **8**).

In centrally located lung cancers, DWI has been shown to be able to accurately differentiate postobstructive consolidation from central lung carcinoma, which is important in the planification of radiotherapy.[53] In another series, the differentiation of central lung cancer from postobstructive lobar collapse was superior with DWI compared with either T2-weighted sequences or enhanced CT (**Fig. 10**).[54]

Other potential applications of DWI in lung cancer, still to be fully explored, are monitoring treatment response after chemotherapy or radiation, distinguishing posttherapeutic changes from residual active tumor, and the detection of recurrent cancer (**Fig. 11**). DWI has also been used in other organs to predict response to treatment of cancer before and soon after therapy, which has still to be investigated for lung cancer.[2] In the same direction, Okuma and colleagues[55] evaluated prospectively 17 patients with 20 malignant lung lesions that underwent CT-guided radiofrequency ablation. DWI with ADC calculation was performed immediately before and 3 days after treatment. The posttreatment ADC of the lesions without local progression was significantly higher than that of the lesions with local progression. However, this difference could not be demonstrated for the pretreatment ADC quantification.

Staging of NSCLC with DWI

Currently, PET and PET-CT are considered the most accurate noninvasive techniques in the

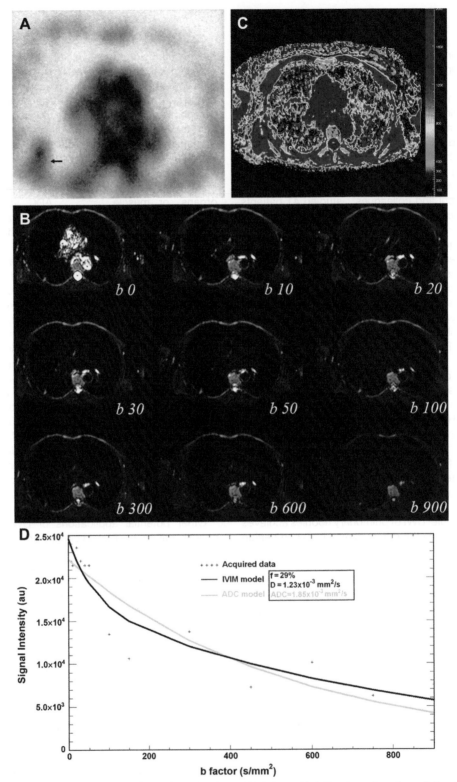

Fig. 8. Bronchioalveolar carcinoma. (*A*) Fluorodeoxyglucose PET shows ill-defined uptake of a peripheral lesion in right upper lobe (*arrow*), which was not considered suspicious for malignancy. (*B*) IVIM-DWI sequence at 3-T magnet with multiple b values (only shown 9) depicts the nodule as moderately hyperintense with high b values. (*C*) Parametric map of D confirms the lesional restricted diffusion. (*D*) Comparison of signal decay within the lesion using either the IVIM model estimation (*black line*) or the conventional ADC estimation from the mono-exponential model (*gray line*). The ADC value is that of 1.85×10^{-3} mm²/s, in the range of a benign lesion. However, if one applies the bicompartimental model of DWI, one can calculate the lesional value of D, 1.23×10^{-3} mm²/s, in the range of a malignant lesion. In this case, the effect of the perfusion contribution to the ADC estimation may cause a false-positive, as was the PET.

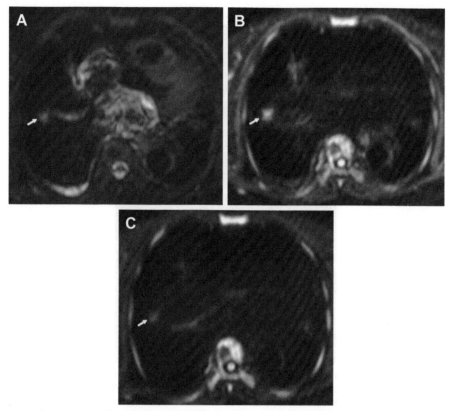

Fig. 9. Benign pulmonary nodule. Respiratory-triggered SS EPI DWI sequence with SPIR on a 1.5-T magnet with b values of 0 (*A*), 150 (*B*), and 600 s/mm^2 (*C*) demonstrates a spiculated nodule in right lung (*arrows*) with progressive loss of signal while increasing the diffusion-weighting. An ADC value of 1.9 × 10^{-3} mm^2/s suggests a benign lesions, as confirmed clinically in 6 years of imaging follow-up.

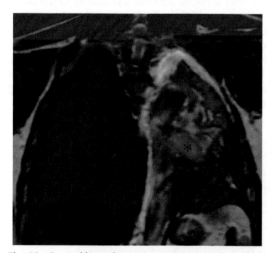

Fig. 10. Central bronchogenic carcinoma with postobstructive consolidation. Coronal fusion image of a T2 TSE image and a SS EPI DWI sequence with a b value of 1000 s/mm^2 allows a good depiction of the epidermoid carcinoma as an area of restricted diffusion (*asterisk*) surrounded by postobstructive consolidation, which does not demonstrate hyperintensity on DWI.

N-staging of NSCLC, although they lack specificity because of concurrent inflammatory lymphadenitis.[56] The morphology and size criteria used by CT and MR imaging in hilar and mediastinal node staging have also demonstrated their limitations.[57] Although STIR turbo-SE sequence has shown is ability to distinguish between benign and malignant mediastinal lymph nodes, its use is still limited in daily clinical practice.[58]

DWI is able to differentiate between benign and malignant adenopathies in the neck and head.[59] In a similar fashion, Nomori and colleagues[60] demonstrated that DWI was significantly more accurate than PET in the N-staging of NSLC, because of less overstaging and fewer false-positives in the former (**Fig. 12**). The detectable size of node metastases for both methods was 4 mm. They used a maximum b value of 1000 s/mm^2 and a threshold ADC value of 1.6 × 10^{-3} mm^2/s. In this series, inflammatory lymphadenitis usually showed increased fluorodeoxyglucose uptake but not restricted diffusion, which justifies the difference in false-positive results

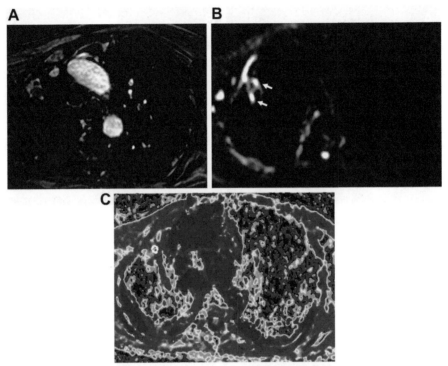

Fig. 11. Recurrent poorly differentiated adenocarcinoma. A 64 year-old man with antecedent of NSCLC, treated 2 years before, and in clinical complete response. (*A*) Axial postcontrast THRIVE shows a spiculated lesion with heterogeneous enhancement. (*B*) IVIM-DWI sequence with a b value of 900 mm²/s depicts the nodule with focal areas of hyperintensity (*arrows*). (*C*) Parametric map of D confirms the restricted diffusion. Lesional D value, at the place where the ROI is positioned, was that of 1.5×10^{-3} mm²/s, consistent with recurrent lesion.

between both techniques (**Fig. 13**). Most of the false-positive results on DWI were caused by lymph nodes with granulation tissue of tuberculosis or nontuberculosis origin, which are also a cause of false-positives on PET-CT.

Other series have confirmed the potential of DWI in the characterization of mediastinal node involvement of NSCLC using either visual assessment[57] or ADC measurements.[61] In all of these series, the presence of susceptibility and chemical shift artifacts was not a limitation to obtaining acceptable ADC maps. A potential problem when using DWI for mediastinal imaging may be to correctly locate the lymph nodes, because of its intrinsic low spatial resolution of DWI sequences. The use of fusion software allows the overlay of anatomic and DWI sequences, partially solving this problem.

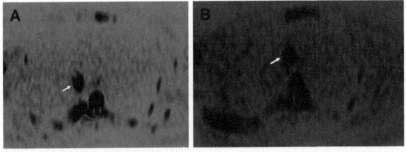

Fig. 12. Metastatic adenopathies of poorly differentiated lung adenocarcinoma. (*A, B*) Free breathe SS EPI DWI sequence with SPIR on a 1-T magnet with a b value of 800 s/mm² at two different levels demonstrates a mass with restricted diffusion in the superior segment of the right inferior lobe corresponding to a pulmonary adenocarcinoma (*red arrow*) (*A*) and metastatic right hilar (*white arrow* on *A*) and right paratracheal adenopathies (*white arrow* on *B*).

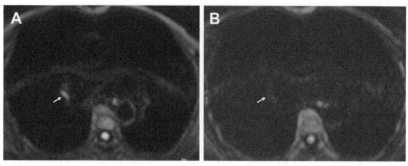

Fig. 13. Lymphadenitis in a patient with bronchioalveolar carcinoma (same case as **Fig. 8**). Respiratory-triggered SS EPI DWI sequence with SPIR on a 3-T magnet with b values of 300 s/mm^2 (*A*) and 900 s/mm^2 (*B*) demonstrates absence of restricted diffusion of a small right hilar lymph node (*arrows on both images*), which was confirmed as benign lymphadenitis on pathologic analysis. Notice the presence of fat signal overlap in both images, although consistent fat suppression was reached.

The detectable size of metastatic thoracic lymph node with the current available technology is around 4 to 5 mm for both DWI and PET-CT. Therefore, lymph node dissection may not be reduced for patients with N0 stage diagnosed by DWI or PET-CT, because node metastases inferior to this size are not uncommon. **Table 3** summarizes the technical characteristics of the DWI sequences used in the evaluation of mediastinal lymph nodes.

In contrast to these results, in series using WB-DWI MR imaging approach with a DWIBS sequence, the accuracy of the N-staging of lung cancer has not been as favorable as PET-CT. Lichy and colleagues[62] evaluated the performance of WB-DWI MR imaging for tumor detection compared with PET-CT. They included in their series three patients with lung cancer and 11 metastatic thoracic lymph nodes detected on PET-CT, of which WB-DWI MR imaging could only detect one. More recently, Chen and colleagues[33] analyzed in 56 patients the performance of WB-DWI MR imaging and PET-CT in the N- and M-staging of NSCLC. They obtained significant differences in the accuracy of lymph node metastases detection, favoring PET-CT. In the evaluation of hilar and mediastinal node metastases, they had two false-negative cases not detected by WB-DWI MR imaging that corresponded to lymph nodes with a size less of 10 mm, and only one with PET-CT. In the same series, WB-DWI MR imaging missed six node metastases in the neck and presented four false-positive cases in the same region. In contrast, PET-CT had only one false-negative and another false-positive in the same area. The evaluation of the neck region was problematic because of parallel girdle-like artifacts, which frequently obscured the metastatic lymph nodes.

In the same series by Chen and colleagues,[33] similar results were found in the M-staging of NSCLC for WB-DWI MR imaging and PET-CT, although better detection rates were achieved with the last technique. Ohno and colleagues[30] stated that WB-DWI MR imaging should be used alone with morphological whole-body sequences to improve the diagnostic accuracy of this technique, because WB-DWI MR imaging, including only a DWIBS sequence, showed a significantly worse specificity and accuracy for M-stage assessment of NSCLC with the inclusion of brain metastases than either morphological WB imaging, with or without DWIBS sequence or PET-CT (**Fig. 14**). Most of the false-positives and false-negatives with both techniques corresponded to brain and pulmonary lesions. Chen and colleagues[33] did not used conventional MR imaging sequences in their series, which may justify the differences in results compared with the report by Ohno and colleagues.[30] Neither performed ADC quantifications, which may also leave room for further improvements in the accuracy of WB-DWI MR imaging.

Mediastinum

As previously reported in other anatomic regions, Koşucu and colleagues[63] demonstrated that DWI and ADC measurements allowed one to distinguish between benign and metastatic lymph nodes of SCLC and NSCLC. In a similar manner, Sakurada and colleagues[64] demonstrated that the ADC values of node metastases of esophageal cancer unexpectedly were significantly higher than that of nonmetastatic lymph nodes, although there was an overlap in the ADCs of both groups. The higher ADC values of node metastases may

Table 3
Resume of technical parameters of DWI sequences used in the published series evaluating mediastinal lymph nodes

	Seq type/Parallel Acceleration Factor	B values (s/mm²)	TR/TE (ms)	Resolution (mm³)	Synchronization	Fat Suppression	Image Evaluation
Hasegawa et al[57]	SS EPI/factor 2	1000	5037/68	3.3 × 3.3 × 5	Free breathing	STIR	Visual inspection
Nomori et al[60]	SS EPI/not available	0–1000	5900/60	3.6 × 3.6 × 6	Spin-echo	Not available	ADC
Nakayama et al[61]	SS TSE/not available	50–1000	3000/69	3.5 × 3.6 × 6	Not available	Not available	ADC
Kosucu et al[63]	SS EPI	50–400	3900/76	2.2 × 2.2 × 4	Respiratory triggered	Spectral fat suppression	ADC
Sakurada et al[64]	SS EPI/factor 2	0–1000	10, 191/74	2.7 × 3.9 × 4	Free breathing	STIR	Image overlay and ADC
Lichy et al[62]	SS EPI/factor 2	0–400–1000	3900/76 and 1500/76	2 × 2 × 4	Free breathing and triggered	Spectral fat suppression	ADC
Chen et al[33]	SS EPI/not available	0–1000	Not available	2.8 × 4.5 × 6	Free breathing	Not available	Visual inspection
Ohno et al[30]	SS EPI/none	0–1000	5759/70	2.1 × 4.2 × 8	Not available	STIR	Visual inspection

Abbreviations: Sec type, sequence type; TE, echo time; TR, repetition time.

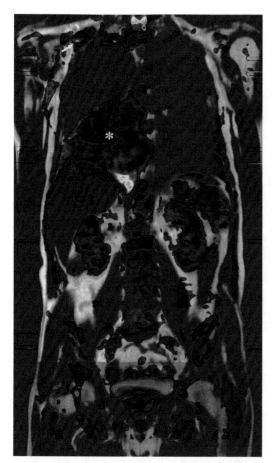

Fig. 14. Staging of lung cancer with WB-DWI MR imaging. Coronal fusion image of a T2-weighted TSE sequence and a DWIBS acquisition (b value of 1000 s/mm²) reveals a huge mass in the inferior lobe of the right lung corresponding to a SCLC (*asterisk*). Metastasis in L2 vertebral body (*green arrow*) and right supraclavicular lymph node metastasis (*yellow arrow*) are depicted as areas of restricted diffusion.

positive predictive value of 94%, negative predictive value of 96%, and area under the curve of 0.938 in the differentiation between benign and malignant tumors. Moreover, there was a significant difference in the ADC value between poorly and well-differentiated malignant tumors of the mediastinum. In this series, the lowest ADC value was that of lymphoma cases, although there was an overlap with ADC of other malignancies, such as thymoma and bronchogenic carcinoma. These results were similar to previous reports using a DWIBS sequence for WB imaging.[66] WB-DWI MR imaging has also been demonstrated to be a feasible technique in the initial staging of lymphoma, including mediastinal involvement, with results as accurate as CT or PET-CT.[67,68] Furthermore, DWI is a potential tool in posttreatment monitoring and early prediction of treatment outcome,[69] being especially interesting in pediatric and pregnant patients (**Fig. 16**).

Pleural Disease

There is scarce experience in the use of DWI for pleural pathology. Baysal and colleagues[70] could accurately differentiate between exudative and transudative pleural effusion using a DWIBS sequence with the body coil and a maximum b value of 1000 s/mm². They proposed a cutoff ADC value of 3.38×10^{-3} mm²/s to obtain a sensitivity of 90.6% and specificity of 85% (see **Fig. 7; Fig. 17**). In a more recent report by Inan,[71] the ADCs of the exudative lesions were also significantly lower than those of transudative ones. In this series, the DWI sequence was performed with a four-element phased-array coil using spectral fat saturation with inversion recovery technique and obtaining b values of 0, 500, and 1000 s/mm². The signal intensity of transudative effusions tend to be isointense and exudative effusions hyperintense compared with muscle.[71]

None of the three distinct histologic subtypes of MPM (epithelial, sarcomatoid, and biphasic) can be distinguished from each other by current imaging modalities.[72] This differentiation is important because there is a significant difference in prognosis between epithelioid and nonepithelioid (biphasic and sarcomatoid) MPM.[22] DWI has recently demonstrated the ability to differentiate epithelial and sarcomatoid subtypes of MPM in a group of 57 patients, using a 3-T magnet. The authors used a free-breathing SS SE EPI DWI sequence with spectral fat saturation and the generalized autocalibrating partially parallel acquisition (GRAPPA) technique was the parallel imaging technique. They obtained 3 b values (250, 500, and 750 s/mm²) to posterior calculate

be related to areas of microscopic necrosis. Average patient-based sensitivity and specificity for the detection of node metastasis was 77.8% and 55.6%, respectively. They also investigated the role of DWIBS in the detection of thoracic esophageal cancer, with a poor detection rate of 49.4%, the depiction of early tumors being especially problematic (**Fig. 15**).

Razek and colleagues[65] have recently explored the capabilities of DWI to further characterize mediastinal masses using free-breathe SS EPI MR imaging with b factors of 0, 300, and 600 s/mm² and ADC quantification. They evaluated 45 patients with mediastinal tumors, excluding the purely cystic ones. Using a cut-off ADC value of 1.56×10^{-3} mm²/s, they obtained an accuracy of 95%, sensitivity of 96%, specificity of 94%,

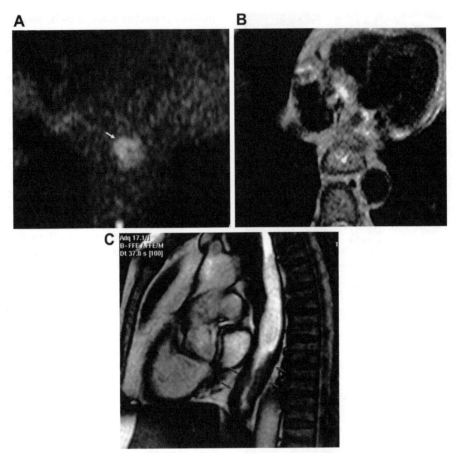

Fig. 15. Esophageal cancer. (*A*) Respiratory-triggered SS EPI DWI sequence with SPIR on a 1.5-T magnet with a b value of 1000 s/mm^2 demonstrates a nodular area of restricted diffusion (*arrow*) corresponding to an esophageal cancer with T2 stage, which was not detectable on the axial T2 TSE image at the same level (*B*). The mural thickening of distal esophagus (*arrows*) is confirmed in an oblique sagittal dynamic balanced field echo acquisition after water swallowing (*C*).

ADC maps. The sarcomatoid subtype showed significantly lower ADC values than the epithelial subtype. The ADC values of biphasic MPM had a wide range of overlap with the ADC values of other subtypes. In the same series, two cases of benign pleural plaque were included, demonstrating a lower ADC value than any type of MPM.

FUTURE DEVELOPMENTS
Cardiac DWI and DTI

Another possibility of DWI is to acquire signal diffusion information from the heart. In DWI of the myocardium, it is a difficult task to completely avoid the macroscopic movement signal, originating in the heartbeat and respiratory motion, from the microscopic movement information provided by DWI and DTI. A deep explanation of the diffusion sequences and DTI reconstruction methods for heart applications is beyond the

scope of this article, but an excellent review can be found in Sosnovik and colleagues.[73] None of those sequences are normally available in commercial scanners. Therefore, to get DWI information of the heart, it is necessary to tune the conventional SE Stejskal–Tanner sequence to the ECG signal by means of synchronization. Conventional DWI sequences for cardiac applications are most commonly synchronized with the systolic part of the heart cycle to improve the reproducibility and to benefit from the increase in thickness of the myocardium in this phase. If a conventional SE Stejskal–Tanner approach is performed, the bulk motion of the heart during systole completely destroys the diffusion signal. For this reason, when using the conventional SE approach, it is desirable to synchronize the DWI acquisition with the diastole reducing the effect of the left ventricle movement. Besides, it is also preferable to use the maximum gradient strength

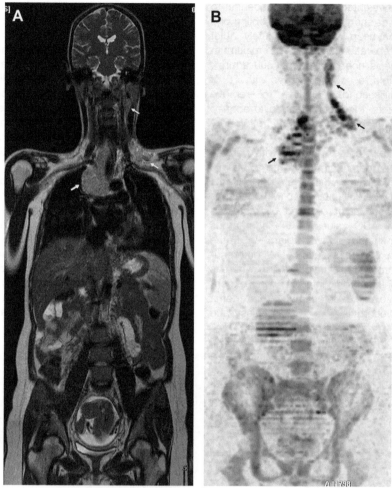

Fig. 16. Staging of Hodgkin's lymphoma in a 24-weeks pregnant woman. (*A*) Coronal TSE T2-weighted image and (*B*) coronal maximum intensity projection (MIP) of a DWIBS sequence with a b value of 1000 s/mm² show disease limited to mediastinum and left laterocervical lymph nodes (*arrows*).

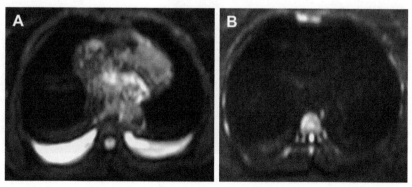

Fig. 17. Transudative pleural effusion in a patient with chronic renal failure. Respiratory-triggered SS EPI DWI sequence with SPIR on a 1.5-T magnet with b values of 0 s/mm² (*A*) and 800 s/mm² (*B*) demonstrates a bilateral pleural effusion, which does not show restriction of diffusion.

in the diffusion-weighted part of the sequence, to make this step as short as possible, enabling one to consider the heart almost completely quiet during this preparation phase. The maximum applied b value is normally around 300 s/mm^2, making it feasible to acquire images with TE of about 40 milliseconds. Finally, to remove breathing artifacts it is recommended to acquire the images with breathholding or respiratory triggered.

In the short existent experience with cardiac DWI, it has been demonstrated to be a feasible method to detect myocardial edema in patients with recent myocardial infarction (MI), because areas of increased signal caused by restricted diffusion, show ADC values in the edematous area lower than in normal myocardium.[74,75] In the series by Laissy and colleagues,[74] DWI differentiated necrotic from viable myocardium, whereas DWI was normal in chronic infarcts. In our experience, DWI is also able to detect myocardial edema in cases of myocarditis (**Fig. 18**), as Laissy and

colleagues anticipated in their paper, and may help to further characterize cardiac and paracardiac masses (**Fig. 19**).

There is a growing interest in the literature to study the microstructure of the heart to separate the different layers of the myocardium using DTI experiments. To acquire this information, it is necessary to perform DWI in at least six different diffusion directions that permit the building of tensor information. In Sosnovik and colleagues[73] a good overview of the reconstruction algorithms can be found. DTI has allowed a better understanding of the three-dimensional organization of myocardial fibers, which is determinant of cardiac torsion, strain, and stress (**Fig. 20**). Nowadays, cardiac DTI is feasible in vivo for animals and humans, although it is still far from being ready for the clinical arena. In vivo DTI of MI has recently revealed a significant increase in trace ADC (mean diffusivity) and a decrease in fractional anisotropy, related to altered myocardial structure, in patients with previous MI at a median interval of 26 days.[76]

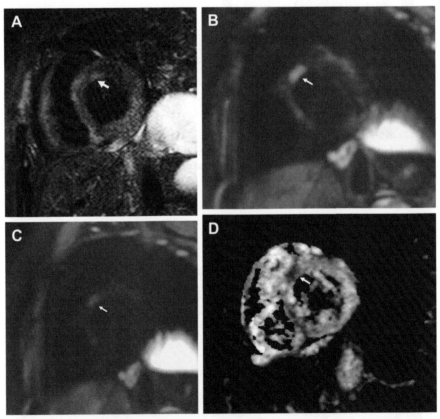

Fig. 18. Detection of myocardial edema in acute myocarditis. (*A*) Short-axis double-inversion black-blood STIR demonstrates an area of myocardial edema in the anteroseptal wall (*arrow*). Respiratory- and cardiac-triggered SS EPI DWI sequences with SPIR on a 1.5-T magnet with b values of 150 s/mm^2 (*B*) and 300 s/mm^2 (*C*) also clearly depict the edematous myocardium as an area of focal hyperintensity (*arrows*). (*D*) On the corresponding ADC map the area of edema demonstrated restricted diffusion (*arrow*).

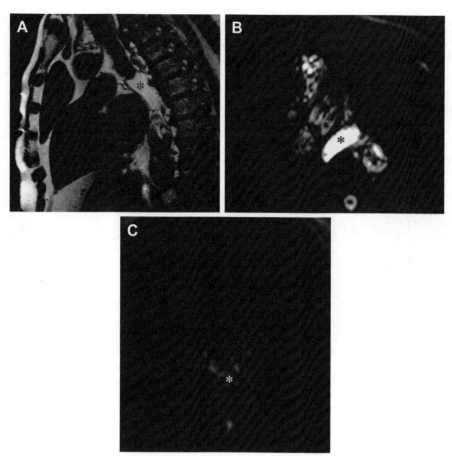

Fig. 19. Bronchogenic cyst. (*A*) Sagittal TSE T2-weighted sequence shows a hyperintense well-defined mass in the posterior mediastinum, which is cystic-appearing (*asterisk*). Respiratory-triggered SS EPI DWI sequence with SPIR on a 1.5-T magnet with b values of 0 s/mm^2 (*B*) and 800 s/mm^2 (*C*) demonstrate absence of restricted diffusion within the mass (*asterisks*), which helps to characterize it as cystic.

In the same study, the alteration of tissue integrity and fiber architecture measured by DTI demonstrated a significant correlation with viable myocardium and regional wall function. Posteriorly, the same researches have shown that DTI may monitor the sequential changes that occur in the transition from recent to chronic MI, with an association between sequential zonal improvement of tissue integrity and fiber architecture remodeling with sequential recovery of zonal wall thickening of the infarcted area.[77] The role of cardiac DTI and DWI in the detection of hyperacute MI and in the monitorization of postinfarction remodeling needs further research.

Hyperpolarized Gases DWI

Functional MR imaging of the lungs with hyperpolarized gases has revolutionized the potential for in vivo lung function measurement in health and disease.[78] Gases, such as ^{129}Xe and more frequently ^{3}He, may be hyperpolarized to be administered into the lungs and imaged with MR imaging, before they return to the thermal equilibrium conditions dictated by the body temperature and the local magnetic field. With the hyperpolarization process of these gases, a very important increase in MR imaging signal is achieved that allows the overcoming of low concentration of gas molecules in airways and may be used for higher spatial or temporal resolution imaging.[79] Their use is still limited to research centers, because the access to hyperpolarization methods and hardware MR imaging requirements limit their spread. The research on imaging of ventilation with ^{3}He is more extended than that with ^{129}Xe, because of higher levels of polarization and higher gyromagnetic ratio, and because it is easily available.[80] In contrast, ^{129}Xe permits a more comprehensive assessment of lung function, because measurement of perfusion and gas exchange is possible because of its solubility in blood and tissues, which are not properties of ^{3}He.[81]

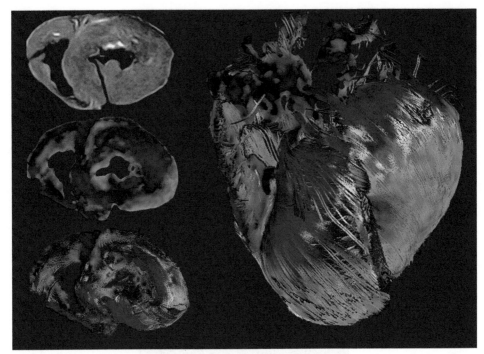

Fig. 20. Ex vivo DTI of a pig heart, using a conventional SE DWI sequence with a b value of 800 s/mm². On the left row, short-axis source and fractional anisotropy images of the heart are presented. On the right, a three-dimensional DTI reconstruction reveals the organization and pathways of the heart fibers. (*Courtesy of* Gerard Blasco, Radiology Department, Hospital Josep Trueta, Girona, Spain.)

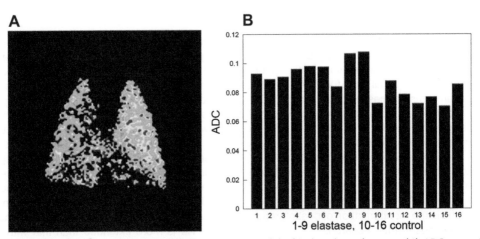

Fig. 21. Hyperpolarized ³He pulmonary diffusion in a rat model of induced emphysema. (*A*) ADC map of a rat lung with emphysema-like disease induced using elastase in left lobe (right-side image in the figure). The emphysema can be considered as mild. (*B*) Graphic of mean ADC value of the entire pulmonary region comparing elastase-treated (*left bars*) with normal (*right bars*) rats, demonstrating higher ADC values in lungs with induced emphysema. The ADC was obtained using four b values between 0 and 2.4 s/cm², and a bipolar sinusoidal diffusion gradient of 1.5-ms diffusion time. The data were accumulated at the end of the expiratory volume after three prewashes with pure ³He and 15 mbar inspiration. (*Courtesy of* Angelos Kyriazis and Jesus Ruiz-Cabello, Research Center of Respiratory Diseases, Complutense University, Madrid, Spain.)

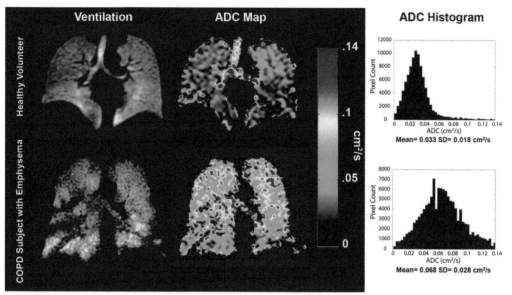

Fig. 22. Hyperpolarized ^{129}Xe pulmonary ventilation and diffusion on a healthy volunteer (*top row*) and subject with COPD (*bottom row*). Multiple ventilation defects and an increase in ADC values are detected in the COPD patient compared with the volunteer. The diffusion alterations are mainly located in both upper lobes. (*Courtesy of* S. Kaushik and B. Driehuys, Center for In Vivo Microscopy, Department of Radiology, Duke University Medical Center, Durham, NC.)

Besides the quantitative MR imaging-derived ventilation, DWI of inhaled hyperpolarized gases has been shown to give information of microstructural pulmonary changes in various diseases, such as asthma or chronic obstructive pulmonary disease (COPD), through measurements of their ADC (**Fig. 21**).[82] This information is obtained by measuring the degree of restriction that suffers the inhaled hyperpolarized gas by the walls of the airways.[83] The MR imaging sequences to monitoring the diffusion information of lung are normally based in a gradient echo or fast gradient echo acquisition where two bipolar gradients, with some separation between them, are included to sensitize DWI. To reduce the T2* decay as much as possible, centric radial or spiral acquisitions are needed.

Studies using ^{3}He have demonstrated increases in ADC in animals and patients with both emphysema and COPD, resulting from the enlargement of the airspaces. Furthermore, increases in ADC have been described in healthy smokers, as an early marker of alveolar breakdown, and also regional differences in ADC values within the same subject indicate different grades of lung destruction.[82,83] Recently, hyperpolarized gases have revealed its potential to categorize COPD ex-smokers.[84] Similar results may be theoretically obtained with ^{129}Xe (**Fig. 22**), although larger studies are needed to validate and extend these data.

SUMMARY

DWI of the chest is technically feasible with state-of-the-art magnets, although it is technically complex. It has a clinical role in lung nodule characterization, lung cancer staging, and the evaluation of pleural and mediastinal pathology, although larger series are needed to validate the existing preliminary data. The evaluation of the IVIM approach in chest pathology may also improve the existing results. Promising applications to be developed are DWI and DTI of the heart and diffusion of hyperpolarized gases.

REFERENCES

1. Kauczor HU, Ley S. Thoracic magnetic resonance imaging 1985 to 2010. J Thorac Imaging 2010; 25(1):34–8.
2. Padhani AR, Liu G, Koh DM, et al. Diffusion-weighted magnetic resonance imaging as a cancer biomarker: consensus and recommendations. Neoplasia 2009;11(2):102–25.
3. Dietrich O. Diffusion-weighted imaging and diffusion tensor imaging. In: Reiser MF, Semmler W, Hricak H,

editors. Magnetic resonance tomography. Berlin: Springer; 2008. p. 130–52.

4. Hahn EL. Spin echoes. Phys Rev 1950;80(4): 580–94.

5. Stejskal EO, Tanner JE. Spin diffusion measurements: spin echoes in the presence of a time-dependent field gradient. J Chem Phys 1965; 42(1):288–92.

6. Reese TG, Weisskoff RM, Smith RN, et al. Imaging myocardial fiber architecture in vivo with magnetic resonance. Magn Reson Med 1995;34:786–91.

7. Reese TG, Wedeen VJ, Weisskoff RM. Measuring diffusion in the presence of material strain. J Magn Reson B 1996;112:253–8.

8. Gamper U, Boesiger P, Kozerke S. Diffusion imaging of the in vivo heart using spin echoes-considerations on bulk motion sensitivity. Magn Reson Med 2007; 57:331–7.

9. Merboldt KD, Hänicke W, Frahm J. Self-diffusion NMR imaging using stimulated echoes. J Magn Reson 1985;64(3):479–86.

10. Taylor DG, Bushell MC. The spatial mapping of translational diffusion coefficients by the NMR imaging technique. Phys Med Biol 1985;30(4): 345–9.

11. Le Bihan D, Breton E, Lallemand D, et al. MR imaging of intravoxel incoherent motions: application to diffusion and perfusion in neurologic disorders. Radiology 1986;161(2):401–7.

12. Turner R, Le Bihan D, Maier J, et al. Echo-planar imaging of intravoxel incoherent motion. Radiology 1990;177(2):407–14.

13. Raya JG, Dietrich O, Reiser MF, et al. Techniques for diffusion-weighted imaging of bone marrow. Eur J Radiol 2005;55(1):64–73.

14. Brockstedt S, Moore JR, Thomsen C, et al. High-resolution diffusion imaging using phase-corrected segmented echo-planar imaging. Magn Reson Imaging 2000;18(6):649–57.

15. Pipe JG, Farthing VG, Forbes KP. Multishot diffusion-weighted FSE using PROPELLER MRI. Magn Reson Med 2002;47(1):42–52 [erratum in: Magn Reson Med 2002;47(3):621].

16. Deng J, Miller FH, Salem R, et al. Multishot diffusion-weighted PROPELLER magnetic resonance imaging of the abdomen. Invest Radiol 2006;41(10):769–75.

17. Pruessmann KP, Weiger M, Scheidegger MB, et al. SENSE: sensitivity encoding for fast MRI. Magn Reson Med 1999;42(5):952–62.

18. Griswold MA, Jakob PM, Heidemann RM, et al. Generalized autocalibrating partially parallel acquisitions (GRAPPA). Magn Reson Med 2002;47(6): 1202–10.

19. Notohamiprodjo M, Dietrich O, Horger W, et al. Diffusion tensor imaging (DTI) of the kidney at 3Tesla–feasibility, protocol evaluation and comparison to 1.5 Tesla. Invest Radiol 2010;45:245–54.

20. Dietrich O, Reiser MF, Schoenberg SO. Artifacts in 3-T MRI: physical background and reduction strategies. Eur J Radiol 2008;65:29–35.

21. Nagy Z, Weiskopf N. Efficient fat suppression by slice-selection gradient reversal in twice-refocused diffusion encoding. Magn Reson Med 2008;60(5): 1256–60.

22. Gill RR, Umeoka S, Mamata H, et al. Diffusion-weighted MRI of malignant pleural mesothelioma: preliminary assessment of apparent diffusion coefficient in histologic subtypes. Am J Roentgenol 2010; 195(2):W125–30.

23. Luciani A, Vignaud A, Cavet M, et al. Liver cirrhosis: intravoxel incoherent motion MR imaging-pilot study. Radiology 2008;249(3):891–9.

24. Kwee TC, Takahara T, Koh DM, et al. Comparison and reproducibility of ADC measurements in breath-hold, respiratory triggered, and free-breathing diffusion-weighted MR imaging of the liver. J Magn Reson Imaging 2008;28(5):1141–8.

25. Kandpal H, Sharma R, Madhusudhan KS, et al. Respiratory-triggered versus breath-hold diffusion-weighted MRI of liver lesions: comparison of image quality and apparent diffusion coefficient values. AJR Am J Roentgenol 2009;192:915–22.

26. Kwee TC, Takahara T, Niwa T, et al. Influence of cardiac motion on diffusion-weighted magnetic resonance imaging of the liver. MAGMA 2009;22: 319–25.

27. Bruegel M, Gaa J, Woertler K, et al. MRI of the lung: value of different turbo spin-echo, single-shot turbo spin-echo, and 3D gradient-echo pulse sequences for the detection of pulmonary metastases. J Magn Reson Imaging 2007;25(1):73–81.

28. Koyama H, Ohno Y, Kono A, et al. Quantitative and qualitative assessment of non-contrast-enhanced pulmonary MR imaging for management of pulmonary nodules in 161 subjects. Eur Radiol 2008; 18(10):2120–31.

29. Frericks BB, Meyer BC, Martus P, et al. MRI of the thorax during whole-body MRI: evaluation of different MR sequences and comparison to thoracic multidetector computed tomography (MDCT). J Magn Reson Imaging 2008;27(3):538–45.

30. Ohno Y, Koyama H, Onishi Y, et al. Non-small cell lung cancer: whole-body MR examination for M-stage assessment-utility for whole-body diffusion-weighted imaging compared with integrated FDG PET/CT. Radiology 2008;248(2):643–54.

31. Komori T, Narabayashi I, Matsumura K, et al. 2-[Fluorine-18]-fluoro-2-deoxy-D-glucose positron emission tomography/computed tomography versus whole-body diffusion-weighted MRI for detection of malignant lesions: initial experience. Ann Nucl Med 2007;21(4):209–15.

32. Takano A, Oriuchi N, Tsushima Y, et al. Detection of metastatic lesions from malignant pheochromocytoma

and paraganglioma with diffusion-weighted magnetic resonance imaging: comparison with 18F-FDG positron emission tomography and 123I-MIBG scintigraphy. Ann Nucl Med 2008;22(5):395–401.

33. Chen W, Jian W, Li H, et al. Whole-body diffusion-weighted imaging vs. FDG-PET for the detection of non-small-cell lung cancer. how do they measure up? Magn Reson Imaging 2010;28:613–20.

34. Koyama H, Ohno Y, Aoyama N, et al. Comparison of STIR turbo SE imaging and diffusion-weighted imaging of the lung: capability for detection and subtype classification of pulmonary adenocarcinomas. Eur Radiol 2010;20(4):790–800.

35. Satoh S, Kitazume Y, Ohdama S, et al. Can malignant and benign pulmonary nodules be differentiated with diffusion-weighted MRI? AJR Am J Roentgenol 2008;191(2):464–70.

36. Liu H, Liu Y, Yu T, et al. Usefulness of diffusion-weighted MR imaging in the evaluation of pulmonary lesions. Eur Radiol 2010;20(4):807–15.

37. Wahidi MM, Govert JA, Goudar RK, et al. Evidence for the treatment of patients with pulmonary nodules: when is it lung cancer? ACCP evidence-based clinical practice guidelines (2nd edition). Chest 2007;132(Suppl 3):94S–107S.

38. Jeong YJ, Lee KS, Jeong SY, et al. Solitary pulmonary nodule: characterization with combined wash-in and washout features at dynamic multi-detector row CT. Radiology 2005;237(2):675–83.

39. Higashi K, Ueda Y, Sakuma T, et al. Comparison of [(18)F]FDG PET and (201)Tl SPECT in evaluation of pulmonary nodules. J Nucl Med 2001;142(10):1489–96.

40. Shioya S, Haida M, Ono Y, et al. Lung cancer: differentiation of tumor, necrosis, and atelectasis by means of T1 and T2 values measured in vitro. Radiology 1988;167(1):105–9.

41. Ohno Y, Koyama H, Takenaka D, et al. Dynamic MRI, dynamic multidetector-row computed tomography (MDCT), and coregistered 2-[fluorine-18]-fluoro-2-deoxy-D-glucose-positron emission tomography (FDG-PET)/CT: comparative study of capability for management of pulmonary nodules. J Magn Reson Imaging 2008;27(6):1284–95.

42. Girvin F, Ko JP. Pulmonary nodules: detection, assessment, and CAD. AJR Am J Roentgenol 2008;191(4):1057–69.

43. Uto T, Takehara Y, Nakamura Y, et al. Higher sensitivity and specificity for diffusion-weighted imaging of malignant lung lesions without apparent diffusion coefficient quantification. Radiology 2009;252(1):247–54.

44. Mori T, Nomori H, Ikeda K, et al. Diffusion-weighted magnetic resonance imaging for diagnosing malignant pulmonary nodules/masses: comparison with positron emission tomography. J Thorac Oncol 2008;3(4):358–64.

45. Matoba M, Tonami H, Kondou T, et al. Lung carcinoma: diffusion-weighted MR imaging—preliminary evaluation with apparent diffusion coefficient. Radiology 2007;243(2):570–7.

46. Tanaka R, Horikoshi H, Nakazato Y, et al. Magnetic resonance imaging in peripheral lung adenocarcinoma: correlation with histopathologic features. J Thorac Imaging 2009;24(1):4–9.

47. Kanauchi N, Oizumi H, Honma T, et al. Role of diffusion-weighted magnetic resonance imaging for predicting of tumor invasiveness for clinical stage IA non-small cell lung cancer. Eur J Cardiothorac Surg 2009;35(4):706–10 [discussion:10–1].

48. Ohba Y, Nomori H, Mori T, et al. Is diffusion-weighted magnetic resonance imaging superior to positron emission tomography with fludeoxyglucose F 18 in imaging non-small cell lung cancer? J Thorac Cardiovasc Surg 2009;138(2):439–45.

49. Yamada I, Aung W, Himeno Y, et al. Diffusion coefficients in abdominal organs and hepatic lesions: evaluation with intravoxel incoherent motion echo-planar MR imaging. Radiology 1999;210(3):617–23.

50. Karampinos DC, King KF, Sutton BP, et al. Intravoxel partially coherent motion technique: characterization of the anisotropy of skeletal muscle microvasculature. J Magn Reson Imaging 2010;31(4):942–53.

51. Lemke A, Laun FB, Klau M, et al. Differentiation of pancreas carcinoma from healthy pancreatic tissue using multiple b-values: comparison of apparent diffusion coefficient and intravoxel incoherent motion derived parameters. Invest Radiol 2009;44(12):769–75.

52. Koh DM. Collins DJ. Diffusion weighted MRI in the body: applications and challenges in oncology. AJR Am J Roentgenol 2007;188:1622–35.

53. Baysal T, Mutlu DY, Yologlu S. Diffusion-weighted magnetic resonance imaging in differentiation of postobstructive consolidation from central lung carcinoma. Magn Reson Imaging 2009;27(10):1447–54.

54. Qi LP, Zhang XP, Tang L, et al. Using diffusion-weighted MR imaging for tumor detection in the collapsed lung: a preliminary study. Eur Radiol 2009;19(2):333–41.

55. Okuma T, Matsuoka T, Yamamoto A, et al. Assessment of early treatment response after CT-guided radiofrequency ablation of unresectable lung tumours by diffusion-weighted MRI: a pilot study. Br J Radiol 2009;82(984):989–94.

56. Henzler T, Schmid-Bindert G, Schoenberg SO, et al. Diffusion and perfusion MRI of the lung and mediastinum. Eur J Radiol 2010. [Epub ahead of print].

57. Hasegawa I, Boiselle PM, Kuwabara K, et al. Mediastinal lymph nodes in patients with non-small cell lung cancer: preliminary experience with diffusion-weighted MR imaging. J Thorac Imaging 2008;23(3):157–61.

58. Ohno Y, Hatabu H, Takenaka D, et al. Metastases in mediastinal and hilar lymph nodes in patients with non-small cell lung cancer: quantitative and qualitative assessment with STIR turbo spin-echo MR imaging. Radiology 2004;231(3):872–9.

59. King AD, Ahuja AT, Yeung DK, et al. Malignant cervical lymphadenopathy: diagnostic accuracy of diffusion-weighted MR imaging. Radiology 2007; 245(3):806–13.

60. Nomori H, Mori T, Ikeda K, et al. Diffusion-weighted magnetic resonance imaging can be used in place of positron emission tomography for N staging of non-small cell lung cancer with fewer false-positive results. J Thorac Cardiovasc Surg 2008;135(4): 816–22.

61. Nakayama J, Miyasaka K, Omatsu T, et al. Metastases in mediastinal and hilar lymph nodes in patients with non-small cell lung cancer: quantitative assessment with diffusion-weighted magnetic resonance imaging and apparent diffusion coefficient. J Comput Assist Tomogr 2010;34(1):1–8.

62. Lichy MP, Aschoff P, Plathow C, et al. Tumor detection by diffusionweighted. MRI and ADC-mapping—initial clinical experiences in comparison to PET-CT. Invest Radiol 2007;42:605–13.

63. Koşucu P, Tekinbaş C, Erol M, et al. Mediastinal lymph nodes: assessment with diffusion-weighted MR imaging. J Magn Reson Imaging 2009;30(2): 292–7.

64. Sakurada A, Takahaara T, Kwee TC, et al. Diagnostic performance of diffusion-weighted MRI in esophageal cancer. Eur Radiol 2009;19:1461–9.

65. Razek AA, Elmorsy A, Elshafey M, et al. Assessment of mediastinal tumors with diffusion-weighted single-shot echo-planar MRI. J Magn Reson Imaging 2009; 30:535–40.

66. Li S, Xue HD, Li J, et al. Application of whole body diffusion-weighted MR imaging for diagnosis and staging of malignant lymphoma. Chin Med Sci J 2008;23:138–44.

67. Lin C, Luciani A, Itti E, et al. Whole-body diffusion-weighted magnetic resonance imaging with apparent diffusion coefficient mapping for staging patients with diffuse large B-cell lymphoma. Eur Radiol 2010;20(8):2027–38.

68. Kwee TC, van Ufford HM, Beek FJ, et al. Whole-body MRI, including diffusion-weighted imaging, for the initial staging of malignant lymphoma: comparison to computed tomography. Invest Radiol 2009;44(10):683–90.

69. Huang MQ, Pickup S, Nelson DS, et al. Monitoring response to chemotherapy of non-Hodgkin's lymphoma xenografts by T(2)-weighted and diffusion-weighted MRI. NMR Biomed 2008;21(10): 1021–9.

70. Baysal T, Bulut T, Gökirmak M, et al. Diffusion-weighted MR imaging of pleural fluid: differentiation of transudative vs exudative pleural effusions. Eur Radiol 2004;14(5):890–6.

71. Inan N, Arslan A, Akansel G, et al. Diffusion-weighted MRI in the characterization of pleural effusions. Diagn Interv Radiol 2009;15(1):13–8.

72. Gill RR, Gerbaudo VH, Sugarbaker DJ, et al. Current trends in radiologic management of malignant pleural mesothelioma. Semin Thorac Cardiovasc Surg 2009;21(2):111–20.

73. Sosnovik DE, Wang R, Dai G, et al. Diffusion MR tractography of the heart. J Cardiovasc Magn Reson 2009;11:47–61.

74. Laissy JP, Serfaty JM, Messika-Zeitoun D, et al. Cardiac diffusion MRI of recent and chronic myocardial infarction: preliminary results. J Radiol 2009; 90(4):481–4.

75. Okayama S, Uemura S, Saito Y. Detection of infarct-related myocardial edema using cardiac diffusion-weighted magnetic resonance imaging. Int J Cardiol 2009;133(1):20–1.

76. Wu MT, Tseng WY, Su MY, et al. Diffusion tensor magnetic resonance imaging mapping the fiber architecture remodeling in human myocardium after infarction: correlation with viability and wall motion. Circulation 2006;114(10):1036–145.

77. Wu MT, Su MY, Huang YL, et al. Sequential changes of myocardial microstructure in patients postmyocardial infarction by diffusion-tensor cardiac MR: correlation with left ventricular structure and function. Circ Cardiovasc Imaging 2009;2(1):32–40.

78. Van Beek EJ, Wild JM, Kauczor HU, et al. Functional MRI of the lung using hyperpolarized 3-helium gas. J Magn Reson Imaging 2004;20:540–54.

79. Hopkins SR, Levin DL, Emami K, et al. Advances in magnetic resonance imaging of lung physiology. J Appl Physiol 2007;102(3):1244–54.

80. Patz S, Hersman FW, Muradian I, et al. Hyperpolarized 129Xe MRI: a viable functional lung imaging modality? Eur J Radiol 2007;64(3):335–44.

81. Driehuys B, Möller HE, Cleveland ZI, et al. Pulmonary perfusion and xenon gas exchange in rats: MR imaging with intravenous injection of hyperpolarized 129Xe. Radiology 2009;252(2):386–93.

82. Fain SB, Panth SR, Evans MD, et al. Early emphysematous changes in asymptomatic smokers: detection with 3He MR imaging. Radiology 2006;239(3): 875–83.

83. Wang C, Altes TA, Mugler JP, et al. Assessment of the lung m in patients with asthma using hyperpolarized 3He diffusion MRI at two time scales: comparison with healthy subjects and patients with COPD. J Magn Reson Imaging 2008;28(1):80–8.

84. Mathew L, Kirby M, Etemad-Rezai R, et al. Hyperpolarized 3He magnetic resonance imaging: preliminary evaluation of phenotyping potential in chronic obstructive pulmonary disease. Eur J Radiol 2009. [Epub ahead of print].

Diffusion Magnetic Resonance Imaging of the Breast

Fernanda Philadelpho Arantes Pereira, MD[a,b,]*,
Gabriela Martins, MD[a,c],
Raquel de Vasconcellos Carvalhaes de Oliveira, MSc[d]

KEYWORDS

- Breast cancer • Breast tumor
- Magnetic resonance imaging (MRI)
- Diffusion-weighted imaging (DWI)
- Apparent diffusion coefficient (ADC) • b-value
- Chemotherapy • Diffusion tensor imaging (DTI)

Magnetic resonance (MR) imaging has been increasingly used for accurate diagnosis of both primary and recurrent breast cancers, particularly in cases in which mammography and breast sonography are inconclusive or yield discrepancies. In addition, MR imaging may improve the analysis of the local extent of breast cancer by revealing multifocal and multicenter tumor growth in patients scheduled for conservative breast surgery. Although the high sensitivity of breast MR imaging has proved to be advantageous for preoperative patients, the limited specificity of this imaging method continues to be a significant problem, particularly in patients referred for further clarification and delineation of inconclusive findings obtained using conventional breast imaging techniques.[1]

MR imaging has high sensitivity (89%–100%), but lacks specificity for characterization of breast tumors.[2–6] An overlap between MR imaging findings for benign and malignant lesions persists, resulting in variable specificity (50%–90%).[4,7–9] This phenomenon can be caused by false-positive results related to the menstrual cycle, hormonal therapy, proliferative alterations, fibroadenomas, and papillomas. As a result of this confounding overlap, in some cases it is not possible to make a differential diagnosis between benign and malignant lesions from conventional MR imaging features.[10,11] In addition to morphologic and kinetic analyses, molecular characterization has been expected to be useful for the diagnosis of breast disease. Hence, several studies have investigated the role of advanced MR imaging techniques, such as diffusion-weighted imaging (DWI), in improvement of the specificity of MR imaging for the evaluation of breast lesions.[10,12–18]

DWI has been used in neurologic imaging for some time, but has only recently been applied to breast imaging.[8,12–14,19,20] However, recent developments in MR imaging technology have enabled the clinical application of DWI to the entire body, which has shown great promise for the detection and characterization of most tumor types. Through imaging of alterations in the microscopic motion of water molecules, DWI can yield novel quantitative

The authors have nothing to disclose.

[a] Department of Breast Imaging, Clínica de Diagnóstico por Imagem (CDPI), Av. Ataulfo de Paiva 669, Leblon, Rio de Janeiro 22440-032, Brazil

[b] Department of Radiology, Federal University of Rio de Janeiro, Rua Professor Rodolpho Paulo Rocco 255, Cidade Universitária, Rio de Janeiro 21941-913, Brazil

[c] Department of Breast MR Imaging, Multi-imagem Ressonância Magnética, Rua Saddock de Sa 266, Ipanema, Rio de Janeiro 22411-040, Brazil

[d] Clinic Epidemiology Department, Instituto de Pesquisa Evandro Chagas (IPEC), Fundação Oswaldo Cruz (Fiocruz), Av. Brasil 4365, Manguinhos, Rio de Janeiro 21040-900, Brazil

* Corresponding author. Rua Corcovado 57/502, Jardim Botânico, Rio de Janeiro 22460-050, Brazil.
E-mail address: fephila@gmail.com

Magn Reson Imaging Clin N Am 19 (2011) 95–110
doi:10.1016/j.mric.2010.09.001

and qualitative information reflecting cellular changes that can provide unique insights into tumor cellularity.[21] With respect to breast DWI, a potential role for the apparent diffusion coefficient (ADC), a quantitative measure that is directly proportional to the diffusion of water and inversely proportional to the tumor cellular density,[22] has been reported to be useful for characterizing breast tumors and distinguishing malignant tissues from benign tissues.[13,17,18,23]

CLINICAL APPLICATIONS OF DIFFUSION IMAGING

Despite improvements in the detection of breast cancer as a result of the widespread application of mammography and ultrasound, breast lesions remain difficult to diagnose and characterize. The primary advantage of MR imaging of the breast is improvement of the detection and characterization of multiple and/or small lesions, even in dense fibroglandular breast tissue. However, the low specificity of MR imaging remains a significant problem.[24]

DWI has been increasingly recognized as a promising quantitative method for use in differential diagnosis of enhancing lesions in breast MR imaging.[25] Based on the principles of DWI, visualization and quantification of the random motions of molecules, this technique can be used to analyze tissue microstructure in vivo. Compared with contrast-enhanced techniques, which can reveal the vasculature and perfusion, this new approach to assess tissue characteristics can provide additional diagnostic information to improve differential diagnosis. In general, the DWI technique is faster than dynamic contrast-enhanced MR imaging. Consequently, this imaging method can easily be added to a standard breast MR imaging protocol.

DWI of Normal Breast Tissue

In diffusion-weighted images, the normal breast gland has a high signal in images acquired with low b-values and low signal in images acquired with high b-values. Ideally, the background signal for the breast gland should be suppressed to emphasize the tumor signal and to avoid the T2 shine-through effect.[26]

A trend toward a decreased ADC has been observed during the second week of the menstrual cycle, and an increased ADC during the final week before menstruation.[27] Variations in the ADC occur in the breast as a result of normal hormonal fluctuations associated with the menstrual cycle. The reduced ADC in the second week is correlated with reduced water content in the breast, and the increased ADC during the week before menstruation has been attributed to increases in secretion activity, stromal edema, and water volume in the extracellular matrix. Normal breast ADC values seem to vary by only 5.5% across the different menstrual phases.[27] However, no statistically significant influence of the menstrual cycle on the ADC values for the breast has been reported. Because contrast-enhanced breast MR imaging is recommended to be performed in the second week of the menstrual cycle,[28] a similar recommendation may be optimal for DWI. In women with less dense breasts, the ADC values for breast tissue may be artificially reduced as a result of partial volume effects of fat tissue.[20] The mean ADC values in normal breast tissue vary from 1.51×10^{-3} to 2.37×10^{-3} mm^2/s for sequences acquired with b-values ranging from 0 to 1074 s/mm^2.[14,16,23,29–32]

Diffusion of Water in Malignant and Benign Tissues

In biologic tissues, microscopic water molecular motion is induced by both intravascular water movement (flow) and an extravascular component (diffusion).[33] With respect to the extravascular component, the state of the extracellular space is the most important factor that regulates diffusion. If a tissue is made up of tightly packed cells, as occurs in a malignant tumor, the extracellular space is reduced, and diffusion of water is decreased. This phenomenon results in a higher DWI signal intensity, restricted signal intensity on the ADC map, and a lower ADC value (**Fig. 1**). In contrast, in benign lesions in which the cells are more separated, the extracellular space is larger, diffusion of water is less restricted, and the ADC value is higher.[20,34] Tumor cellularity is inversely correlated with the ADC value, and malignant breast tumors exhibit higher cellularity and lower ADC values than benign breast tumors.

Specificity and Sensitivity of DWI

There seems to be a consensus in the literature regarding the ability of DWI of the breast to differentiate between malignant and benign breast lesions. Many studies have shown that lower ADC values are associated with breast cancer tissues compared with normal breast tissues or benign tumors.[7,10,12,13,15,16,19,25,29,31,34,35] A meta-analysis of 12 articles reported that the ADC values for benign breast tumors ranged from 1.41×10^{-3} to 2.01×10^{-3} mm^2/s, and those of malignant breast tumors ranged from 0.9×10^{-3} to 1.61×10^{-3} mm^2/s. Variations in ADC values may be present across different studies as a result of technical differences. For example, studies analyzed in the

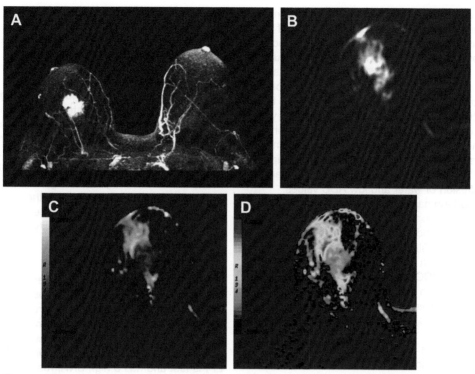

Fig. 1. 49-year-old woman with IDC of the right breast. (A) Axial maximum intensity projection of a contrast-enhanced T1-weighted three-dimensional spoiled gradient-echo image, first phase, subjected to subtraction technique. (B) Axial diffusion-weighted image. (C) Axial black-and-white and (D) colored ADC maps obtained using b-values of 0 and 750 s/mm² show enhancement of a highly suspicious mass, evident as increased loss of signal on the ADC black-and-white map and blue on the ADC colored map, which indicate restricted diffusion.

meta-analysis used different b-values, varying from 0 to 1074 s/mm², yet a significant difference in the ADC values was identified between malignant and benign lesions, with a pooled sensitivity of 89.1% (range, 85%–91%) and a pooled specificity of 77% (range, 69%–84%) for an ADC cutoff of 1.1 to 1.6 × 10⁻³ mm²/s.[34]

The literature also shows that increased positive predictive value (PPV) can be achieved by incorporating an ADC threshold into breast MR imaging assessment. In a study by Partridge and colleagues,[18] in which DWI was acquired using b-values of 0 and 600 s/mm², application of an ADC threshold of 1.8 × 10⁻³ mm²/s for 100% sensitivity produced a PPV of 47%, compared with 37% for MR imaging alone. This methodology would have avoided biopsy for 33% of benign lesions without missing any cancers.

Correlation of the ADC with Tumor Histology

Several investigators have described an inverse correlation between tumor cellularity and ADC values, and have suggested that further associations with the proliferation rate and tumor aggressiveness may be assumed.[12,25,32,35] ADC values for the noninvasive malignant lesion, ductal carcinoma in situ (DCIS), were found to be significantly higher than those of invasive cancer, but lower than those of benign lesions, consistent with the less aggressive, but malignant, nature of these lesions.[25] In another study, high-grade DCIS was shown to be associated with a significantly lower ADC value than low-grade DCIS.[23] These and other results suggest that there is a significant correlation between tumor ADC values and tumor histology.[12,14,35–37] Conversely, others investigators have found that no correlation exists between the ADC and breast cancer histology and that no statistically significant difference is present between the ADC values associated with invasive ductal carcinoma (IDC) and DCIS.[32,38] Therefore, further studies are needed to critically evaluate the clinical usefulness of the mean ADC for tumor grading.

False-positive and False-negative Results of DWI

Several benign lesion subgroups exhibit a remarkable overlap with malignant lesions. According to previous reports,[12,21,39] the diffusion of water molecules is not only restricted in environments containing high cellularity but also in cases of intracellular and extracellular edema, high viscosity regions in abscesses and hematomas, coagulated blood or proteinaceous debris within ducts and cysts, and areas with a high degree of fibrosis. Similar to decreases in extracellular space, these conditions can impede the movement of water molecules. Inflammatory changes also favor high cellularity, granulomatous inflammatory elements, fibrous components, and hemosiderin capabilities.[38] These benign conditions can also lead to low diffusion of water and low ADC values.

Fibroadenomas would be expected to have high rates of diffusion and ADC values as a result of stromal myxoid changes and consequently increased mobility of water.[16,38] However, fibroadenomas with a predominant fibrous component have lower ADC values. In addition, fibrocystic disease, which is characterized by varying degrees of fibrosis and proliferation, can be associated with ADC values in the range of malignant lesions.[25,35,39]

With respect to false-negative results, the mucinous colloid carcinoma, which is characterized by the presence of extracellular mucus in the absence of increased cellularity, has been reported to have high ADC values.[17,25,35,39] For this reason, further information, such as irregular margins, is required for reliable diagnosis.

Occasionally, DCIS and malignant phyllodes tumor with bleeding present with high ADC values as a result of the strong effects of magnetic susceptibility.[31,36] Malignant phyllodes tumor can have high ADC values as a result of cystic areas inside the tumor.[17] Similarly, scirrhous carcinomas may be associated with high ADC values and may, consequently, be misdiagnosed as benign in nature.

Papillary cancer has a mean ADC value similar to that of papilloma, a reflection of the similarity between benign and malignant papillary lesions, and it is speculated that hemorrhage is the differentiating factor between malignant and benign intraductal papillomas.[31,36] Papillomas can also have low ADC values as a result of high cellularity.[17,25,36]

Technical Issues Associated with DWI

Initial results from studies characterizing DWI seem promising, but the considerable heterogeneity between studies and the lack of a complete understanding of the factors that influence this heterogeneity represent significant obstacles in the use of this diagnostic tool. For example, variations between studies could be caused by the use of different protocols. Therefore, standardization of DWI parameters and postprocessing methods is necessary to achieve uniform results and to make interstudy comparisons on the diagnostic accuracy of DWI for breast cancer possible.

Effects of the magnetic strength on DWI

MR imaging scanners operating at 3 T are widely used in the clinic and provide higher signal-to-noise ratio (SNR) and greater spatial resolution than 1.5-T scanners. Small cancers are more clearly visible by DWI at 3 T compared with 1.5 T. However, higher magnetic strengths are also accompanied by an increase in susceptibility artifacts and nonuniformity of the magnetic field, which can cause image distortions. With the application of parallel imaging techniques, these artifacts can be reduced, and the image quality is markedly improved.[37,40,41]

Diffusion-weighted techniques

No consensus exists among different research groups regarding the optimal diffusion-weighted technique for the breast. Most groups perform DWI by an echo-planar imaging (EPI) approach.[10,12–14,29,35,39,40,42,43] However, other groups apply fast spin-echo technique. Although EPI is fast and has a high SNR, results using this technique can be distorted by susceptibility and chemical shift artifacts, as well as by breathing and other motion artifacts.[11,36,37] Distortion can be decreased by improving the homogeneity of the magnetic field using manual shimming or parallel imaging. However, EPI remains limited by noise, and thicker slices are generally used compared with contrast-enhanced T1 imaging.

Determination of the optimum b-value

For clinical MR imaging scanners, the diffusion sensitivity can easily be altered by changing the parameter known as the b-value. Diffusion images are produced using at least 2 different b-values, and the loss of signal between these images is proportional to the amount of diffusion. Images acquired with low b-values are less diffusion-weighted because they use less of a gradient. The diffusion sensitivity is also more affected by microperfusion when low b-values are used, which leads to higher ADC values.[23] On the other hand, high b-value images are strongly diffusion-weighted, highlighting signals from malignant tumors and eliminating signals from normal tissues, but have a lower SNR and, consequently, more image distortion.[26]

The presence of the T2 shine-through effect, in which molecules with long T2 relaxation times produce high signal intensities on diffusion-weighted images, and the high signal intensity of the surrounding normal breast parenchyma can limit lesion visibility on images obtained using lower b-values. For a given level of a basic T2-dependent signal, a lesion with a lower ADC value requires a higher b-value than a lesion with a higher ADC value to compensate for the T2-dependent signal and avoid T2 shine-through.[26]

DWI is typically performed using at least 2 b-values to enable meaningful interpretation of the results. In theory, the inherent error of ADC calculations can be reduced by the use of more b-values. However, the more b-values used, the longer time the DWI sequence requires.[17] Moreover, no consensus exists as to how many and which b-values should be used for breast DWI.

Pereira and colleagues[17] found no statistically significant difference between the ADC values obtained using different b-value combinations for differentiation of benign and malignant lesions. However, the ADC values calculated using b-values of 0 and 750 s/mm^2 were slightly better than the other combinations analyzed. These findings suggest that higher b-values are useful for distinguishing benign from malignant lesions, and that the use of multiple b-values in the DWI sequence is unnecessary, saving examination time. Consistent with these results, a study by Bogner and colleagues[23] found that a combined b-value protocol of 50 and 850 s/mm^2 resulted in optimum ADC determination and DWI quality at 3.0 T. ADC calculations performed using multiple b-values were not significantly more precise than those performed with only two.

Effect of the contrast medium

DWI is generally performed before contrast administration, but it has been reported that it can also be performed after contrast. When DWI is performed after contrast, a reduction in the ADC value is usually expected. Yuen and colleagues[33] reported a mean ADC value reduction of 23% for performance after contrast, and this reduction was generally higher in tumors with relatively high ADC values (>1.3 $\times$ 10^{-3} mm^2/s).[44] Investigators have postulated that the contrast causes suppression of the microperfusion effect, leading to a reduction in the ADC value.

Pathologic studies have revealed that microvessel counts are higher for malignant tumors compared with benign tumors,[33] representing a factor that could potentially increase the ADC values of malignant breast tumors.[23] This phenomenon is referred to as the microperfusion effect. Considering the suppressive effect of contrast on microperfusion, postcontrast ADC values may purely reflect tumor cellularity in these cases. Thus, postcontrast ADC may be a more reliable indicator than precontrast ADC for reflection of the malignant potential of tumors. On the other hand, Rubesova and colleagues[13] and Baltzer and colleagues[25] did not find a significant difference in ADC values obtained before and after contrast injection.

Postprocessing

The placement of the region of interest (ROI) is crucial for proper analysis of DWI results.[10,13] First, it is important to localize the lesion on diffusion-weighted images and on the ADC map and to determine the location at which the lesion is best visualized. In most previous studies, the ROI was placed directly on the ADC map. The subtracted images of the dynamic contrast-enhanced sequence can also be referenced to the ROI placement. The ROI should cover the tumor, avoiding areas of hemorrhage or necrosis. In previous studies, ROIs of variable areas have been used, ranging from 8 mm^2 to more than 100 mm^2.[19,29,35,44] The optimal number and type of ROIs remain to be determined. Further studies are needed to characterize the optimal ROI parameters for measurement of ADC values that best reflect the characteristics of tumors.

DWI Limitations

Movement artifacts

Application of DWI to the breast has previously been limited by movement artifacts. Patient movement during the acquisition of the diffusion-weighted sequences can lead to inaccurate ADC values.[10] In addition, longer acquisition times caused by the use of a greater number of b-values can lead to patient motion. Therefore, improvement of patient comfort to reduce motion, respiratory gating, and the use of alternative pulse sequences or postprocessing techniques to reduce eddy current-based distortions may help to improve the quality of clinical breast DWI data.[18,45]

Lesion visibility and size

Even under optimal circumstances, DWI can fail to categorize breast lesions because of the limited spatial resolution and capability of recognizing some lesions on ADC maps, particularly lesions smaller than 1 cm.[7] When lesions cannot be visualized on diffusion-weighted images, the precise localization of the ROI on the ADC map cannot be determined. Studies focused on lesion visibility in DWI compared with contrast-enhanced breast MR imaging detected 89% to 100% of all lesions,[10,12,25,29,42] and good visibility was obtained for 89% to 95.3% of lesions.[10,25,42] However, less visible lesions were reported being either small or benign. Another recent study compared the lesion visibility in DWI results with those of subtracted contrast-enhanced images.[42] Approximately 68.9% of lesions showed the same level of visibility on DWI as on subtraction images, 20.3% of lesions showed good, but inferior, visibility, and 10.8% of lesions showed poor visibility. All lesions were depicted on diffusion-weighted images.

The critical problem is that breast lesions must be detected as a prerequisite for differential diagnosis. However, current studies have reported a lower to equal lesion detection rate for DWI compared with dynamic contrast-enhanced MR imaging.[10,12,25,29,42] These findings may be at least partially a result of the DWI technique used, because the distortion of EPI remains a major problem for accurate measurement of the ADC, particularly for small lesions.[11,34,36,37]

Nonmasslike enhancement

Another factor that can affect ADC values is the architecture of tumors. According to the American College of Radiology Breast Imaging Reporting and Data System (BI-RADS) lexicon, pathologic growth conditions in the breast can be described as mass or nonmasslike enhancement.[46] Guo and colleagues[12] and Sinha and colleagues[16] found that the mean ADC value is inversely proportional to the cell density. Therefore, as nonmasslike enhancement lesions can form large and noncompact lesions, with normal parenchyma in the center of the tumor, a lesser restriction of the diffusion processes may occur in these tumors compared with mass lesions (**Fig. 2**). This phenomenon has been reported for several pathologic and normal states, including noninvasive ductal carcinomas, lobular carcinoma in situ, atypical ductal hyperplasia, papillomas, hormonal changes, and fibrocystic disease.[47]

These results indicate that ADC measurements have a limited ability to differentiate between benign and malignant nonmasslike enhancement lesions. ADC values for malignant lesions may be in the range of benign lesions in these cases.[25] Therefore, a higher ADC value cutoff may be required for nonmasslike enhancement lesions compared with mass lesions. Yabuuchi and colleagues[47] suggested that an ADC value of less than 1.3×10^{-3} mm^2/s was a significant factor for indication of malignancy for nonmasslike enhancement lesions. In contrast, Baltzer and colleagues[42] found that ADC measurements failed to be of diagnostic value for these lesions. Further investigation is needed to analyze the precise diagnostic potential of DWI for diagnosis of nonmasslike enhancement lesions.

ANALYSIS OF DWI AT OUR INSTITUTION

A preliminary study in our institution[17] confirmed the usefulness of DWI for the differential diagnosis of benign and malignant breast lesions. In addition, this study revealed no significant statistical difference between ADC values obtained using different b-value combinations, although b-values of 0 and 750 s/mm^2 performed slightly better at differentiating between benign and malignant breast lesions than the other combinations analyzed. However, a further study using a larger population was needed to improve the statistical power and to fortify the previous results.

Study Population

From August 2007 to March 2010, 156 women with 178 breast mass-type lesions were prospectively enrolled in the study. The study was approved by our institutional review board, and all patients provided informed consent. Exclusion criteria included benign cysts, patient movement, sequences with susceptibility and chemical shift artifacts, lesions not visible on the DWI sequence, and neoadjuvant treatment before MR imaging. From these criteria, 40 lesions from 34 patients were excluded. As a result, the study included 122 patients (age range, 22–86 years; mean age, 46.9 years) with 138 breast lesions.

On histopathologic examination, 81 malignant lesions were identified, including IDC (n = 64), invasive lobular carcinoma (ILC; n = 6), DCIS (n = 4), tubular carcinoma (n = 2), mucinous colloid carcinoma (n = 2), medullary carcinoma (n = 1), adenoid cystic carcinoma (n = 1), and malignant phyllodes tumor (n = 1). The median size of the malignant lesions was 2.1 cm (range, 0.8–11.2 cm).

A total of 57 benign lesions were identified, 19 of which showed histopathologic results, which included fibroadenoma (n = 14), papilloma (n = 2), epidermoid cyst (n = 1), nodular adenosis (n = 1), and ductal ectasia with stroma fibrosis (n = 1). The authors also included 38 lesions classified as BI-RADS [46] category 2 by MR imaging to increase the number of samples of benign lesions for use in identification of more reliable and representative ADC values. The diagnoses were defined by the consensus of 2 experienced breast radiologists with 12 and 9 years of experience, respectively. Benign lesions were followed up for at least 1 year by mammography, sonography, or MR imaging, with no significant modifications in the imaging patterns. The median size of benign lesions was 1.2 cm (range, 0.6–11.4 cm).

MR Imaging Acquisition, Analysis and Data Collection

All MR imaging examinations, including DWI, were performed on a 1.5-T MR System with a bilateral

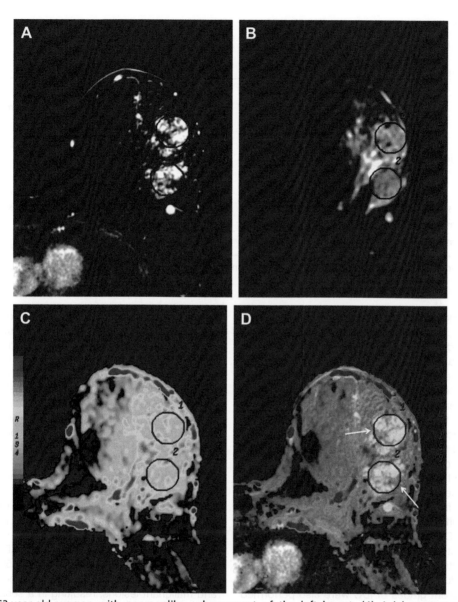

Fig. 2. 62-year-old woman with nonmasslike enhancement of the left breast. (*A*) Axial contrast-enhanced T1-weighted three-dimensional spoiled gradient-echo image, first phase, subjected to subtraction technique. (*B*) Axial diffusion-weighted image. (*C*) Axial colored ADC map obtained using b-values of 0 and 750 s/mm². (*D*) Fusion axial contrast-enhanced T1-weighted subjected to subtraction technique and axial colored ADC map reveal a nonmasslike enhancement lesion classified as highly suspicious by conventional MR imaging. Because nonmasslike enhancement lesions form large but noncompact lesions, a lesser restriction of the diffusion processes may occur, evident as yellow, and not blue, on the ADC colored map. Note that even using the subtracted image as reference to the ROI placement, there are still no enhancing areas, which may not represent tumor inside the ROIs (*white arrows*).

8-channel breast coil. DWI was performed using an axial single-shot EPI sequence centered on the lesion (**Table 1**). Standard sequences, including pre- and postcontrast sequences, were acquired before DWI.

All images were transferred to a workstation, and the DWI sequence was postprocessed using commercial software to obtain black-and-white and color ADC maps. Color maps used a color scheme, ranging from blue (diffusion restriction) to red (no diffusion restriction). The ADC maps of each lesion were calculated using 5 b-values (0, 250, 500, 750, and 1000 s/mm²) and also using the b 0 s/mm² value in combination with the other b-values (0 and 250 s/mm², 0 and 500 s/mm², 0 and 750 s/mm², 0 and 1000 s/mm²).

Table 1
Protocol used for the DWI study at our institution

Parameter	Value
Sequence	DWI single-shot EPI
TR/TE	1800 ms/93.8 ms (minimum TE)
FOV	360 mm
Matrix	160×192
Slice thickness/interval	5 mm/0 mm
NEX	16
rBW	25 kHz
b-values	0, 250, 500, 750, 1000 s/mm^2
Scan time	224 s
Scan time for b-value	56 s

Abbreviations: FOV, field of view; NEX, number of excitations; rBW, receive band width; TE, echo time; TR, repetition time.

DWI and ADC maps are typically noisy and were therefore viewed in conjunction with contrast-enhanced images. To achieve standardized conditions for analysis and to avoid contamination of the data by adjacent structures, 2 similar circular ROIs with a median area of 49 mm^2 (range, 16–536 mm^2) were individually placed within the target lesion in the same location for the 5 ADC maps described earlier, and the average ADC was acquired for each b-value combination. Apparent necrotic or cystic components were avoided by referring to conventional MR images.

The median ADC values were correlated with imaging findings and histopathologic diagnoses. The cutoff ADC value and the sensitivity and specificity of DWI to differentiate between benign and malignant lesions were calculated for all b-value combinations. Comparisons between the median ADC values for noninvasive ductal carcinoma and different grades of IDC were also performed for all b-value combinations. *P*-values less than .05 were considered statistically significant.

Results

The median ADC values obtained using 5 b-values and b 0 s/mm^2 value in combination with the other b-values were significantly lower for malignant breast lesions (median, 0.82–1.19; interquartile range [IQR] 0.72–1.4 $\times$ 10^{-3} mm^2/s) than for benign lesions (median, 1.38–1.71; IQR 1.22–1.93 $\times$ 10^{-3} mm^2/s) (*P*<.001, **Table 2**).

All of the b-value combinations used to calculate the ADC resulted in high sensitivity and specificity for the differentiation of benign and malignant lesions (**Table 3**). The only significant difference that occurred between the different b-value combinations was for the combination of b 0 and 250 s/mm^2, which exhibited a significantly lower area under the curve (AUC) compared with the other combinations (*P* = .019). No significant differences were observed between the other b-value combinations (*P*>.05). Consistent with previous findings, the ADC values calculated using b-values of 0 and 750 s/mm^2 were still slightly better than the other b-value combinations. Based on a cutoff value of 1.24 $\times$ 10^{-3} mm^2/s for ADCs calculated using b-values of 0 and 750 s/mm^2, 4 of 57 benign lesions (two fibroadenomas, one papilloma, and one nodular adenosis) and 7 of 81 malignant lesions (3 IDC, one ILC, 2 mucinous colloid carcinomas, and one malignant phyllodes tumor) were misdiagnosed, resulting in a sensitivity of 91.4% and a specificity of 93%. The ADC values calculated using b-values of 0 and 250 s/mm^2 yielded the poorest differentiation between benign and malignant lesions, resulting in a sensitivity of 81.5% and a specificity of 87.7%, based on a cutoff value of 1.47 $\times$ 10^{-3} mm^2/s.

With respect to the different benign histologic types, for the b-value combination of 0 and 750 s/mm^2, the median ADC values for fibroadenoma, papilloma, epidermoid cyst, nodular adenosis, and ductal ectasia with stroma fibrosis were 1.46 $\times$ 10^{-3} mm^2/s, 1.22 $\times$ 10^{-3} mm^2/s, 1.32 $\times$ 10^{-3} mm^2/s, 0.99 $\times$ 10^{-3} mm^2/s, and 1.99 $\times$ 10^{-3} mm^2/s, respectively. With respect to the different malignant histologic types, for the b-value combination of 0 and 750 s/mm^2, the median ADC values for IDC, ILC, DCIS, tubular carcinoma, mucinous colloid carcinoma, medullary carcinoma, adenoid cystic carcinoma, and malignant phyllodes tumor were 0.91 $\times$ 10^{-3} mm^2/s, 0.94 $\times$ 10^{-3} mm^2/s, 0.91 $\times$ 10^{-3} mm^2/s, 0.84 $\times$ 10^{-3} mm^2/s, 1.59 $\times$ 10^{-3}

Table 2
ADC values by b-value combination for benign and malignant lesions

b-Value Combinations (s/mm²)	ADC values (×10⁻³ mm²/s)					
	Benign Lesions (n = 57)		Malignant Lesions (n = 81)		
	Median	IQR	Median	IQR	P-value
0, 250, 500, 750, and 1000	1.45	1.30−1.58	0.907	0.76−1.01	<0.001
0 and 250	1.71	1.56−1.93	1.190	1.04−1.40	<0.001
0 and 500	1.59	1.44−1.77	1.010	0.90−1.19	<0.001
0 and 750	1.51	1.34−1.64	0.931	0.83−1.03	<0.001
0 and 1000	1.38	1.22−1.55	0.820	0.72−0.94	<0.001

mm^2/s, 0.86×10^{-3} mm^2/s, 0.93×10^{-3} mm^2/s, and 1.84×10^{-3} mm^2/s, respectively.

No statistically significant difference was evident between the median ADC values for noninvasive ductal carcinoma and the different grades of IDC using any of the b-value combinations. For the b-value combination of 0 and 750 s/mm², the median ADC value for DCIS was 0.91×10^{-3} mm²/s, and the median ADC values for IDC grades I, II, and III were 0.92×10^{-3} mm²/s, 0.88×10^{-3} mm²/s, and 1.02×10^{-3} mm²/s, respectively (P = .426).

Comments

The present results confirmed the findings of our previous study.[17] Both studies showed that the median ADC value for benign lesions was significantly lower than that of malignant lesions for all b-value combinations analyzed. Moreover, no statistically significant difference was observed between ADC values calculated using most of the b-value combinations analyzed, although the ADC calculated using b-values of 0 and 750 s/mm²

was slightly better than the others. These findings suggest that higher b-values can be useful for distinguishing benign from malignant lesions and that use of multiple b-values in DWI sequences is unnecessary.

Based on the diagnostic criteria used in this study, only two fibroadenomas (14.2%) and 4 invasive carcinomas (5.7%) were not appropriately classified using the ADC. These results indicate that DWI can effectively discriminate between fibroadenomas and invasive carcinomas (**Figs. 3 and 4**). This capability could likely prove to be useful for lesion characterization, because fibroadenomas have characteristics that overlap with malignant lesions in both sonography and dynamic contrast-enhanced MR imaging studies.[16,48,49] In our series, 5 fibroadenomas were misdiagnosed as suspect by MR imaging, but 3 of these lesions were correctly diagnosed as benign by DWI.

The primary limitations of our study were similar to those reported in the literature, including poor quality data as a result of patient movement and

Table 3
Sensitivity and specificity of the ADC in differentiation of benign from malignant lesions for each b-value combination

b-Value Combinations (s/mm²)	Cutoff (×10⁻³ mm²/s)[a]	Sensitivity (%)	95% CI[b]	Specificity (%)	95% CI[b]	AUC[c]
0, 250, 500, 750, and 1000	1.17	90.1 (73/81)	81.4−95.6	94.7 (54/57)	85.4−98.9	0.929
0 and 250	1.47	81.5 (66/81)	73.0−90.0	87.7 (50/57)	79.2−96.2	0.891
0 and 500	1.34	91.4 (74/81)	85.3−97.5	91.2 (52/57)	83.8−98.6	0.928
0 and 750	1.24	91.4 (74/81)	85.3−97.5	93.0 (53/57)	86.4−99.6	0.941
0 and 1000	1.12	91.4 (74/81)	85.3−97.5	91.2 (52/57)	83.8−98.6	0.943

Numbers in parentheses indicate number of lesions.

[a] ADC cutoff value.

[b] Confidence interval.

[c] Area under the curve, represents the probability that the ADC value accurately characterizes a breast lesion as malignant or benign according to the cutoff value.

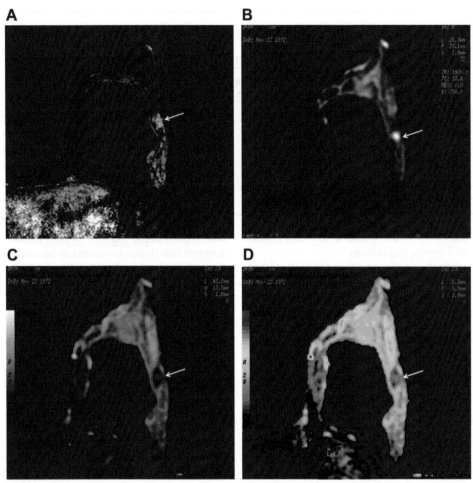

Fig. 3. 35-year-old woman with IDC of the left breast. (*A*) Axial contrast-enhanced T1-weighted three-dimensional spoiled gradient-echo image, in late phase. (*B*) Axial diffusion-weighted image. (*C*) Axial black-and-white and (*D*) colored ADC maps obtained using b-values of 0 and 750 s/mm² reveal a 1.1-cm mass (*white arrows*) classified as probably benign by conventional MR imaging. Note the low signal on the ADC black-and-white map and the blue on the ADC colored map, which indicates a malignant lesion.

difficulty visualizing some lesions on DWI, particularly small lesions. Limited ADC value measurements resulting from motion artifacts (10.1%) or from lack of visibility of the lesion on DWI, even after correlation with contrast-enhanced images (7.9%), resulted in exclusion of these cases. However, generally, good lesion visibility (92.1%) was obtained in the present study, and 8 of the 14 nonvisible lesions (57.1%) were smaller than 1 cm.

Despite these limitations, our results and the results of others suggest that DWI of the breast can provide additional information for the characterization of mass breast lesions in a rapid and straightforward manner. Furthermore, combination of ADC measurements with dynamic studies that interpret enhancement patterns, which exhibit good sensitivity but variable specificity for characterizing lesions, can increase the overall

accuracy of MR imaging, reducing the number of unnecessary invasive procedures. In our study, the overall specificity of MR imaging increased from 82.4% to 93% with the use of DWI.

POTENTIAL APPLICATIONS OF DIFFUSION IMAGING

Our results indicate that DWI can serve as a powerful tool for differentiating benign from malignant breast lesions. In addition to this use, DWI also shows potential for use in several additional diagnostic and therapeutic applications, including monitoring of neoadjuvant chemotherapy (NAC), evaluation of peritumor tissues, and assessment of axillary lymph nodes. These promising novel applications of DWI are discussed in the following sections.

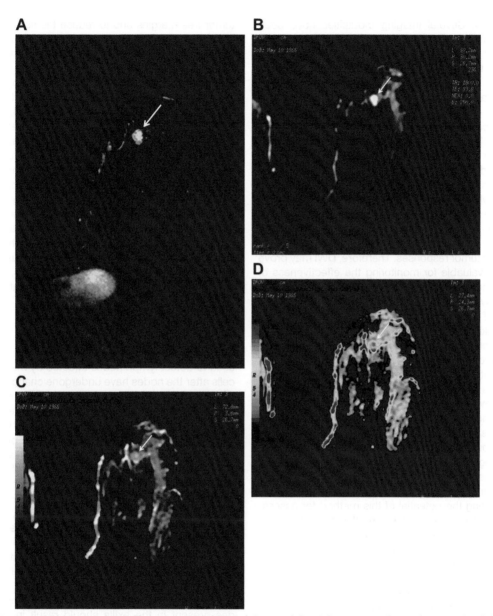

Fig. 4. 43-year-old woman with fibroadenoma of the left breast. (*A*) Axial contrast-enhanced T1-weighted three-dimensional spoiled gradient-echo image, first phase, subjected to subtraction technique. (*B*) Axial diffusion-weighted image. (*C*) Axial black-and-white and (*D*) colored ADC maps obtained using b-values of 0 and 750 s/mm^2 reveal a 1.3-cm mass (*white arrows*) classified as suspicious by conventional MR imaging. Note the high signal on the ADC black-and-white map and the red on the ADC colored map, which suggest that the lesion is benign.

Application of DWI to Monitoring of NAC

NAC is used to achieve tumor shrinkage, allowing breast conservation surgery for a proportion of patients with locally advanced breast cancer. Large clinical trials assume that the degree of response of the primary tumor to NAC is correlated with patient survival.[50] However, 20% to 25% of all patients with breast cancer do not respond to chemotherapy. Identification of surrogate biomarkers able to predict therapeutic outcomes earlier or more accurately than the current methods would be valuable for individualized tailoring of treatment and would allow for more cost-effective use of resources.[51]

Imaging modalities can be used to track tumor changes in response to a particular chemotherapy regimen. Several imaging modalities have been used to assess the extent of response to primary breast cancer treatment. MR imaging is considered to be the best available choice for evaluating the tumor and its response to the administered treatment as a result of the higher accuracy of this technique compared with the traditional methods of physical examination and mammography.[52]

A role for DWI in monitoring and predicting early breast tumor responses to NAC has previously been described.[21,30,51,53] Chemotherapy treatment results in cell lysis and loss of cell membrane integrity, which results in an increase in extracellular space and a concomitant increase in diffusion of water. Based on these effects, interest is growing in the measurement of changes in diffusion to detect tumor responses. Therefore, DWI may prove to be valuable for monitoring the effectiveness of treatment and for assessing changes caused by cell swelling and apoptosis rather than the application of conventional radiologic response indicators.

Pickles and colleagues[53] reported that a significant increase in the ADC occurred before a decrease in tumor size measured by MR imaging in a cohort of patients with invasive breast cancer examined before and after the first and second NAC cycles. The increase in the ADC value at the first cycle time point was significant, but the decrease in the longest diameter at the second cycle time point was only of borderline significance. Sharma and colleagues[30] found a statistically significantly larger increase in the ADC after the first chemotherapy cycle in responders compared with nonresponders, indicating the potential of this method for assessment of early responses. At this time point, no change in tumor size was evident for either group. These results underscore the potential usefulness of DWI for assessing treatment responses at early time points, before changes in tumor size.

A comparison between the ability of MR imaging and DWI to detect residual tumors revealed accuracy rates of 89% and 96%, respectively, which were not found to be statistically significant.[54] DWI exhibited, at minimum, equivalent accuracy levels to contrast-enhanced MR imaging for monitoring NAC. Therefore, use of DWI to visualize residual breast cancer without the need for contrast medium could be advantageous.

Application of DWI to Evaluation of Peritumor Tissues

Conservative surgery has become a well-established alternative to mastectomy for treatment of breast cancer. However, for conservative surgery to be successful, it is necessary to remove an adequate volume of breast tissue to achieve tumor-free margins and to reduce the risk of local recurrence without compromising the cosmetic outcome. Therefore, accurate determination of the transition boundary between the tumor and normal tissue is critical for deciding the surgical scope.

A previous study was designed to analyze changes in ADC values in peritumor tissues using DWI.[55] This study was based on the hypothesis that genetic and molecular alterations precede phenotypic changes in peritumor tissues. Therefore, DWI may be able to detect alterations earlier than conventional MR imaging. These investigators revealed that the ADC value of malignant lesions was statistically lower than that of peritumor tissues. They also found that the ADC values increased gradually from the innermost to the outermost layers of peritumor tissues. These results suggest that DWI can be used to predict the involvement of peritumor tissues, which could be highly beneficial for surgery preparation.

Application of DWI to Assessment of Axillary Lymph Nodes

Preliminary studies have shown that diffusion can be used to detect lymph nodes affected by malignant cells after the nodes have undergone changes and increases in cellularity that lead to diffusion restriction and low ADC values.[21] In a retrospective feasibility study, DWI was evaluated as a potential tool for characterization of pelvic lymph nodes in patients with prostate cancer.[56] The results from this study showed that there was a highly significant difference between the mean ADC values of malignant versus benign lymph nodes. Use of a cutoff of 1.30×10^{-3} mm^2/s resulted in good accuracy (85.6%), sensitivity (86.0%), and specificity (85.3%) for differentiation between malignant and benign lymph nodes using ADC values. These findings indicate that DWI is an accurate technique for the analysis of pelvic lymph nodes.

One could predict that metastasis to lymph nodes present in the axilla should result in similar effects on the ADC, specifically restricted diffusion and corresponding low ADC values. However, further studies are necessary to investigate the usefulness of DWI for characterization of malignant axillary lymph nodes. In addition, characterization of the necessary lymph nodal invasion level required to restrict diffusion and reduce the ADC value is needed for clinical applications. It also remains unclear whether DWI can accurately diagnose small metastases.

Use of DWI for Cancer Screening in Clinical Practice

The usefulness of DWI in clinical practice remains to be determined. DWI is often used as a supportive tool when results from conventional MR imaging are unclear. Applications using DWI for assessment of the response to NAC are also under development. Therefore, DWI has primarily been used for diagnostic purposes. However, the power of DWI for evaluation of high-risk patients who undergo screening MR imaging remains unknown.

The objectives of cancer screening are to improve the prognosis of patients with cancer and to reduce mortality. The accurate and timely detection of cancer is crucial to decreasing cancer-related mortality. High-risk groups are likely to be given priority for screening. Insufficient objective data are available to evaluate the effectiveness of DWI for cancer screening, and future studies in this area are needed. DWI can be predicted to be a useful screening tool because of its short scan time, cost-effectiveness, and high sensitivity.[36,37]

Use of DWI as a Stand-alone Technique

Because DWI does not require the injection of any contrast agent, it could possibly be of value as a stand-alone technique in severely ill patients, who cannot tolerate extended examinations. Furthermore, in patients with impaired renal function, the risk of nephrogenic systemic fibrosis is avoided using this technique.[25]

An initial investigation focused exclusively on malignant lesions showed a high rate of sensitivity for a contrast-free diagnostic approach combining DWI and short T1 inversion recovery imaging.[25,43] However, before such an approach could be introduced into the clinical routine, a possible incremental increase in value of contrast-free breast MR imaging over conventional methods must be validated. Knowledge regarding the diagnostic usefulness of ADC values compared with standard morphologic and dynamic descriptors remains limited. In a recent investigation, quantitative diffusivity measurements resulted in high, but nonetheless clearly inferior, diagnostic parameters compared with routine breast MR imaging.[25,42] Therefore, further studies are needed to quantitatively compare the accuracy of contrast-free and contrast-enhanced MR imaging of the breast.

Diffusion Tensor Imaging: An Extension of DWI

Diffusion tensor imaging (DTI) extends standard DWI, characterizing diffusion in at least 6 directions, to measure the full diffusion tensor and to characterize the motion of water in greater detail. In addition to the ADC value, DTI enables calculation of the degree of diffusion anisotropy (or directionality).[57] Therefore, information obtained by DTI for normal and altered breast tissue may also be useful for detecting disease and assessing local invasion.

In the brain, diffusion anisotropy measures have been useful for elucidating organization and development of white matter and for identifying abnormalities.[57] With recent advancements in MR imaging technology, DTI has also enabled unique microstructural characterization of normal and abnormal tissues in other areas of the body. The general assumption in previous studies has been that water diffusion in breast tissue is isotropic, with equal mobility in all directions. However, in more organized breast tissues, such as the parenchyma, which has a network of branching ducts and associated periductal fibrous stroma that extends radially and posteriorly from the nipple, it is possible that water molecules tend to follow a less restricted path and diffuse preferentially along or parallel to the ducts.[57] This phenomenon may result in anisotropic diffusion in normal breast tissue that can be detected by DTI.

Partridge and colleagues[57] found low to moderate diffusion anisotropy in normal fibroglandular tissue. Fractional anisotropy (FA) measurements differed between breast regions and were generally higher in the outer posterior region. This observation may reflect microstructural differences in the fibroglandular tissue. A higher concentration of smaller tapering ducts and terminal ductolobular units in the peripheral breast could influence diffusion directionality and increase posterior FA measurements in this region. Characterization of these influences on DTI measurements may be important for clinical interpretation of DTI results and standardization of techniques. Future studies are necessary to assess the clinical usefulness of DTI for breast imaging by comparing diffusion anisotropy in breast tumors and normal tissue. DTI may be able to detect disruptions in the normal anisotropy of water diffusion in the breast caused by cancer growth and may lead to new indices for identification of breast cancer.

SUMMARY

Diffusion sequences can be used for characterization and differentiation of malignant and benign breast lesions. Use of DWI as a diagnostic tool can increase the specificity of breast MR imaging and can reduce the number of false-positive results and associated unnecessary biopsies. In addition, DWI can be performed without significantly increasing examination time and can easily be introduced into the standard breast MR imaging protocol. Furthermore, novel applications for DWI are under development, including monitoring of the response to NAC, evaluation of peritumor tissues, assessment of axillary lymph nodes, and characterization of the advanced DTI technique. Although DWI is not currently recommended as a stand-alone diagnostic tool, future studies without injection of contrast agents may support the use of DWI in this capacity.

The performance of DWI under different conditions and at different field strengths must be better characterized to define a universal protocol. In addition, determination of the diagnostic criteria is also important, such as the threshold ADC value for quantitative diagnosis and the signal intensity for qualitative diagnosis. Potential pitfalls related to the diagnosis of nonmass-type enhancement lesions and small mass-type lesions, as well as movement artifacts, should be taken into consideration.

REFERENCES

1. Kuhl CK. Current status of breast MR imaging. Part II. Clinical applications. Radiology 2007;244(3): 672–91.
2. Kuhl CK. The current status of breast MR imaging. Part I. Choice of technique, image interpretation, diagnostic accuracy, and transfer to clinical practice. Radiology 2007;244(2):356–78.
3. Schnall MD, Blume J, Bluemke DA, et al. Diagnostic architectural and dynamic features at breast MR imaging: multicenter study. Radiology 2006;238(1): 42–53.
4. Macura KJ, Ouwerkerk R, Jacobs MA, et al. Patterns of enhancement on breast MR images: interpretation and imaging pitfalls. Radiographics 2006;26(6): 1719–34.
5. Wierner JI, Schilling KJ, Adami C, et al. Assessment of suspected breast cancer by MRI: a prospective clinical trial using a combined kinetic and morphologic analysis. AJR Am J Roentgenol 2005;184(3): 878–86.
6. Bedrosian I, Mick R, Orel SG, et al. Changes in the surgical management of patients with breast carcinoma based on preoperative magnetic resonance imaging. Cancer 2003;98(3):468–73.
7. Marini C, Iacconi C, Giannelli M, et al. Quantitative diffusion-weighted MR imaging in the differential diagnosis of breast lesion. Eur Radiol 2007;17(10): 2646–55.
8. Kuhl CK, Mielcareck P, Klaschik S, et al. Dynamic breast MR imaging: are signal intensity time course data useful for differential diagnosis of enhancing lesions? Radiology 1999;211(1):101–10.
9. Fischer U, Kopka L, Grabbe E. Breast carcinoma: effect of preoperative contrast-enhanced MR imaging on the therapeutic approach. Radiology 1999;213(3):881–8.
10. Wenkel E, Geppert C, Schulz-Wendtland R, et al. Diffusion weighted imaging in breast MRI: comparison of two different pulse sequences. Acad Radiol 2007;14(9):1077–83.
11. Sinha S, Sinha U. Functional magnetic resonance of human breast tumors: diffusion and perfusion imaging. Ann N Y Acad Sci 2002;980:95–115.
12. Guo Y, Cai YQ, Cai ZL, et al. Differentiation of clinically benign and malignant breast lesions using diffusion-weighted imaging. J Magn Reson Imaging 2002;16(2):172–8.
13. Rubesova E, Grell AS, De Maertelaer V, et al. Quantitative diffusion imaging in breast cancer: a clinical prospective study. J Magn Reson Imaging 2006; 24(2):319–24.
14. Woodhams R, Matsunaga K, Iwabuchi K, et al. Diffusion-weighted imaging of malignant breast tumors: the usefulness of apparent diffusion coefficient (ADC) value and ADC map for the detection of malignant breast tumors and evaluation of cancer extension. J Comput Assist Tomogr 2005;29(5): 644–9.
15. Kuroki Y, Nasu K, Kuroki S, et al. Diffusion-weighted imaging of breast cancer with the sensitivity encoding technique: analysis of the apparent diffusion coefficient value. Magn Reson Med Sci 2004;3(2): 79–85.
16. Sinha S, Lucas-Quesada FA, Sinha U, et al. In vivo diffusion-weighted MRI of the breast: potential for lesion characterization. J Magn Reson Imaging 2002;15(6):693–704.
17. Pereira FPA, Martins G, Figueiredo E, et al. Assessment of breast lesions with diffusion-weighted MRI: comparing the use of different b values. AJR Am J Roentgenol 2009;193(4):1030–5.
18. Partridge SC, De Martini WB, Kurland BF, et al. Quantitative diffusion-weighted imaging as an adjunct to conventional breast MRI for improved positive predictive value. AJR Am J Roentgenol 2009;193(6):1716–22.
19. Yabuuchi H, Matsuo Y, Okafuji T, et al. Enhanced mass on contrast-enhanced breast MR imaging: lesion characterization using combination of dynamic contrast-enhanced and diffusion-weighted MR images. J Magn Reson Imaging 2008;28(5): 1157–65.
20. Kelcz F. Diffusion weighted imaging of breast – promises and problems. Eur Radiol 2009;19(Suppl 4): S856–8.
21. Koh DM, Collins DJ. Diffusion-weighted MRI in the body: applications and challenges in oncology. AJR Am J Roentgenol 2007;188(6):1622–35.
22. Paran Y, Bendel P, Margalit R, et al. Water diffusion in the different microenvironments of breast cancer. NMR Biomed 2004;17(4):170–80.
23. Bogner W, Gruber S, Pinker K, et al. Diffusion-weighted MR for differentiation of breast lesions at

3.0 T: how does selection of diffusion protocols affect diagnosis? Radiology 2009;253(2):341−51.

24. Kuhl CK. Concepts for differential diagnosis in breast MR imaging. Magn Reson Imaging Clin N Am 2006;14(3):305−28.

25. Baltzer PAT, Dietzal M, Vag T, et al. Diffusion weighted imaging − useful in all kinds of lesions? A systematic review. Eur Radiol 2009;19(Suppl 4):S765−9.

26. Geijer B, Sundgren PC, Lindgren A, et al. The value of b required to avoid T2 shine-through from old lacunar infarcts in diffusion-weighted imaging. Neuroradiology 2001;43(7):511−7.

27. Partridge SC, McKinnon GC, Henry RG, et al. Menstrual cycle variation of apparent diffusion coefficients measured in the normal breast using MRI. J Magn Reson Imaging 2001;14(4):433−8.

28. Kuhl CK, Bieling HB, Gieseke J, et al. Healthy premenopausal breast parenchyma in dynamic contrast-enhanced MR imaging of the breast: normal contrast medium enhancement and cyclical-phase dependency. Radiology 1997;203(1):137−44.

29. Park MJ, Cha ES, Kang BJ, et al. The role of diffusion-weighted imaging and the apparent diffusion coefficient (ADC) values for breast tumors. Korean J Radiol 2007;8(5):390−6.

30. Sharma U, Danishad KK, Seenu V, et al. Longitudinal study of the assessment by MRI and diffusion-weighted imaging of tumor response in patients with locally advanced breast cancer undergoing neoadjuvant chemotherapy. NMR Biomed 2009;22(1):104−13.

31. Woodhams R, Matsunaga K, Kan S, et al. ADC mapping of benign and malignant breast tumors. Magn Reson Med Sci 2005;4(1):35−42.

32. Yoshikawa MI, Ohsumi O, Sugata S, et al. Comparison of breast cancer detection by diffusion-weighted magnetic resonance imaging and mammography. Radiat Med 2007;25(5):218−23.

33. Yuen S, Yamada K, Goto M, et al. Microperfusion-induced elevation of ADC is suppressed after contrast in breast carcinoma. J Magn Reson Imaging 2009;29(5):1080−4.

34. Tsushima Y, Takahashi-Taketomi A, Endo K. Magnetic resonance (MR) differential diagnosis of breast tumors using apparent diffusion coefficient (ADC) on 1.5-T. J Magn Reson Imaging 2009;30(2):249−55.

35. Hatakenaka M, Soeda H, Yabuuchi H, et al. Apparent diffusion coefficients of breast tumors: clinical application. Magn Reson Med Sci 2008;7:23−9.

36. Razek AA, Gaballa G, Denewer A, et al. Diffusion-weighted MR imaging of the breast. Acad Radiol 2010;17(3):382−6.

37. Kuroki Y, Nasu K. Advances in breast MRI: diffusion-weighted imaging of the breast. Breast Cancer 2008;15(3):212−7.

38. Belli P, Constantini M, Bufi E, et al. Diffusion-weighted imaging in breast lesion evaluation. Radiol Med 2010;115(1):51−69.

39. Woodhams R, Kakita S, Hata H, et al. Diffusion-weighted imaging of mucinous carcinoma of the breast: evaluation of apparent diffusion coefficient and signal intensity in correlation with histologic findings. AJR Am J Roentgenol 2009;193(1):260−6.

40. Matsuoka A, Minato M, Harada M, et al. Comparison of 3.0 and 1.5-tesla diffusion-weighted imaging in the visibility of breast cancer. Radiat Med 2008;26(1):15−20.

41. Lo GG, Ai V, Chan JK, et al. Diffusion-weighted magnetic resonance imaging of breast lesions: first experiences at 3.0T. J Comput Assist Tomogr 2009;33(1):63−9.

42. Baltzer PA, Renz DM, Herrmann KH, et al. Diffusion-weighted imaging (DWI), in MR mammography (MRM): clinical comparison of echo planar imaging (EPI) and half-Fourier single-shot turbo spin echo (HASTE) diffusion techniques. Eur Radiol 2009;19(7):1612−20.

43. Kuroki-Suzuki S, Kuroki Y, Nasu K, et al. Detecting breast cancer with non-contrast MR-imaging: combining diffusion-weighted and STIR imaging. Magn Reson Med Sci 2007;6(1):21−7.

44. Kim SH, Cha ES, Kim HS, et al. Diffusion-weighted imaging of breast cancer: correlation of the apparent diffusion coefficient value with prognostic factors. J Magn Reson Imaging 2009;30(3):615−20.

45. Le Bihan D, Poupon C, Amadon A, et al. Artifacts and pitfalls in diffusion MRI. J Magn Reson Imaging 2006;24(3):478−88.

46. American College of Radiology (ACR). ACR BIRADS: magnetic resonance imaging. In: Ikeda DM, Hylton NM, editors. ACR breast imaging reporting and data system, breast imaging atlas. Reston (VA): American College of Radiology; 2003. p. 111−4.

47. Yabuuchi H, Matsuo Y, Kamitani T, et al. Non-mass-like enhancement on contrast-enhanced breast MR imaging: lesion characterization using combination of dynamic contrast-enhanced and diffusion-weighted MR images. Eur J Radiol 2010;75(1):126−32.

48. Stomper PC, Winston JS, Herman S, et al. Angiogenesis and dynamic MR imaging gadolinium enhancement of malignant and benign breast lesions. Breast Cancer Res Treat 1997;45(1):39−46.

49. Hochman MG, Orel SG, Powell CM, et al. Fibroadenomas: MR imaging appearances with radiologic−histopathologic correlation. Radiology 1997;204(1):123−9.

50. Ma B, Meyer CR, Pickles MD, et al. Voxel-by-voxel functional diffusion mapping for early evaluation of breast cancer treatment. Inf Process Med Imaging 2009;21:276–87.

51. Turnbull LW, Ma B, Meyer CR, et al. Diffusion changes in chemotherapy of breast cancer: the earliest sign? Eur Radiol 2009;19(Suppl 4): S948–9.

52. Iacconi C, Giannelli M, Marini C, et al. The role of mean diffusivity (MD) as a predictive index of the response to chemotherapy in locally advanced breast cancer: a preliminary study. Eur Radiol 2010;20(2):303–8.

53. Pickles MD, Gibbs P, Lowry M, et al. Diffusion changes precede size reduction in neoadjuvant treatment of breast cancer. Magn Reson Imaging 2006;24(7):843–7.

54. Woodhams R, Kakita S, Hata H, et al. Identification of residual breast carcinoma following neoadjuvant chemotherapy: diffusion-weighted imaging—comparison with contrast-enhanced MR imaging and pathologic findings. Radiology 2010; 254(2):357–66.

55. Yili Z, Xiaoyan H, Hongwen D, et al. The value of diffusion-weighted imaging in assessing the ADC changes of tissues adjacent to breast carcinoma. BMC Cancer 2009;9:18.

56. Eiber M, Beer AJ, Holzapfel K, et al. Preliminary results for characterization of pelvic lymph nodes in patients with prostate cancer by diffusion-weighted MR-imaging. Invest Radiol 2010;45(1):15–23.

57. Partridge SC, Murthy RS, Ziadloo A, et al. Diffusion tensor magnetic resonance imaging of the breast. Magn Reson Imaging 2010;28(3):320–8.

Diffusion-Weighted Magnetic Resonance Imaging in the Upper Abdomen: Technical Issues and Clinical Applications

Leonardo K. Bittencourt, MD[a],*, Celso Matos, MD[b],
Antonio C. Coutinho Jr, MD[c]

KEYWORDS

- Diffusion-weighted imaging • Magnetic resonance
- Upper abdomen • Liver

Diffusion-weighted imaging (DWI) is a modality that assesses the random movement of water molecules within different physical media through the use of magnetic resonance (MR) imaging. In a totally unrestricted environment, water movement is completely random, a phenomenon known as Brownian motion or free diffusion.[1,2] In biologic tissues, this movement is impeded by interactions with molecules and cellular structures. The data generated with DWI allows for an indirect estimate of information concerning tissue composition, cell density, microperfusion, and even cell membrane viability.

Historically, the DWI sequence found its first clinical application in the early diagnosis of acute ischemic stroke.[3] To date, it has been widely used in the neuroimaging setting. Application of the technique was until recently limited to brain studies because of its low signal/noise ratio (SNR) and high susceptibility to movement and paramagnetic artifacts.

DWI of the abdomen and pelvis in routine clinical practice is a recent achievement, owing to a new generation of scanners with higher magnetic fields (3.0 T vs 1.5 T), higher gradient amplitudes, echo planar and parallel image acquisition protocols, better movement-correction solutions, and new phased-array multichannel surface coils.

With growing interest from the scientific community, many centers have now integrated DWI into their abdominal MR protocols, owing to its potential to detect, characterize, and even provide follow-up parameters for neoplastic and inflammatory conditions. Nevertheless, although strong evidence has increasingly supported these assumptions, the technique still lacks measurement reproducibility and standardization across different scanners/vendors, sequence designs, acquisition parameters, and follow-up features.

This article reviews imaging strategies for DWI in the upper abdomen that are currently used, describes the routine clinical protocols and variants

The authors have nothing to disclose.
[a] Clínica de Diagnóstico por Imagem, Carlos Bittencourt Diagnóstico por Imagem and Department of Radiology, Rio de Janeiro Federal University (UFRJ), Av. Das Américas, 4666, Centro Medico, Sala 325, Rio de Janeiro 22649-900, Brazil
[b] Department of Radiology, Hospital Erasme, Université Libre de Bruxelles, 808 Route de Lennik, 1070 Brussels, Belgium
[c] Clínica de Diagnóstico por Imagem and Fatima Digittal, Av. Das Américas, 4666, Centro Medico, Sala 325, Rio de Janeiro 22649-900, Brazil
* Corresponding author.
E-mail address: lkayat@gmail.com

Magn Reson Imaging Clin N Am 19 (2011) 111–131
doi:10.1016/j.mric.2010.09.002

that have been reported, reviews the most common and established clinical applications, and lists possible avenues of investigation and future indications.

RATIONALE FOR ABDOMINAL DWI

Standard anatomic MR imaging is based solely on contrast differences between proton density, T1, and T2 among structures and tissues. Although these distinctions enable some tissue characterization (eg, water vs fat, white matter vs gray-matter), they give no information about tissue integrity and cellularity, and may not always reflect early alterations with sufficient contrast resolution for recognition with the naked eye.

DWI is deemed to be a functional modality because impedance of water molecule diffusion partially reflects tissue cellularity[4–6] and the presence of intact cellular membranes.[5] Therefore, tissues associated with restricted diffusion include tumors, inflamed tissues/abscesses, fibrotic tissues, hematomas, and cytotoxic edema. Conversely, unimpeded diffusion is found in tissues with low cellularity, disrupted cell membranes, and fluid cystic content. The basic physics involved and the measurement parameters are addressed elsewhere in this issue.

In the abdomen, the additional information provided by DWI examinations may be extremely useful because many neoplastic and inflammatory lesions have a low contrast in relation to background tissues/organs on conventional sequences, thus enabling better detection through DWI. Furthermore, the quantitative information provided by apparent diffusion coefficient (ADC) measurements is believed to correlate with tissue cellularity, potentially allowing for lesion characterization. Also, alterations in microscopic cytoarchitecture and vascularization may precede changes in macroscopic morphologic measurements, underscoring the potential for DWI in follow-up after chemoradiation therapy. Patients with impaired renal function or those who are allergic to gadolinium chelates may benefit from DWI, precluding the use of endovenous paramagnetic agents.

FINE-TUNING DWI PARAMETERS FOR THE UPPER ABDOMEN

To achieve good diagnostic DWI sequences in the abdomen, one has to overcome the intrinsic limitations of the technique, as well as a series of known pitfalls and artifacts related to this region of interest.

Low SNR, which is inherent to the method, is the first limitation. It may be resolved by using high magnetic field imaging (1.5 vs 3.0 T), low echo

time values (<100 ms), an increased number of excitations, low matrix resolution (eg, 128×128 at 1.5 T and 256×256 at 3.0 T), a thickening of the slices (of ≥6 mm), and a large field of view. Also, faster imaging techniques, such as parallel imaging, allow the acquisition of b-values in multiple directions, which enables signal averaging that further increases SNR.

The choice of an adequate set of b-values is a topic of much debate among institutions and investigators, because each b-value adds a considerable fraction of acquisition time, but too few b-values compromise tissue characterization and accurate ADC measurement. There are ongoing studies to examine the balance of this relationship and determine the best set of b-values for most organs in the human body. In addition, some propose 2 different sequences in the same examination, one with 2 b-values (usually 0 and 10–100 s/mm^2) for lesion detection and another with multiple b-values (6–12 b-values, of 0–1600 s/mm^2, depending on the institution) for accurate ADC calculation and lesion characterization.

Another major limitation of DWI is the increased susceptibility to motion and magnetic artifacts, which can be managed by respiratory and cardiac triggering, breath-hold acquisition, and fast imaging techniques. Although breath-hold sequences are less prone to motion artifacts, their quantitative ADC analyses are considered to be less accurate and have generally lower values than those provided by respiratory-triggered sequences.[7] Another strategy, described by Takahara and colleagues,[8] relies on free-breathing acquisition with multiple numbers of excitations and signal averaging, which claims to increase SNR and enable more accurate ADC measurement. Susceptibility to magnetic artifacts is intrinsic to the echo planar sequence and evidence shows that iron deposits or metal devices may lead to restricted diffusion. However, this same artifact may be useful because the use of superparamagnetic iron oxide (SPIO)–based contrast media on echo planar sequences can be used for the further detection and characterization of liver lesions.[9]

Ghosting from respiratory movements and chemical-shift artifacts is resolved by the robust fat-suppression techniques that are now available. T1 effects can be minimized by using high repetition time values (usually >2500 ms, which is 3 times the T1 of a typical liver metastasis). And T2 shine-through effects are dealt with by applying high b-values (>1000 s/mm^2) or by interpreting the ADC map in conjunction with the raw diffusion-weighted images.

DWI, being a functional MR modality, is a technique that relies more on contrast than on resolution. Therefore, when fine-tuning an acquisition protocol, a high SNR and a low influence of artifacts or T1/T2 effects should be pursued rather than striving for in-plane resolution. Good spatial resolution can be more easily achieved through conventional anatomic sequences, which are then fused with DWI information through simple postprocessing applications.

DWI IN THE UPPER ABDOMEN: HOW WE DO IT?

DWI is routinely performed at our institution during abdominal MR examinations, regardless of the indication. Although previous studies have shown that performing DWI after the administration of gadopentetate dimeglumine does not seem to affect ADC calculations in the liver,[10] there seems to be a slight decrease on the ADC at brain studies.[11,12] Therefore, we try to perform the acquisition before contrast material administration.

The two imaging strategies used are summarized in **Table 1**. The first strategy relies on a two b-value (0 and 1000 s/mm^2) breath-hold acquisition and is used either when there is no suspected focal lesion to characterize, or when the indication is unclear/nonspecific. The region of interest ranges from the liver to the lower renal poles and comprises widely-spaced thick slices. Once the acquisition time reaches approximately 29 seconds, the benefits gained from occasional unsuspected lesion detection or characterization by this sequence outweigh the extra time that is needed.

The second strategy is used for known or evident lesion characterization and involves a respiration-triggered sequence with 4 b-values (0, 100, 500, and 1000 s/mm^2) and narrowly-spaced thin slices, which are optimized for the region of interest. This approach benefits from the detection capabilities of bright- and dark-blood low b-values and enables an acceptable routine ADC calculation without compromising the overall examination time. These strategies are also roughly in accordance with the protocols suggested by other groups.[13] Images can then be postprocessed on general workstation applications to generate fusion maps with anatomic and postcontrast images that resemble those obtained in positron emission tomography (PET) and computed tomography (CT) examinations.[8]

CLINICAL APPLICATIONS OF UPPER ABDOMINAL DWI
Liver

No organ in the abdomen has received more attention in the DWI literature than the liver. Many different applications and clinical settings have been investigated for both focal and diffuse liver lesions. Several publications have reported the usefulness of DWI for liver lesion detection.[14–21] Most of these focused on the value of low b-value images (50–100 s/mm^2) compared with T2-weighted (T2w), fat-suppressed T2w, and postgadolinium T1-weighted (T1w) images. This distinction is because of the black-blood effect inherent in low b-values, which suppresses the background signal of vessels in the liver parenchyma while maintaining the signal intensity of focal lesions (**Fig. 1**). Moreover, there is reduced blurring with spin echo (SE) echo planar DWI compared with T2w turbo SE or half-Fourier turbo SE (HASTE).[22] Coenegrachts and colleagues[17] showed a higher conspicuity of hemangiomas and metastases with respiratory-triggered low b-value DWI compared with conventional unenhanced MR imaging. Zech and colleagues[21] compared DWI (b-value = 50 s/mm^2) with fat-suppressed T2w images, and observed better image quality and a better sensitivity for lesion detection with DWI (83% vs 61%). When Bruegel and colleagues[19] compared respiratory-triggered DWI with 5 different either fat-suppressed T2w or short tau inversion recovery (STIR) sequences for the diagnosis of hepatic metastases at 1.5 T, they found that DWI showed greater accuracy (0.91–0.92 vs 0.47–0.67, respectively), and an even more pronounced advantage compared with T2w images in the examination of metastatic lesions smaller than 1 cm in diameter. The combination of these results, especially when combined with other similar studies already published, has led to the claim that low b-value DWI outperforms both fat-suppressed T2w and STIR in the detection of focal liver lesions (**Figs. 2 and 3**). Consequently, many centers, including ours, have removed fat-suppressed T2w sequences from their routine protocols to invest extra time in enhancing DWI parameters.[20,23] However, the left liver lobe is a notoriously weak spot for DWI in the detection of focal lesions because of cardiac motion artifacts (**Fig. 4**).[16]

Regarding contrast media and DWI, there is evidence to suggest that DWI has a better diagnostic accuracy in the detection of colorectal metastases in conjunction with mangafodipir trisodium (MnDPDP),[24] better performance in association with SPIO in the detection of hepatocellular carcinoma (HCC) compared with SPIO-enhanced MR imaging,[9] and no significant difference in performance on a per lesion basis compared with gadolinium-enhanced T1w.[25] These data support the use of DWI as an alternative to gadolinium chelates, or other contrast media, in patients with severe renal dysfunction or in those at risk for nephrogenic systemic fibrosis.

Table 1
Acquisition parameters for DWI on 1.5 T and 3.0 T

Parameter	1.5 T		3 T	
	Breath-hold Acquisition	Respiratory-triggered Acquisition	Breath-hold Acquisition	Respiratory-triggered Acquisition
Field of view (right–left × anteroposterior in mm)	400 × 400	360 × 347	400 × 400	360 × 360
Matrix size (phase × frequency encoding)	128 × 128	164 × 164	130 × 130	164 × 164
Repetition time (ms)	2600	2800	2100	1500
Echo time (ms)	80	81	70	74
Echo planar imaging factor	128	158	130	164
Phase-encoding direction	Anteroposterior	Anteroposterior	Anteroposterior	Anteroposterior
Parallel imaging acceleration factor	2	2	2	2
Number of averages/excitations/signals acquired	2	5	1	2
Slice thickness (mm)	6.5	5.0	7.0	5.0
Slice spacing (mm)	2.27	0.50	2.80	0.75
Number of slices	20	20	20	20
Direction of motion probing gradients	Phase, frequency, and slice (3-scan trace)	Phase, frequency, and slice (3-scan trace)	Phase, frequency, and slice (3-scan trace)	Phase, frequency, and slice (3-scan trace)
Fat suppression	Yes	Yes	Yes	Yes
b-values (s/mm^2)	0, 1000	0, 100, 500, 1000	0, 1000	0, 100, 500, 1000
Acquisition time (min:s)	00:29	03:28	00:29	03:52

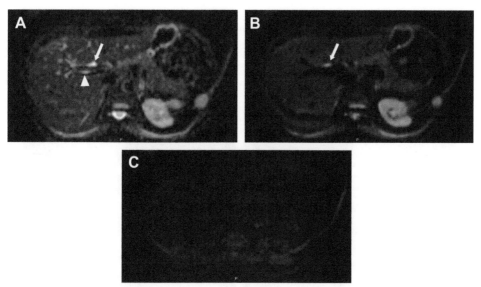

Fig. 1. The influence of the b-value on the signal intensities of liver structures: (*A*) b-value = 0 s/mm², showing both blood vessels (*arrowhead*) and biliary ducts (*arrow*) with high signal intensity, overlaid on liver parenchyma with intermediate signal intensity. When the b-value is equal to 0, there is maximum overall SNR but also a maximal T2 shine-through effect; (*B*) with a b-value of 100 s/mm², structures with blood flow have a dark signal caused by their markedly unimpeded diffusion (the so-called black-blood effect). Resting or slow-flowing fluids, such as within the biliary ducts (*arrow*) or simple cysts, retain high signal intensities, as do most benign and malignant focal lesions, which is useful for lesion detection; and (*C*) with a b-value of 1000 s/mm², fluid structures and most benign lesions have dark signal intensities. On high b-values, the diffusion weighting is maximized and the T2 shine-through effect is minimized, but at the expense of a significantly low SNR when compared with low b-values.

The most straightforward approach for characterizing focal liver lesions relies on visual assessment of high b-value (≥500 s/mm²) images, that may help distinguish between cystic and solid lesions, the latter usually retaining high signal intensity compared with the background liver on increases in the b-values (**Fig. 5**). A more sophisticated and less subjective approach based on quantitative ADC measurements may also be used to differentiate between benign and malignant lesions, owing to the generally lower ADC values in the latter, probably resulting from greater cellularity (**Fig. 6**). Although an average ADC cutoff of between 1.4×10^{-3} and 1.6×10^{-3} mm/s² may provide sensitivity as high as 74% to 100% and specificity in the range of 77% to 100% in the distinction between benign and malignant liver lesions,[20,26–31] other published ADC values show

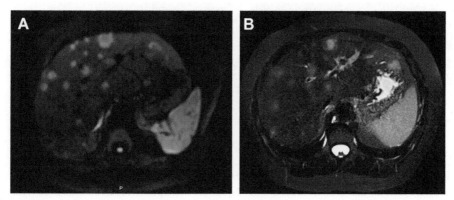

Fig. 2. The usefulness of low b-value images in the detection of liver lesions. In this 62-year-old female patient with metastatic pancreatic adenocarcinoma, the low b-value images (*A*), b = 100 s/mm², depicted more lesions with smaller dimensions and better conspicuity than did fat-suppressed T2w images (*B*).

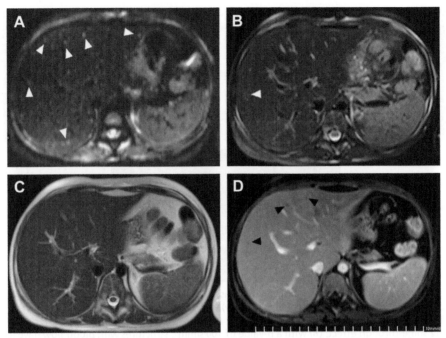

Fig. 3. An 18-year-old female patient with acute myeloid leukemia presented with sepsis: (*A*) the low b-value images (b = 50 s/mm²) depicted several millimetric hyperintense foci that were diffusely distributed in the liver parenchyma (*arrowheads*), which were better displayed using DWI than using fat-suppressed T2w images (*arrowhead* in *B*), T2w images (*C*), or delayed-phase postgadolinium T1w (*arrowheads* in *D*). These lesions were deemed to be suspicious for liver microabscesses, probably caused by fungal infection. The blood cultures were positive for *Candida albicans* and the patient eventually died of the infection and sepsis.

much wider variation, in the range of 0.94×10⁻³ to 2.85×10⁻³ mm/s² for metastases and 0.69×10⁻³ to 2.28×10⁻³ mm/s² for normal liver parenchyma.[13,17,18,30–34] Detailed tables that compare the ADC values of different focal liver lesions can be found in the cited references. As noted, there is considerable overlap between the ADC values of solid benign hepatic lesions, such as focal nodular hyperplasia or adenoma, and those of malignant lesions, such as metastases and HCC (**Fig. 7**). Also, cystic, necrotic, or mucinous components in a malignant lesion may increase ADC values, which can generate false-negatives when DWI data alone are considered (**Fig. 8**). In contrast, abscesses or inflammatory lesions show low ADC values, because of their inflammatory and viscous contents, potentially generating false-positives. Furthermore, every

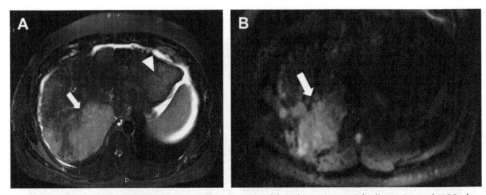

Fig. 4. Motion artifacts on the left liver lobe. In this 42-year-old male patient with disseminated HCC, there were 2 bulky lesions detected on fat-suppressed T2w images (*arrow* and *arrowhead* in *A*), but only the one in the right liver lobe was detected using DWI (*arrow* in *B*). The left liver is completely blurred from motion artifacts, caused by its proximity to the heart.

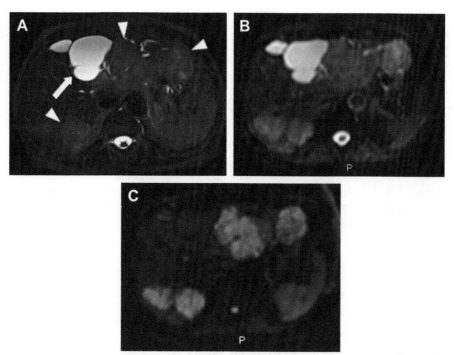

Fig. 5. Lesion characterization using DWI based on visual assessment. In this 74-year-old female patient with metastatic pancreatic adenocarcinoma, the fat-suppressed T2w image (*A*) shows a markedly hyperintense cystic lesion on segment IV (*arrow*) and 3 ill-defined, mildly hyperintense solid lesions on segments II and VII (*arrowheads*). The cystic lesion is also hyperintense on low b-value DWI (*B*, b = 0 s/mm^2), but shows a significant signal drop on high b-value images (*C*, b = 1000 s/mm^2). In contrast, the metastatic lesions are mildly hyperintense on low b-value images (*B*), but retain high signal intensity in comparison with the background on high b-value images (*C*).

study group uses their own scanning protocols, with different manufacturers, different field strength scanners, different b-value sets, breath-hold or respiratory-triggered techniques, different ADC calculation algorithms, and different measurement

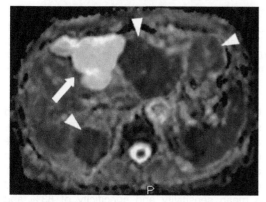

Fig. 6. The ADC map from the same patient as in **Fig. 5**, depicting the metastatic lesions as dark areas (*arrowheads*), with a mean ADC of 0.95 ($\pm$0.01)$\times$ 10^{-3} mm/s^2. The cystic lesion (*arrow*) is shown as a bright area and has a mean ADC of 2.50 ($\pm$0.07)$\times$ 10^{-3} mm/s^2.

techniques, making it difficult to integrate results across studies and propose a standardized ADC evaluation. Therefore, DWI alone is currently not suitable for stand-alone characterization of focal liver lesions, but it may show better accuracy when used in conjunction with contrast-enhanced and conventional MR imaging sequences.

In the clinical setting of diffuse liver disease, a noninvasive alternative has long been sought for liver biopsy for the diagnosis and monitoring of fibrosis and nonalcoholic fatty liver disease. Among other techniques, DWI has shown some usefulness in these applications, because hepatic steatosis and collagen deposition in fibrosis may be associated with a consequent reduction in ADC.[5] Moreover, ADC values in the liver have been found to be reduced in patients with cirrhosis.[27,29,35-38] Nevertheless, although most studies have shown good performance of ADC measurement in distinguishing moderate and severe (F2–F3) from mild (F0–F1) fibrosis[37,38] with ADC cutoff values in the range of 1.53$\times$10^{-3} to 1.60$\times$10^{-3} mm/s^2, there is still a significant overlap of ADC values for the various degrees of

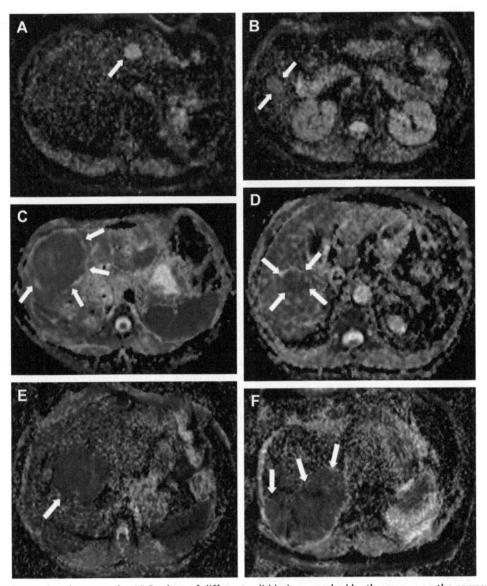

Fig. 7. Comparison between the ADC values of different solid lesions, marked by the arrows on the corresponding images: (*A*) hemangioma (ADC 2.38 $\pm$ 0.24$\times$10^{-3} mm/s^2); (*B*) another hemangioma (1.42 $\pm$ 0.16$\times$10^{-3} mm/s^2); (*C*) focal nodular hyperplasia (1.23 $\pm$ 0.7$\times$10^{-3} mm/s^2); (*D*) hepatocellular adenoma (0.91 $\pm$ 0.14$\times$10^{-3} m/s^2); (*E*) intrahepatic cholangiocarcinoma (0.92 $\pm$ 0.09$\times$10^{-3} mm/s^2); and (*F*) hepatocellular carcinoma (0.88 $\pm$ 0.14$\times$ 10^{-3} mm/s^2).

fibrosis,[39] inflammation, and fatty deposition. Thus, DWI should currently be considered an ancillary method for the assessment of diffuse liver disease, requiring further studies and technical implementations.

Gallbladder and Biliary Ducts

The bile ducts and gallbladder generally exhibit contents with high diffusivity and high ADC values, resembling those of simple hepatic cysts. Thus far, few studies have evaluated biliary tract diseases

through DWI, and most such studies have focused selectively on malignant processes (**Fig. 9**). Sugita and colleagues[40] retrospectively evaluated the usefulness of high b-value DWI in the detection of gallbladder carcinoma in 29 patients with focal gallbladder wall thickening. They achieved a mean sensitivity and specificity of 83% and 100%, respectively, finding a mean ADC value of 1.28 ($\pm$0.41)$\times$10^{-3} mm/s^2 for gallbladder adenocarcinoma, as opposed to 1.92 ($\pm$0.21)$\times$10^{-3} mm/s^2 for control gallbladder lesions (ie, chronic cholecystitis, adenomyomatosis, and polyps).

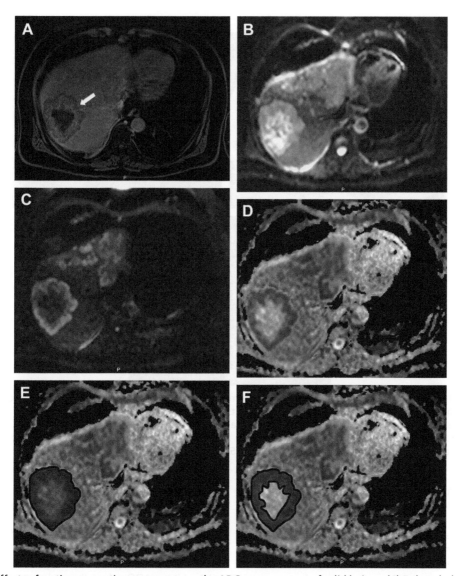

Fig. 8. Effects of cystic or necrotic components on the ADC measurement of solid lesions. (*A*) Delayed-phase post-gadolinium fat-suppressed T1w image depicting a large mass with central necrosis or cystic degeneration in a 57-year-old male patient with metastatic colonic carcinoma (*arrow*). The lesion shows high signal intensity on DWI with b = 0 s/mm^2 (*B*), but there is a marked signal drop on the cystic component at b = 1000 s/mm^2, whereas the peripheral solid component remains with high signal intensity (*C*). The ADC map (*D*) shows a ringlike dark area, corresponding to the enhancing solid component. In these cases, adequate region of interest placement and measurement standardization are essential because, although the ADC of the whole lesion shaded area in (*E*) was 1.82 ($\pm$0.57)$\times$10^{-3} mm/s^2, the ADC value that measured only on the solid component (*shaded area in F*) was as low as 1.20 ($\pm$0.25)$\times$10^{-3} mm/s^2.

Likewise, Cui and Chen[41] studied the value of DWI compared with magnetic resonance cholangio-pancreatography findings in the diagnosis of extrahepatic cholangiocarcinoma, achieving a 94.3% sensitivity, a 100% specificity, and an overall rate of correct diagnosis of 96.4%. Moreover, DWI correctly diagnosed cases of common bile duct calculi and cholangitis. An ADC value of 1.31 ($\pm$0.29)$\times$10^{-3} mm/s^2 was proposed for extrahepatic cholangiocarcinoma, whereas chol-angiolithiasis showed an ADC of 0.48 ($\pm$0.22)$\times$ 10^{-3} mm/s^2. There were no quantitative data that could enable distinction between cholangitis and cholangiocarcinoma.

In our experience, DWI has proved useful as a complimentary method in the diagnosis of intrahe-patic inflammatory biliary conditions, most notably for ascending cholangitis (**Fig. 10**). This usefulness

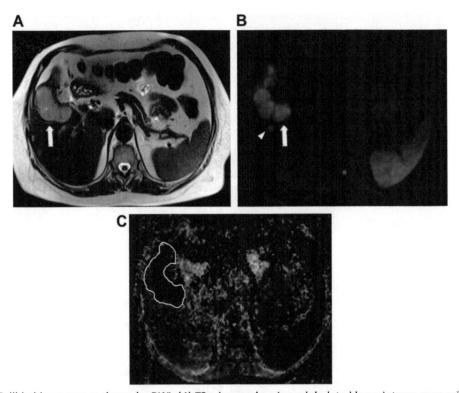

Fig. 9. Gallbladder cancer as shown by DWI. (*A*) T2w image showing a lobulated hyperintense mass originating from the gallbladder fossa and infiltrating the adjacent liver parenchyma (*arrow*), which is also seen as a hyperintense lesion on high b-value diffusion-weighted images (*arrow* in *B*). Note the satellite nodule (*arrowhead* in *B*), which was not seen on the T2w images. On the ADC map (*C*), the lesion shows low signal intensity and the ADC value inside the white outline was 0.84 ($\pm$0.15)$\times10^{-3}$ mm/s^2.

can be appreciated in high b-value images as tracking linear hyperintensities along the portal branches, occasionally with accompanying abscesses. This same principle could be further investigated to predict periductal-infiltrating spread for intrahepatic cholangiocarcinoma.

Adrenal Glands

When imaging the adrenal glands, the most frequent clinical question is whether a focal lesion is an adenoma or a malignant neoplasm. This issue has been studied extensively with both unenhanced and contrast-enhanced CT, as well as chemical-shift MR imaging, gadolinium-enhanced MR imaging, and MR spectroscopy. Currently, tailored CT protocols or chemical-shift MR imaging constitute the mainstay of diagnostic imaging modalities, owing to robust density measurements and high sensitivity for fat detection, respectively.

Nevertheless, several investigators have evaluated the usefulness of DWI in the characterization of adrenal masses, with 2 groups finding no statistically significant difference between the ADC values of adenomas and adrenal malignancies,[42,43]

and 1 group showing only a marginal difference between the ADC values of adenomas and nonadenomatous solid masses.[44] On one of those studies,[43] the median ADC values of lipid-rich adenomas did not differ from those of lipid-poor ones. However, pheochromocytomas tend to show higher ADC values than adenomas or metastatic tumors,[42] a feature that may turn out to be helpful in appropriate clinical settings.

Kidneys

There is a high degree of urgency to pursue application of DWI in the evaluation of focal and diffuse kidney disease, especially in patients showing impaired renal function. Contrast-enhanced examinations in such patients either risk nephrogenic systemic fibrosis caused by gadolinium-chelates, or nephrotoxicity, which is related to iodinated contrast media. A variety of studies have shown DWI to be valuable in diffuse renal disease,[45–47] renal artery stenosis,[48] infection,[49] kidney transplantation,[50] and urinary obstruction.[51,52]

The normal ADC values vary considerably across studies, depending on equipment, imaging acquisition

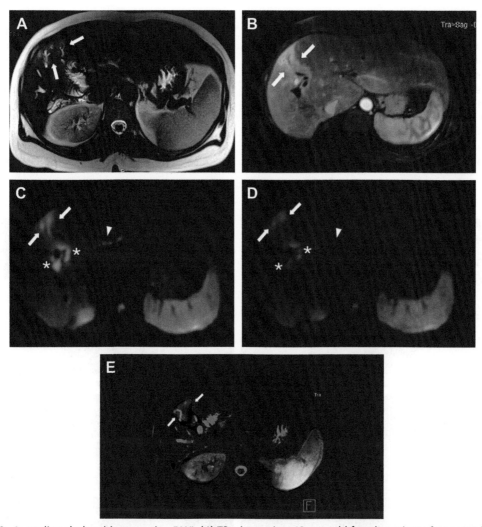

Fig. 10. Ascending cholangitis seen using DWI. (*A*) T2w image in a 48-year-old female patient after enterobiliary anastomosis, showing an ill-defined, mildly hyperintense, peripheral triangular area on segment V (*arrows*), surrounding dilated small intrahepatic biliary branches. On the arterial phase after gadolinium injection (*B*), there is an early enhancement of this same area (*arrows*). Diffusion-weighted images with low and high b-values (*C* and *D*, respectively) also show high signal intensity in this area (*arrows*), but additionally depict subtle linear hyperintensities along more proximal biliary branches (*asterisks* in *C* and *D*). This finding was believed to represent inflammatory content, suggesting ascending cholangitis. The main left biliary duct (*arrowhead* in *C*), which is seen as a hyperintense structure in (*C*), shows marked signal drop in (*D*), indicating simple fluid content. The diagnosis was confirmed and the patient was discharged as asymptomatic after treatment. (*E*) The fused image containing the high b-value sequence (*orange*) overlaid on fat-suppressed T2w images is a way of showing with greater certainty that the anatomic findings from conventional sequences (*arrows*) match the functional findings of DWI.

parameters, hydration status[53] and, most of all, the chosen set of b-values.[45,46,54] Average ADC values range between 1.63×10^{-3} and 5.76×10^{-3} mm/s^2. Moreover, the cortex shows higher overall ADC values than the medulla.[51,55] Because of the tubular microstructure of the medulla, the kidney is also subject to evaluation based on diffusion tensor imaging for corticomedullary differentiation, since the medulla has a higher fractional anisotropy than the cortex,[56]

although these applications are beyond the scope of this article.

Diffusely compromised kidneys may have lower ADC values than normal kidneys. Namimoto and colleagues[45] showed that the ADC values in the cortex and the medulla of patients with either chronic or acute renal failure were lower than those of healthy patients, although this discrepancy was more pronounced in chronic renal failure, especially in the cortex. Likewise, in one study, it was shown that the cortical ADC value had a negative linear correlation with serum creatinine levels and a positive linear correlation with glomerular filtration rate (GFR).[47] In contrast, another study[57] found that patients with a low estimated GFR tended to have lower ADC values, but found no significant correlation between mean ADC value and estimated GFR.

Ischemic conditions, caused by kidney infarction or renal artery stenosis,[48] and infectious conditions, such as acute pyelonephritis,[55] both show areas of restricted diffusion in the involved parenchyma. These areas occur at the same spots where perfusion defects are seen on contrast-enhanced images.

With the development of targeted therapies and new antiangiogenic drugs for renal cell carcinoma (RCC), there is growing interest in the accurate characterization of renal masses through imaging. All of the studies that have addressed this issue[58–63] have shown that solid or malignant

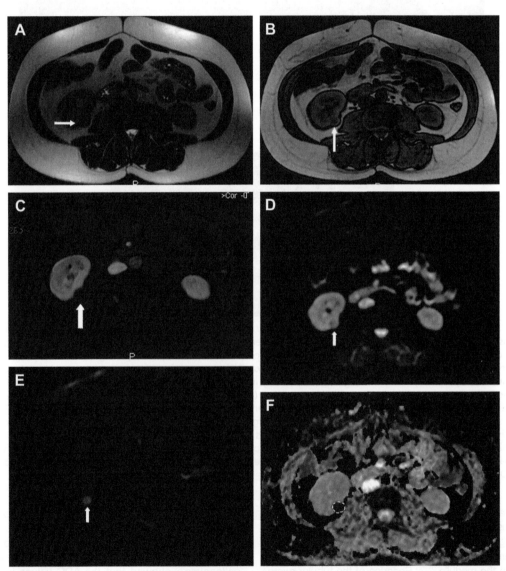

Fig. 11. Papillary RCC. This 49-year-old female patient had an incidental solid renal lesion detected in a previous ultrasound scan. In the T2w images (*A*) there is a discrete hypointense round mass (*arrow*), which shows no chemical-shift artifacts or signal drop at opposed-phase T1W images (*B*) and exhibits mild enhancement on the late phase after gadolinium (*C*). Using DWI, the lesion is hypointense to the renal parenchyma on low b-values (*D*), but maintains high signal intensity with high b-values (*E*). The measured ADC (*F*) was $0.71\ (\pm0.07)\times10^{-3}\ \mathrm{mm^2/s}$.

lesions generally have restricted diffusion and lower ADC values than cystic or benign lesions. Although most studies could confidently differentiate simple cysts from RCC and normal parenchyma (**Figs. 11** and **12**), no single study could distinguish between different solid lesions solely based on ADC values, and there was considerable overlap between measurements. Taouli and colleagues[62] accomplished an area under the curve (AUC) of 0.854, a sensitivity of 90%, and a specificity of 83% in the differentiation between RCC and oncocytoma, using an ADC cutoff of 1.66×10^{-3} mm/s^2. This finding is promising because, although oncocytomas are benign, they constitute an important cause of partial or total nephrectomy because of their resemblance to RCCs when imaged. Conversely, a recent study[63] showed a significant difference between the ADC values of clear cell and non−clear cell RCCs

$(1.59 \pm 0.55 \times 10^{-3}$ mm/s^2 vs $6.72 \pm 1.85 \times 10^{-3}$ mm/s^2). This difference may help in the selection of patients who would benefit most from therapies that target the tyrosine-kinase receptors bound by vascular endothelial growth factor, which are more effective in clear-cell RCCs.

When evaluating complex cystic lesions through DWI for the characterization of malignancy, it is important to measure the ADC values of the solid components, if they are present, because ADC measurements in the whole lesion may be equivocally high, thus generating false-negatives (**Fig. 13**). Measuring ADC values in the fluid components is also useful, but mostly for the characterization of benign lesions, because simple fluid content will show unimpeded diffusion, while proteic or hemorrhagic content will show mildly restricted diffusion, and inflammatory content (ie, abscesses) will show markedly restricted

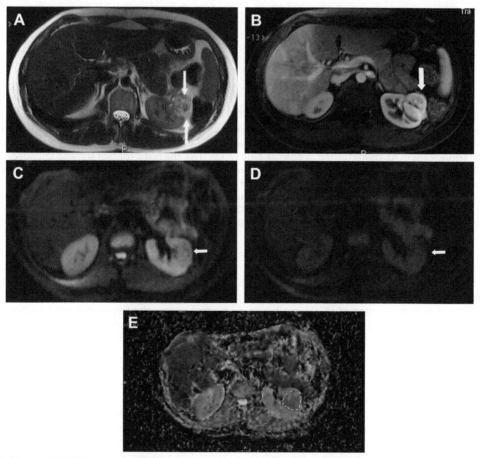

Fig. 12. Clear-cell RCC (compare with **Fig. 11**) in a case of an incidental renal mass in a 39-year-old female patient. The T2w images (*A*) show a heterogeneous partially defined solid mass (*arrows*), with early and intense enhancement on the arterial phase after gadolinium (*B*). The mass was hypointense to the renal parenchyma on low b-values (*C*), but seemed almost isointense with high b-values (*D*). The measured ADC (*E*) was 1.46 ($\pm$0.11) $\times$ 10^{-3} mm/s^2. In both cases, the renal parenchyma had ADC values greater than 1.80×10^{-3} mm/s^2.

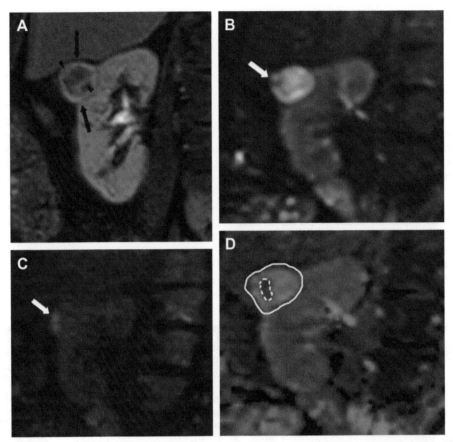

Fig. 13. Cystic RCC: importance of the region of interest placement on ADC measurements. This 79-year-old female patient presented with a complex cystic renal mass (*arrows* in *A*) with thick enhancing septa and a mural nodule (*arrowheads* in *A*), characterized as Bosniak type IV. On DWI, the cystic content showed unimpeded diffusion, with high signal intensity when low b-values were used (*B*) and low signal intensity when high b-values were used (*B*). Conversely, the mural nodule (*arrow* in *B* and *A*) showed restricted diffusion, with evident hyperintensity when high b-values were used (*C*). When measuring the ADC (*D*), if the whole lesion was included in the region of interest, the value was as high as 2.31 ($\pm$0.33)$\times10^{-3}$ mm/s^2. In contrast, if only the mural nodule was considered, the ADC values dropped to 1.70 ($\pm$0.19)$\times10^{-3}$ mm/s^2.

diffusion, although quantitative data with regards to specific ADC values are still lacking. In addition, Zhang and colleagues[61] have shown that ADC values on the necrotic portion of RCCs are lower than those of simple cysts (2.21 $\pm$ 0.63$\times10^{-3}$ mm/s^2 vs 3.26 $\pm$ 0.61$\times10^{-3}$ mm/s^2).

Pancreas

The reported ADC values for the normal pancreas range between 1.02$\times10^{-3}$ and 1.94$\times10^{-3}$ mm/s^2.[64] The head and body of the pancreas seem to exhibit slightly higher ADC values than the tail. Different investigators have evaluated the usefulness of DWI in the diagnosis and characterization of pancreatic carcinoma (PC) and, in most studies, the ADC values of PC had a tendency to be lower than those of a normal pancreas or of benign lesions (**Fig. 14**).[64–68] By using a cutoff value of 1.4$\times10^{-3}$ mm/s^2, ADC measurements have proved useful for the differentiation of PC from normal pancreatic tissue, but not for other benign or inflammatory lesions.[67–69] The measurement of the ADC also enables differentiation between PC and mass-forming pancreatitis.[67,70]

Neuroendocrine (ie, islet cell) tumors also pose a diagnostic challenge for routine imaging techniques, either because of their often small dimensions or their markedly hypervascular pattern of contrast enhancement. In this context, DWI has shown similar diagnostic performance to conventional MR sequences.[71] It is hypothesized to be superior with small (0.5–1.0 cm) or nonhypervascular lesions (**Fig. 15**).[72]

Some researchers have tried to differentiate between cystic pancreatic lesions based on ADC

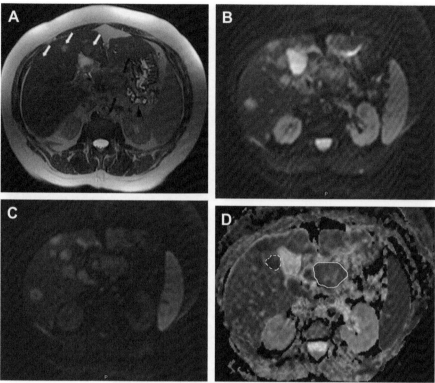

Fig. 14. Pancreatic adenocarcinoma in a 62-year-old female patient. In T2w images (*A*), there is an ill-defined heterogeneous solid mass on the pancreatic body (*black arrows*), determining obstruction, and upstream dilatation of the main pancreatic duct (*arrowhead*). Liver metastases (*white arrows*) are also evident. Using DWI, both the pancreatic mass and the liver metastases show high signal intensity with low b-values (*B*) and retain high signal intensity with high b-values (*C*). The diffusion-weighted images seem to detect more liver metastases than the T2w sequence of practically the same location. The ADC values (*D*) measured for the pancreatic mass and the metastases are 1.19 ($\pm$0.14)$\times$10^{-3} mm/s^2 and 0.84 ($\pm$0.06)$\times$10^{-3} mm/s^2 respectively.

values or DWI characteristics,[73] but the results have been controversial. The ADC values of different lesions show substantial overlap, that is particularly troubling when trying to distinguish between pancreatic pseudocysts and mucinous cystic neoplasms, which is a common clinical question.

Acute pancreatitis and acute exacerbations in chronic pancreatitis (**Fig. 16**) show an overall tendency toward increased diffusion and ADC values relative to normal parenchyma. This increased diffusion is probably caused by the presence of increased vascular permeability and edema. However, chronic pancreatitis shows lower ADC values than the normal pancreas, possibly because of the replacement of normal pancreatic parenchyma with fibrous tissue and/or reduced exocrine function that may reduce diffusible tissue water.[74]

Autoimmune pancreatitis (AIP) is a form of chronic pancreatitis characterized by extensive fibrosis of the exocrine pancreas, along with the infiltration of lymphocytes and plasmocytes. Although pancreatic exocrine function is typically limited, the peripancreatic tissues are typically spared. Taniguchi and colleagues[75] showed that the ADC values of AIP are consistently lower than those of both chronic pancreatitis and normal pancreatic tissue. More interestingly, it was verified that the ADC values in AIP patients increased with steroid treatment (**Fig. 17**), suggesting that DWI may also be useful for monitoring treatment response in AIP cases.

Spleen

The literature on splenic DWI is sparse, with no single recent article specifically addressing splenic diseases. The spleen has the lowest mean ADC value among the abdominal organs, ranging from 0.87 ($\pm$0.11)$\times$10^{-3} mm/s^2 to 1.44 ($\pm$0.26)$\times$10^{-3} mm/s^2.[60,76] Also, it is known that enlarged

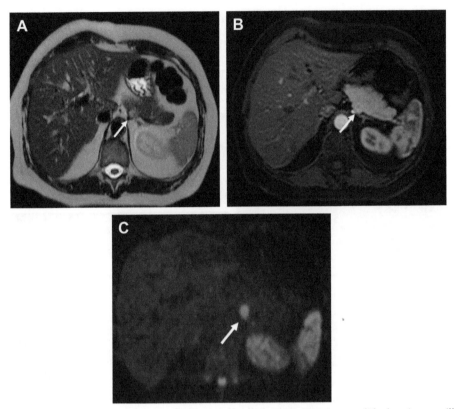

Fig. 15. Pancreatic neuroendocrine tumor diagnosed through DWI. T2w image (*A*) showing an ill-defined, slightly hyperintense focal lesion on the posterior aspect of the pancreatic body (*arrow*), that was not visible in the arterial phase after gadolinium injection (*B*). In high b-value DWI (*C*) the lesion is well seen as a hyperintense focus, in keeping with restricted diffusion. The diagnosis of a hypovascular neuroendocrine tumor was surgically confirmed.

spleens in cirrhotic patients show increased mean ADC values ($5.63 \pm 1.85 \times 10^{-3}$ mm/s^2),[60] probably because of edema and congestion. Regarding the characterization of focal lesions, an isolated case report by Ertan and colleagues[76] suggested that increased ADC values within contrast-enhancing splenic lesions may correlate with a vascular cause.

Another interesting application for DWI would be for the characterization of accessory spleens (**Fig. 18**), especially when they are intrapancreatic

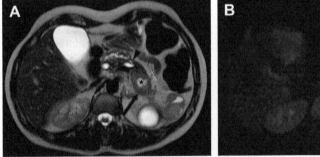
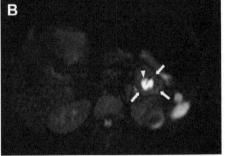

Fig. 16. Chronic pancreatitis with superimposed acute pancreatitis. (*A*) T2w image of a patient with chronic pancreatitis presenting with abdominal pain, showing an irregularly dilated main pancreatic duct (*arrowhead*). There is mild parenchymal hyperintensity on the tail (*arrow*), and an irregular cystic area (*asterisk*) is noted. High b-value DWI (*B*) reveals high signal intensity involving the pancreatic tail (*arrows*), representing a focus of acute pancreatitis. The cystic lesion shows markedly restricted diffusion (*arrowhead*), probably related to focal necrosis or a pseudocyst.

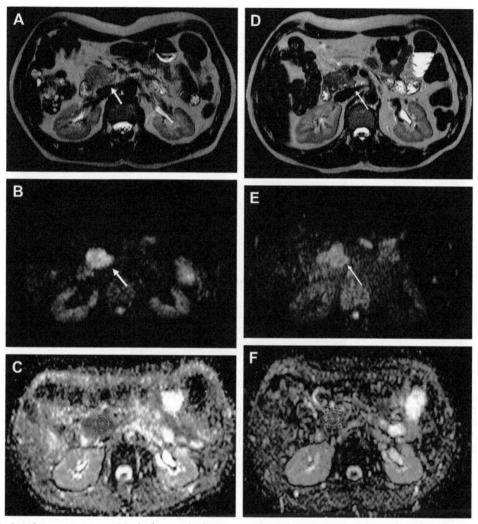

Fig. 17. Autoimmune pancreatitis, before and after treatment. In pretreatment T2w images (*A*), the pancreatic head appears mildly enlarged and slightly hyperintense (*arrow*). High b-value DWI (*B*) shows markedly high signal intensity on the same area (*arrow*), with an ADC value of 0.96×10^{-3} mm/s^2 (*C*). Two weeks after corticotherapy, the T2w image (*D*) shows partial regression on the pancreatic head swelling, with lower signal intensity (*arrow*). The high b-value DWI (*E*) remains with correspondingly high signal intensity (*arrow*), although with an increase on the ADC value (*F*), which has risen to 1.09×10^{-3} mm/s^2.

or in uncommon locations, because the inherent restricted diffusion in an accessory spleen would be similar to that of the original organ.

FUTURE PERSPECTIVES

As MR technology evolves, with stronger gradients, new phased-array coils, more robust fat-suppression techniques, and better movement-correction solutions, so too does DWI, which benefits from a higher SNR and better lesion conspicuity. This evolution may enhance the results of future studies, enabling better measurements and even automated lesion segmentation.

Also, because of the enormous variability observed among acquisition protocols, image postprocessing, and ADC measurements, an increased number of joint initiatives for standardization protocols is anticipated.[77]

Furthermore, there has been a recent surge of interest in the literature in multiple b-value DWI with biexponential fit following the principle of intravoxel incoherent motion, which generates information regarding both tissue perfusion and diffusion.[28,78–81] Although further detail on this

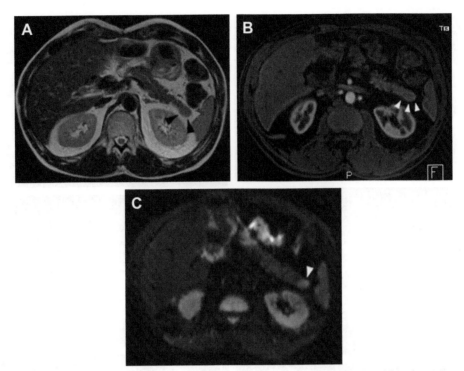

Fig. 18. Intrapancreatic ectopic spleen seen using DWI. (*A*) T2w image of a 55-year-old male patient showing a discrete solid mass at the tip of the pancreatic tail, slightly hyperintense to the pancreas (*arrowheads*). Usually, intrapancreatic ectopic spleens can be identified easily in the arterial phase after gadolinium (*B*), showing an enhancement pattern similar to that of the original spleen, but, in this case, there was no characteristic hyper-enhancement in the mass (*arrowheads*). Using DWI (*C*), the nodule appeared hyperintense with high b-values (*arrowhead*), always resembling the signal intensity of the spleen. The lesion showed no significant growth in successive follow-up examinations and was, therefore, characterized as an ectopic spleen.

topic is beyond the scope of this article, readers are invited to follow the references that describe this promising technique.

SUMMARY

This article describes the current understanding and application of DWI in the upper abdomen. DWI is now a well-established technique for body imaging. There is consistent evidence of its usefulness for the detection of lesions in solid organs and also of its potential to differentiate cystic lesions from solid lesions. Although it is still not possible to confidently characterize different types of solid lesions based solely on ADC values, greater diagnostic confidence is achieved when ADC values are combined with the findings of standard MR sequences.

In conclusion, we support the view that DWI should be a routine component of every abdominal MR examination. Increased dissemination of the technique will contribute to its improvement and, consequently, to better patient care.

REFERENCES

1. Stejskal EO, Tanner JE. Spin diffusion measurements: spin echoes in the presence of a time-dependent field gradient. J Chem Phys 1965;42(1):288.
2. Le Bihan D, Breton E, Lallemand D, et al. MR imaging of intravoxel incoherent motions: application to diffusion and perfusion in neurologic disorders. Radiology 1986;161(2):401–7.
3. Warach S, Chien D, Li W, et al. Fast magnetic resonance diffusion-weighted imaging of acute human stroke. Neurology 1992;42(9):1717–23.
4. Neil JJ. Measurement of water motion (apparent diffusion) in biological systems. Concepts Magn Reson 1997;9(6):385–401.
5. Qayyum A. Diffusion-weighted imaging in the abdomen and pelvis: concepts and applications. Radiographics 2009;29(6):1797–810.
6. Pagani E, Bizzi A, Di Salle F, et al. Basic concepts of advanced MRI techniques. Neurol Sci 2008; 29(Suppl 3):290–5.
7. Kwee TC, Takahara T, Koh DM, et al. Comparison and reproducibility of ADC measurements in

breathhold, respiratory triggered, and free-breathing diffusion-weighted MR imaging of the liver. J Magn Reson Imaging 2008;28(5):1141–8.

8. Takahara T, Imai Y, Yamashita T, et al. Diffusion weighted whole body imaging with background body signal suppression (DWIBS): technical improvement using free breathing, STIR and high resolution 3D display. Radiat Med 2004;22(160): 275–82.

9. Nishie A, Tajima T, Ishigami K, et al. Detection of hepatocellular carcinoma (HCC) using super para-magnetic iron oxide (SPIO)-enhanced MRI: Added value of diffusion-weighted imaging (DWI). J Magn Reson Imaging 2010;31(2):373–82.

10. Chiu FY, Jao JC, Chen CY, et al. Effect of intravenous gadolinium-DTPA on diffusion-weighted magnetic resonance images for evaluation of focal hepatic lesions. J Comput Assist Tomogr 2005;29(2): 176–80.

11. Yamada K, Kubota H, Kizu O, et al. Effect of intra-venous gadolinium-DTPA on diffusion-weighted images: evaluation of normal brain and infarcts. Stroke 2002;33(7):1799–802.

12. Firat A, Şanli B, Karakaş H, et al. The effect of intra-venous gadolinium-DTPA on diffusion-weighted imaging. Neuroradiology 2006;48(7):465–70.

13. Taouli B, Koh DM. Diffusion-weighted MR imaging of the liver. Radiology 2010;254(1):47–66.

14. Okada Y, Ohtomo K, Kiryu S, et al. Breath-hold T2-weighted MRI of hepatic tumors: value of echo planar imaging with diffusion-sensitizing gradient. J Comput Assist Tomogr 1998;22(3):364–71.

15. Moteki T, Sekine T. Echo planar MR imaging of the liver: comparison of images with and without motion probing gradients. J Magn Reson Imaging 2004; 19(1):82–90.

16. Nasu K, Kuroki Y, Nawano S, et al. Hepatic metas-tases: diffusion-weighted sensitivity-encoding versus SPIO-enhanced MR imaging. Radiology 2006;239(1):122–30.

17. Coenegrachts K, Delanote J, Ter Beek L, et al. Improved focal liver lesion detection: comparison of single-shot diffusion-weighted echo planar and single-shot T2 weighted turbo spin echo techniques. Br J Radiol 2007;80(955):524–31.

18. Low RN, Gurney J. Diffusion-weighted MRI (DWI) in the oncology patient: value of breathhold DWI compared to unenhanced and gadolinium-enhanced MRI. J Magn Reson Imaging 2007;25(4): 848–58.

19. Bruegel M, Gaa J, Waldt S, et al. Diagnosis of hepatic metastasis: comparison of respiration-triggered diffusion-weighted echo-planar MRI and five t2-weighted turbo spin-echo sequences. AJR Am J Roentgenol 2008;191(5):1421–9.

20. Parikh T, Drew SJ, Lee VS, et al. Focal liver lesion detection and characterization with diffusion-weighted MR imaging: comparison with standard breath-hold T2-weighted imaging. Radiology 2008; 246(3):812–22.

21. Zech CJ, Herrmann KA, Dietrich O, et al. Black-blood diffusion-weighted EPI acquisition of the liver with parallel imaging: comparison with a standard T2-weighted sequence for detection of focal liver lesions. Invest Radiol 2008;43(4):261–6.

22. Hussain SM, De Becker J, Hop WC, et al. Can a single-shot black-blood T2-weighted spin-echo echo-planar imaging sequence with sensitivity encoding replace the respiratory-triggered turbo spin-echo sequence for the liver? An optimization and feasibility study. J Magn Reson Imaging 2005; 21(3):219–29.

23. van den Bos IC, Hussain SM, Krestin GP, et al. Liver imaging at 3.0 T: diffusion-induced black-blood echo-planar imaging with large anatomic volumetric coverage as an alternative for specific absorption rate–intensive echo-train spin-echo sequences: feasibility study. Radiology 2008;248(1):264–71.

24. Koh DM, Brown G, Riddell AM, et al. Detection of colorectal hepatic metastases using MnDPDP MR imaging and diffusion-weighted imaging (DWI) alone and in combination. Eur Radiol 2008;18(5): 903–10.

25. Hardie AD, Naik M, Hecht EM, et al. Diagnosis of liver metastases: value of diffusion-weighted MRI compared with gadolinium-enhanced MRI. Eur Radiol 2010;20(6):1431–41.

26. Namimoto T, Yamashita Y, Sumi S, et al. Focal liver masses: characterization with diffusion-weighted echo-planar MR imaging. Radiology 1997;204(3): 739–44.

27. Kim T, Murakami T, Takahashi S, et al. Diffusion-weighted single-shot echoplanar MR imaging for liver disease. AJR Am J Roentgenol 1999;173(2): 393–8.

28. Yamada I, Aung W, Himeno Y, et al. Diffusion coef-ficients in abdominal organs and hepatic lesions: evaluation with intravoxel incoherent motion echo-planar MR imaging. Radiology 1999;210(3): 617–23.

29. Taouli B, Vilgrain V, Dumont E, et al. Evaluation of liver diffusion isotropy and characterization of focal hepatic lesions with two single-shot echo-planar MR imaging sequences: prospective study in 66 patients. Radiology 2003;226(1):71–8.

30. Bruegel M, Holzapfel K, Gaa J, et al. Characteriza-tion of focal liver lesions by ADC measurements using a respiratory triggered diffusion-weighted single-shot echo-planar MR imaging technique. Eur Radiol 2008;18(3):477–85.

31. Gourtsoyianni S, Papanikolaou N, Yarmenitis S, et al. Respiratory gated diffusion-weighted imaging of the liver: value of apparent diffusion coefficient measurements in the differentiation between most

commonly encountered benign and malignant focal liver lesions. Eur Radiol 2008;18(3):486–92.

32. Goshima S, Kanematsu M, Kondo H, et al. Diffusion-weighted imaging of the liver: optimizing b value for the detection and characterization of benign and malignant hepatic lesions. J Magn Reson Imaging 2008;28(3):691–7.

33. Holzapfel K, Bruegel M, Eiber M, et al. Characterization of small (≤10 mm) focal liver lesions: value of respiratory-triggered echo-planar diffusion-weighted MR imaging. Eur J Radiol 2010;76(1): 89–95.

34. Kandpal H, Sharma R, Madhusudhan KS, et al. Respiratory-triggered versus breath-hold diffusion-weighted MRI of liver lesions: comparison of image quality and apparent diffusion coefficient values. AJR Am J Roentgenol 2009;192(4):915–22.

35. Amano Y, Kumazaki T, Ishihara M. Single-shot diffusion-weighted echo-planar imaging of normal and cirrhotic livers using a phased-array multicoil. Acta Radiol 1998;39(4):440–2.

36. Aube C, Racineux PX, Lebigot J, et al. Diagnosis and quantification of hepatic fibrosis with diffusion weighted MR imaging: preliminary results. J Radiol 2004;85(3):301–6.

37. Koinuma M, Ohashi I, Hanafusa K, et al. Apparent diffusion coefficient measurements with diffusion-weighted magnetic resonance imaging for evaluation of hepatic fibrosis. J Magn Reson Imaging 2005;22(1):80–5.

38. Taouli B, Tolia AJ, Losada M, et al. Diffusion-weighted MRI for quantification of liver fibrosis: preliminary experience. AJR Am J Roentgenol 2007;189(4):799–806.

39. Boulanger Y, Amara M, Lepanto L, et al. Diffusion-weighted MR imaging of the liver of hepatitis C patients. NMR Biomed 2003;16(3):132–6.

40. Sugita R, Yamazaki T, Furuta A, et al. High b-value diffusion-weighted MRI for detecting gallbladder carcinoma: preliminary study and results. Eur Radiol 2009;19(7):1794–8.

41. Cui XY, Chen HW. Role of diffusion-weighted magnetic resonance imaging in the diagnosis of extrahepatic cholangiocarcinoma. World J Gastroenterol 2010;16(25):3196–201.

42. Tsushima Y, Takahashi-Taketomi A, Endo K. Diagnostic utility of diffusion-weighted MR imaging and apparent diffusion coefficient value for the diagnosis of adrenal tumors. J Magn Reson Imaging 2009; 29(1):112–7.

43. Miller FH, Wang Y, McCarthy RJ, et al. Utility of diffusion-weighted MRI in characterization of adrenal lesions. AJR Am J Roentgenol 2010; 194(2):W179–85.

44. Kilickesmez O, Inci E, Atilla S, et al. Diffusion-weighted imaging of the renal and adrenal lesions. J Comput Assist Tomogr 2009;33(6):828–33.

45. Namimoto T, Yamashita Y, Mitsuzaki K, et al. Measurement of the apparent diffusion coefficient in diffuse renal disease by diffusion-weighted echo-planar MR imaging. J Magn Reson Imaging 1999;9(6):832–7.

46. Fukuda Y, Ohashi I, Hanafusa K, et al. Anisotropic diffusion in kidney: apparent diffusion coefficient measurements for clinical use. J Magn Reson Imaging 2000;11(2):156–60.

47. Xu Y, Wang X, Jiang X. Relationship between the renal apparent diffusion coefficient and glomerular filtration rate: preliminary experience. J Magn Reson Imaging 2007;26(3):678–81.

48. Yildirim E, Kirbas I, Teksam M, et al. Diffusion-weighted MR imaging of kidneys in renal artery stenosis. Eur J Radiol 2008;65(1):148–53.

49. Chan JH, Tsui EY, Luk SH, et al. MR diffusion-weighted imaging of kidney: differentiation between hydronephrosis and pyonephrosis. Clin Imaging 2001;25(2):110–3.

50. Thoeny HC, Zumstein D, Simon-Zoula S, et al. Functional evaluation of transplanted kidneys with diffusion-weighted and bold MR imaging: initial experience1. Radiology 2006;241(3):812–21.

51. Thoeny HC, De Keyzer F, Oyen RH, et al. Diffusion-weighted MR imaging of kidneys in healthy volunteers and patients with parenchymal diseases: initial experience. Radiology 2005;235(3):911–7.

52. Thoeny HC, Binser T, Roth B, et al. Noninvasive assessment of acute ureteral obstruction with diffusion-weighted MR imaging: a prospective study1. Radiology 2009;252(3):721–8.

53. Müller MF, Prasad PV, Bimmler D, et al. Functional imaging of the kidney by means of measurement of the apparent diffusion coefficient. Radiology 1994;193(3):711–5.

54. Ichikawa T, Haradome H, Hachiya J, et al. Diffusion-weighted MR imaging with single-shot echo-planar imaging in the upper abdomen: preliminary clinical experience in 61 patients. Abdom Imaging 1999; 24(5):456–61.

55. Kim S, Naik M, Sigmund E, et al. Diffusion-weighted MR imaging of the kidneys and the urinary tract. Magn Reson Imaging Clin N Am 2008;16(4):585–96.

56. Ries M, Jones RA, Basseau F, et al. Diffusion tensor MRI of the human kidney. J Magn Reson Imaging 2001;14(1):42–9.

57. Toya R, Naganawa S, Kawai H, et al. Correlation between estimated glomerular filtration rate (eGFR) and apparent diffusion coefficient (ADC) values of the kidneys. Magn Reson Med Sci 2010;9(2):59–64.

58. Cova M, Squillaci E, Stacul F, et al. Diffusion-weighted MRI in the evaluation of renal lesions: preliminary results. Br J Radiol 2004;77(922):851–7.

59. Squillaci E, Manenti G, Di Stefano F, et al. Diffusion-weighted MR imaging in the evaluation of renal tumours. J Exp Clin Cancer 2004;23(1):39–46.

60. Yoshikawa T, Kawamitsu H, Mitchell DG, et al. ADC measurement of abdominal organs and lesions using parallel imaging technique. AJR Am J Roentgenol 2006;187(6):1521–30.

61. Zhang J, Mazaheri Tehrani Y, Wang L, et al. Renal masses: characterization with diffusion-weighted MR imaging—a preliminary experience. Radiology 2008;247(2):458–64.

62. Taouli B, Thakur RK, Mannelli L, et al. Renal lesions: characterization with diffusion-weighted imaging versus contrast-enhanced MR imaging1. Radiology 2009;251(2):398–407.

63. Paudyal B, Paudyal P, Tsushima Y, et al. The role of the ADC value in the characterisation of renal carcinoma by diffusion-weighted MRI. Br J Radiol 2010; 83(988):336–43.

64. Balci NC, Perman WH, Saglam S, et al. Diffusion-weighted magnetic resonance imaging of the pancreas. Top Magn Reson Imaging 2009;20(1):43.

65. Lee SS, Byun JH, Park BJ, et al. Quantitative analysis of diffusion-weighted magnetic resonance imaging of the pancreas: usefulness in characterizing solid pancreatic masses. J Magn Reson Imaging 2008;28(4):928–36.

66. Muraoka N, Uematsu H, Kimura H, et al. Apparent diffusion coefficient in pancreatic cancer: characterization and histopathological correlations. J Magn Reson Imaging 2008;27(6):1302–8.

67. Fattahi R, Balci NC, Perman WH, et al. Pancreatic diffusion-weighted imaging (DWI): comparison between mass-forming focal pancreatitis (FP), pancreatic cancer (PC), and normal pancreas. J Magn Reson Imaging 2009;29(2):350–6.

68. Kartalis N, Lindholm T, Aspelin P, et al. Diffusion-weighted magnetic resonance imaging of pancreas tumours. Eur Radiol 2009;19(8):1981–90.

69. Matsuki M, Inada Y, Nakai G, et al. Diffusion-weighed MR imaging of pancreatic carcinoma. Abdom Imaging 2007;32(4):481–3.

70. Takeuchi M, Matsuzaki K, Kubo H, et al. High-b-value diffusion-weighted magnetic resonance imaging of pancreatic cancer and mass-forming chronic pancreatitis: preliminary results. Acta Radiol 2008;49(4):383–6.

71. Bakir B, Salmaslioglu A, Poyanll A, et al. Diffusion weighted MR imaging of pancreatic islet cell tumors. Eur J Radiol 2009;74(1):214–20.

72. Anaye A, Mathieu A, Closset J, et al. Successful preoperative localization of a small pancreatic insulinoma by diffusion-weighted MRI. JOP 2009;10(5): 528–31.

73. Inan N, Arslan A, Akansel G, et al. Diffusion-weighted imaging in the differential diagnosis of cystic lesions of the pancreas. AJR Am J Roentgenol 2008;191(4): 1115–21.

74. Akisik MF, Sandrasegaran K, Jennings SG, et al. Diagnosis of chronic pancreatitis by using apparent diffusion coefficient measurements at 3.0-T MR following secretin stimulation. Radiology 2009; 252(2):418–25.

75. Taniguchi T, Kobayashi H, Nishikawa K, et al. Diffusion-weighted magnetic resonance imaging in autoimmune pancreatitis. Jpn J Radiol 2009;27(3):138–42.

76. Ertan G, Tekes A, Mitchell S, et al. Pediatric littoral cell angioma of the spleen: multimodality imaging including diffusion-weighted imaging. Pediatr Radiol 2009;39(10):1105–9.

77. Padhani AR, Liu G, Mu-Koh D, et al. Diffusion-weighted magnetic resonance imaging as a cancer biomarker: consensus and recommendations. Neoplasia 2009;11(2):102–25.

78. Le Bihan D, Breton E, Lallemand D, et al. Separation of diffusion and perfusion in intravoxel incoherent motion MR imaging. Radiology 1988;168(2):497–505.

79. Luciani A, Vignaud A, Cavet M, et al. Liver cirrhosis: intravoxel incoherent motion MR imaging - a pilot study. Radiology 2008;249(3):891–9.

80. Lemke A, Laun FB, Klau M, et al. Differentiation of pancreas carcinoma from healthy pancreatic tissue using multiple b-values: comparison of apparent diffusion coefficient and intravoxel incoherent motion derived parameters. Invest Radiol 2009;44(12): 769–75.

81. Zhang JL, Sigmund EE, Chandarana H, et al. Variability of renal apparent diffusion coefficients: limitations of the monoexponential model for diffusion quantification. Radiology 2010;254(3): 783–92.

Pelvic Applications of Diffusion Magnetic Resonance Images

Antonio C. Coutinho Jr, MD[a,b,*],
Arun Krishnaraj, MD, MPH[c], Cintia E. Pires, MD[a],
Leonardo K. Bittencourt, MD[a,d,e],
Alexander R. Guimarães, MD, PhD[c,f]

KEYWORDS

- MR imaging • Pelvic • Diffusion • Neoplasms • Uterus
- Ovaries • Prostate • Rectum

Diffusion-weighted imaging (DWI) is a well-established, powerful imaging technique used in neuroimaging but its value in abdominal and pelvic imaging has only recently been appreciated as a result of improvements in magnetic resonance (MR) imaging technology (eg, stronger diffusion gradients and parallel-imaging sequences). The usefulness of DWI in the abdomen and pelvis is linked to its capacity to more accurately characterize tissues, potentially differentiating malignant from benign entities.

DWI is based on the principle of diffusion of water molecules in an environment. The restriction to flow of water molecules is governed by tissue cellularity (local environment) and the integrity of the cell membrane.[1] Tumors typically display restricted diffusion because of their hypercellularity[2]; however, other types of disease conditions have been associated with restricted diffusion, including cytotoxic edema, abscess, and fibrosis. Tissues with low cellularity or those composed of cells with disrupted membranes allow greater movement of water molecules,[1] which is visualized as decreased signal intensity on DW images and increased signal intensity on corresponding apparent diffusion coefficient (ADC) maps. This unique ability to characterize malignant tumors may obviate contrast material in those patients with renal insufficiency or contrast material allergy.

EXAMINATION OF THE PELVIC REGION USING DWI

DWI is sensitive to the random displacement of water molecules within tissues and is performed by using echo planar imaging (EPI) combined with balanced motion-probing gradients (MPG), which are symmetric and of equal intensity about the 180° refocusing pulse. These MPG exploit the phase offset induced by the random motion of water molecules to discriminate tissues that restrict that motion of water. The intensity of MPG pulses is represented by the b-value (s/mm^2), a measure of the strength of the diffusion-sensitizing gradient. By using multiple b-value MPG, one can map and calculate the ADC.

None of the authors has a financial relationship to disclose.

[a] Clínica de Diagnóstico por Imagem (CDPI), Av das Américas 4666, Sala 325, Rio de Janeiro 22640902, Brazil
[b] Centro de Diagnostico por Imagem da Casa de Saude N. Sra. de Fatima (Fatima Digittal), Rio de Janeiro, Brazil
[c] Division of Abdominal Imaging and Interventional Radiology, Department of Radiology, Massachusetts General Hospital, Harvard Medical School, White 270, Boston, MA 02114, USA
[d] Department of Radiology, Rio de Janeiro Federal University (UFRJ), Rio de Janeiro, Brazil
[e] Carlos Bittencourt Diagnostico por Imagem, Rio de Janeiro, Brazil
[f] Martinos Center for Biomedical Imaging, Department of Radiology, Massachusetts General Hospital, Harvard Medical School, Massachusetts Institute of Technology, Charlestown, MA 02139, USA
* Corresponding author. Clínica de Diagnóstico por Imagem (CDPI), Av das Américas 4666, Sala 325, Rio de Janeiro 22640902, Brazil.
E-mail address: antoniocoutinhojr@yahoo.com.br

Magn Reson Imaging Clin N Am 19 (2011) 133–157
doi:10.1016/j.mric.2010.10.003

Because the DWI sequence is a T2-weighted sequence, the DWI signal is influenced by the T2 of the tissue being imaged. Therefore, the interpretation of DWI must occur concomitant with the ADC image. High-intensity tissues on T2-WI may show increased signal intensity on DWI (the so-called T2 shine-through effect) if also high on ADC. For example, DWI with an intermediate b-value (eg, 500 s/mm^2) shows increased intensity not only in tumors but also in cysts. Thus, DWI with a higher b-value (eg, 800 or 1000 s/mm^2) may be required for the pelvis.

When imaging the abdomen and pelvis optimization of other sequence parameters is crucial because EPI is highly susceptible to distortions in the spatial field caused by air-containing bowel loops. To minimize susceptibility artifacts, shorter echo times (TE) and smaller numbers of echo train lengths (ETLs) are preferable; this can be achieved by the use of parallel-imaging techniques. Unlike sequential acquisitions, parallel imaging is based on the use of coils with multiple small detectors that operate simultaneously to acquire MR data. Each of these detectors contains spatial information that can be used as a substitute for time-consuming phase-encoding steps, thereby allowing both the acquisition time and the ETL to be reduced. In particular, DWI with parallel imaging reduces the number of phase-encoding steps. The effective TE can be shortened and susceptible components of the ETL can be eliminated. This strategy keeps the susceptibility effect to a minimum. Although a wider receiver bandwidth reduces the signal-to-noise ratio (SNR), its use is recommended because it shortens the duration of the MR signal acquisition and reduces susceptibility artifacts.

In our standard protocols for pelvic DWI we use a 3-T magnet unit Magnetom Trio (Siemens, Erlangen, Germany) with a 6-channel body MATRIX and a gradient-recalled echo (GRE) EPI sequence (repetition time [TR] 5000 ms; TE 75 ms; field of view 400 mm; 4 averages; slice thickness 4 mm; interslice gap 1 mm; acquisition matrix 162 × 162; EPI factor 76; and bandwidth 2058 Hz/pixel) with fat suppression (spectral attenuated inversion recovery) and parallel-imaging technique (generalized autocalibrating partially parallel acquisition [GRAPPA] factor of 2) using b-values of 0, 500, and 1000 s/mm^2. Imaging time of DWI is 155 seconds for 30 slices. On a 1.5-T MR imaging scanner (Magnetom Avanto, Siemens, Erlangen, Germany) with a 6-channel torso coil we use a GRE EPI sequence (TR 2600 ms; TE 82 ms; field of view 350 mm; 2 excitations; slice thickness 7 mm; interslice gap 1 mm; acquisition matrix 128 × 128; EPI factor 128; and bandwidth 1302 Hz/pixel) using

b-values of 0 and 1000 s/mm^2 with fat suppression and parallel-imaging technique (GRAPPA factor of 2) with an imaging time of DWI of 60 seconds for 20 slices. On a 1.5-T MR imaging scanner (Philips Intera, Philips Medical Systems, Best, Netherlands) with a 6-channel body coil we use a spin-echo (SE) EPI sequence (TR 2000 ms; TE 71.73 ms; flip angle 90°; field of view 280 mm; 2 excitations; slice thickness 5 mm; interslice gap 0.5 mm; acquisition matrix 128 × 128; ETL 111) with bandwidth of 1.7546 Hz/pixel with fat suppression and parallel-imaging technique (SENSE factor of 2) and an imaging time of DWI of 168 seconds for 23 slices. For a GE Excite system (General Electric Medical Systems, Milwaukee, WI, USA) at 1.5 T we use an SE EPI sequence (TR 5000 ms; TE 93 ms; flip angle 90°; field of view 280 mm; 2 excitations; slice thickness 5 mm; interslice gap 0.5 mm; acquisition matrix 128 × 128;) with bandwidth of 1.953 Hz/pixel with fat suppression and an imaging time of DWI of 4 minutes 30 seconds for 30 slices, 2 b-values (0 and 1000), and 6 directions. DWI is performed in the axial and also in the sagittal plane. The MPG pulses are placed in the x, y, and z axes. Respiratory trigger is not used. Data are then collected using echo planar readout. Fat suppression is added to the DWI to avoid chemical shift artifacts.

Isotropic DW (trace) images are reconstructed for b = 0, 600, 800, and 1000 s/mm^2. From these b-values, ADC maps are computed. ADC measurement is performed on the axial and/or sagittal planes depending on the one that contained the largest region of interest that can be drawn.

INFLAMMATORY LESIONS
Tubo-ovarian Abscess

The MR imaging appearance of a tubo-ovarian abscess (TOA) is classically a hypointense pelvic mass on T1-weighted images with heterogeneous high-signal intensity on T2-weighted images. The innermost portion of the abscess may appear as a thin rim of high-signal intensity on T1-weighted images, reflecting granulation tissue with microscopic hemorrhage.[3]

The signal intensity of the content of the abscess can vary depending on its viscosity or protein concentration. DWI is still an area of ongoing research. However, in our experience, which is in agreement with other investigators,[4] TOA commonly shows restricted diffusion, with increased signal intensity on DW images and decreased signal intensity on ADC maps (Fig. 1). This finding is likely a result of the usual highly viscous content of a TOA. Therefore, DWI could be an alternative to contrast-enhanced

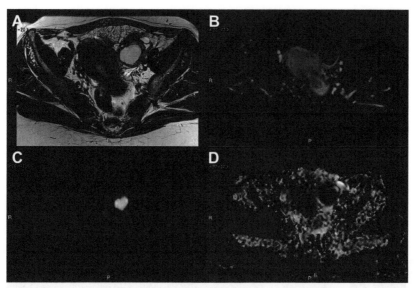

Fig. 1. 25-year-old woman with pelvic pain and vaginal discharge. T2-weighted axial image (*A*) and T1 fat-suppressed (T1FS) postcontrast image (*B*) showing a complex left adnexal cystic lesion. DWI (b = 800) shows hyperintensity within the lesion (*C*) and ADC maps show hypointensity (*D*). Findings are consistent with restricted diffusion. Surgery confirmed a diagnosis of a TOA.

imaging[5] by showing inflammation if there is restricted diffusion (**Fig. 2**).

Similar findings occur in perianal/perirectal and uterine abscess (**Fig. 3**), which also commonly shows increased signal intensity on DW images and markedly decreased signal intensity on ADC maps, and is a useful alternative method to contrast-enhanced imaging.

TUMORS

One of the areas of growing interest with DWI and its applications in the pelvis is its high sensitivity and specificity in distinguishing benign from malignant tumors, because malignancies usually have a larger cell diameter and cellular density than do normal tissue and benign tumors.[6–9] These subjective findings along with the ADC correlate, which is considered to be influenced by nuclear-to-cytoplasm ratio and cellular density,[6–10] assists in this high accuracy. The ADC value has also been reported to correlate with histologic grade of the tumors in cases of malignant neoplasms, in which high-grade tumors tended to show low ADC values.[10]

DWI is not only helpful in differentiating benign from malignant tumors but it is also useful in determining depth of tumor invasion and assessment of metastatic lesions, tumor recurrence, and treatment response.[11]

Endometrial Cancer

On T2-weighted imaging, endometrial cancer is usually shown as thickened endometrium, with low-signal intensity relative to normal endometrium. After intravenous administration of gadolinium, on T1-weighted images, endometrial cancer usually shows lower-signal intensity than normal myometrium, with early enhancement on dynamic imaging when compared with spared endometrium.[6,12,13]

However, conventional MR imaging does not always clearly show the focus of the tumor, because the signal intensity of the endometrial cancer can range from high intensity to low intensity, making it sometimes indistinguishable from normal endometrium or adjacent myometrium.[6] This characteristic is especially notable in cases in which the endometrium is effaced by a leiomyoma or in cases of myometrial involvement by adenomyosis.[12,14]

In this context, many investigators have suggested that fused DW images/T2-weighted images could lead to a more accurate diagnosis and more precise evaluation of the extent of the tumor when compared with isolated conventional MR imaging examination (see **Fig. 2**).[6,12]

Both endometrial cancer (**Fig. 4**) and the normal endometrium (**Fig. 5**) often show increased signal intensity on DWI. The explanation for the high intensity of the normal endometrial tissue on DW images is not yet clear. It has been suggested that increased signal of normal endometrium on DW images could be attributed to abundant water molecules confined within intracellular space of endometrial stromal cells. Therefore, evaluating only the degree of signal intensity on DW images could not precisely differentiate between endometrial

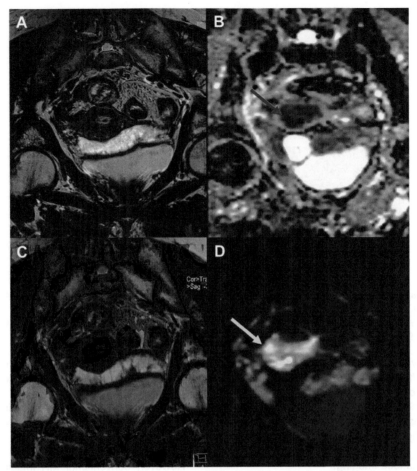

Fig. 2. 53-year-old woman with unusual vaginal bleeding and contrast material allergy, contraindicating dynamic gadolinium-enhanced imaging. T2-weighted image (*A*) and fused DW image/T2-weighted image (*C*) in the coronal plane showing abnormal signal within the endometrial cavity and adjacent myometrium. These lesions show low-signal intensity on ADC map (*B*) (*red arrow*) and hyperintensity on DWI (b = 800) (*D*) (*yellow arrow*), suggesting malignant neoplasm and myometrial invasion. Pathologic examination confirmed endometrial carcinoma with secondary myometrial involvement.

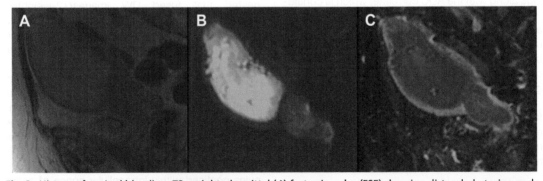

Fig. 3. History of vaginal bleeding. T2-weighted sagittal (*A*) fast spin-echo (FSE) showing distended uterine endometrial cavity with T2 hyperintensity. DWI (b = 400) (*B*) showing hyperintensity in the endometrial cavity and ADC map (*C*) showing hypointensity. Findings are consistent with restricted diffusion. Pathologic diagnosis confirmed pyometra.

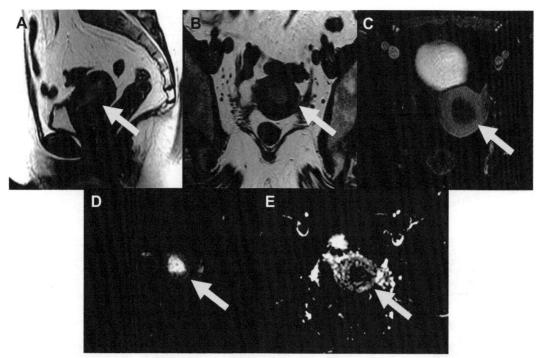

Fig. 4. 63-year-old woman with abnormal vaginal bleeding. T2-weighted sagittal (*A*) and axial (*B*) images show abnormal thickening and loss of T2 hyperintensity within the endometrial cavity (*arrow*). This mass shows heterogeneous early enhancement with rapid washout on T1-weighed high-resolution postcontrast images (*C*), and high signal on DWI (*D*) and low signal on ADC (*E*), with a mean ADC value of 0.93×10^{-3} mm^2/s, consistent with restricted diffusion. Pathologic examination confirmed a diagnosis of endometrial carcinoma.

cancer and the normal endometrium, because the visual assessment of signal intensity is a subjective criterion and can be influenced by the adjustment of the window parameters.[6] However, many studies show that the ADC values of endometrial cancers are significantly lower than those of normal endometrium, which suggests that ADC measurement has a potential ability to differentiate between normal and cancerous tissue in the endometrium. Inada and colleagues,[12] reviewing DW images of endometrial cancer from 23 patients, found a mean ADC value for endometrial cancer of $(0.97 \pm 0.19) \times 10^{-3}$ mm^2/s, which was significantly lower than those of the normal endometrium $(1.52 \pm 0.20) \times 10^{-3}$ mm^2/s and other benign lesions of the myometrium, such as leiomyoma and adenomyosis.

The prognosis of endometrial cancer depends on 3 factors: histologic subtype and grade, tumor stage at diagnosis, including the depth of myometrial invasion, and the presence of lymph node metastases.[6,15,16]

Tamai and colleagues[6] found that the ADC values of endometrial cancer of higher grade tumors showed a tendency to decrease compared with those of lower grade, although there was a considerable overlap among tumors with different grades, thereby making it difficult to estimate the histologic grade based on ADC values.

With regards to determining the depth of myometrial invasion, there is relative concurrence that the boundary between cancer tissue and hypointense normal myometrium could be easily depicted by DW technique, as a result of the remarkably high-signal intensity presented by endometrial cancer relative to the surrounding structures on DW images (see **Fig. 2**).[12,15] Rechichi and colleagues,[15] using a protocol which included spin-echo multishot T2- weighted, dynamic T1-weighted and DW images acquired with b-values of 0 and 500 s/mm^2 to determine the diagnostic accuracy of DW MR imaging in the preoperative assessment of myometrial invasion by endometrial cancer, concluded that T2-weighted imaging performed better than either DW or dynamic MR imaging. However, DWI appeared to be more reliable and to have higher diagnostic performance than dynamic gadolinium-enhanced imaging. Therefore, these investigators concluded that DWI could replace dynamic imaging as an adjunct to routine T2-weighted imaging for preoperative evaluation of endometrial cancer,

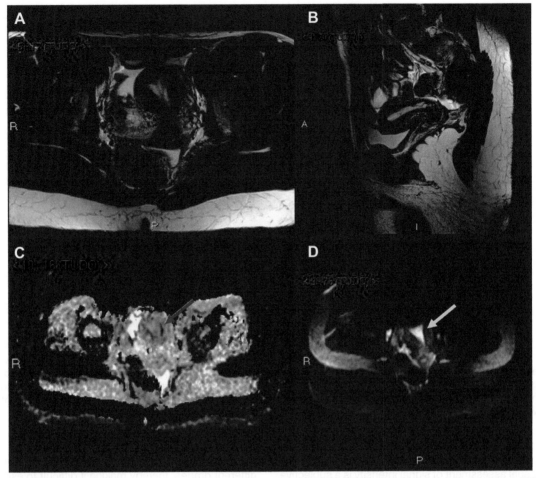

Fig. 5. Normal endometrium on a 29-year-old asymptomatic woman (*A, B*). Note the low-signal intensity on ADC map (*C*) (*red arrow*) and the high-signal intensity on DWI (b = 600) (*D*) (*yellow arrow*). The mean ADC value was 1.61 × 10^{-3} mm^2/s.

especially in those patients for whom contrast agents are contraindicated.

Cervical Cancer

Cervical carcinoma is best defined using T2-weighted imaging, in which it usually presents with intermediate-signal intensity and is seen disrupting the low-signal intensity fibrous stroma.[17] However, small tumors may be more readily identified by their early enhancement after dynamic intravenous administration of gadolinium,[18] and recent data suggest that functional imaging could also play an important role within this context.

The size of the tumor (ie, whether greater or less than 4 cm in diameter) has a great effect on the choice of therapy, and there is good correlation between conventional MR imaging findings and macroscopic measurements.[17] However, the size

of the lesion may be overestimated at T2-weighted imaging because of inflammation or edema.[17,19]

The application of DWI for cervical cancer has been the topic of multiple recent papers, and many investigators suggest it adds usefulness in the delineation of tumor boundaries for therapeutic planning and in determining preoperative staging (**Fig. 6**).

McVeigh and colleagues[20] performed DW MR images (b-value of 600 s/mm^2) in 47 patients with cervical carcinoma and concluded that diffusion in tumor tissues was found to be significantly more restricted than in normal cervical tissue, possibly reflecting greater cell density. The median ADC of cervical cancers was significantly lower than the median ADC of normal cervix stroma, with little overlap between the 2 cases. The average ADC for cancerous tissue in this study was of 1.09 ± 0.20 × 10^{-3} mm^2/s.

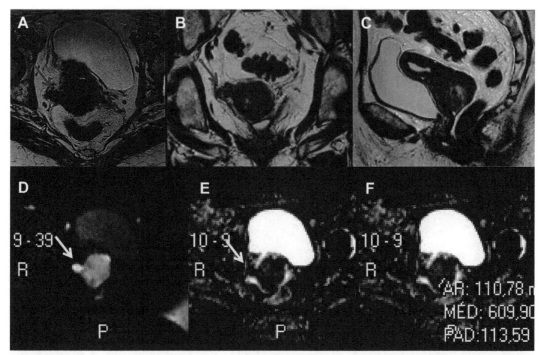

Fig. 6. 85-year-old woman with vaginal bleeding. T2-weighted images (*A, B, C*) show an expansive lesion on the posterior lip of the cervix, extending to the right parametrium (*red arrow*). Note the marked high-signal intensity on DWI (b = 1000) (*D*) and a low ADC value (0.6 × 10⁻³ mm²/s) (*E, F*), consistent with restricted diffusion and malignancy (*yellow arrows*). Pathologic examination confirmed the diagnosis of cervical carcinoma with secondary parametrial involvement.

Naganawa and colleagues[21] also reported that the mean ADC value of cervical cancer lesions was lower than of normal cervical tissue (1.09 × 10⁻³ vs 1.79 × 10⁻³ mm²/s) and showed that it returned to the normal range after chemotherapy and/or radiation therapy. However, this study was limited by its small sample size (n = 12).

These studies suggest that ADC measurement has a potential ability to differentiate between normal and cancerous tissue in the uterine cervix, aiding in the delineation of tumor boundaries, by reducing overestimation caused by inflammation or edema seen at T2-weighted imaging. However, further study is necessary to determine the accuracy of ADC measurement in monitoring the effect of treatment response.

Uterine Leiomyomas x Uterine Sarcomas

Uterine leiomyomas are composed of smooth muscle cells with varying amounts of fibrous connective tissue. Cellular leiomyomas are defined by a greater composition of compact smooth muscle cells (increased cellularity), with little or no collagen, and tend to show contrast enhancement in the early dynamic phase and to

be brighter on T2- and diffusion-weighted images with lower-signal intensity on ADC maps than non-degenerated fibrous leiomyomas.[11,22,23]

Uterine sarcomas also show lower ADC values compared with the normal myometrium, without any overlap, probably because of increased cellular density of the malignant tissues. When compared with sarcomas, degenerated leiomyomas tend to show low-signal intensity on DW images and higher ADC values reflecting the presence of abundant water within these lesions. However, cellular leiomyomas may not be distinguished from sarcomas based on DW images and ADC measurements alone, because both of them usually show high signal in DW with decreased signal intensity on ADC maps.[22]

Takeuchi and colleagues[24] evaluated 34 uterine myometrial lesions including 7 malignant tumors and 27 leiomyomas (6 cellular leiomyomas and 21 degenerated leiomyomas) and measured the ADCs in cellular portions of the lesions. They found that all malignant tumors showed high-signal intensity on DWI with low ADC (0.79 ± 0.26 × 10⁻³), which was significantly lower than that in benign leiomyomas (1.51 ± 0.33 × 10⁻³) (**Figs. 7** and **8**). The ADC in cellular leiomyomas (1.18 ± 0.16 × 10⁻³)

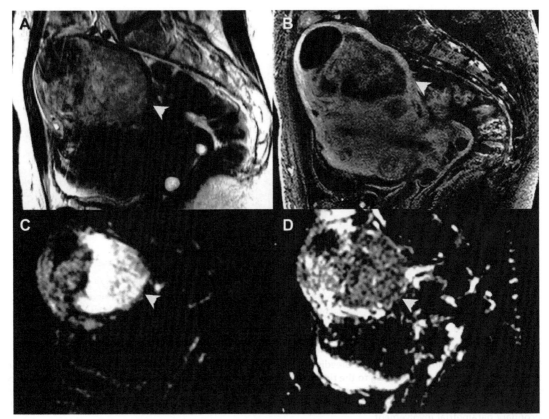

Fig. 7. 50-year-old woman with history of heavy menstrual bleeding, fibroids, and enlarged uterus on examination. T2-weighted sagittal FSE (*A*) showing T2 heterogeneous, hyperintense 10-cm mass along the cephalad, posterior uterus (*arrowhead*) without the usual signal intensity shown by benign fibroids. Postcontrast T1-weighted image in the sagittal plane (*B*) shows heterogeneous, early enhancement of this mass. DWI (b = 400) (*C*) showing hyperintensity and ADC maps (*D*) showing hypointensity consistent with restricted diffusion. The lower ADC value was 0.87 $\times$ 10^{-3} mm^2/s. After resection, this mass was consistent with a leiomyosarcoma arising from fibroid.

was significantly lower than that in degenerated leiomyomas (1.60 $\pm$ 0.30 $\times$ 10^{-3}) and higher than that in malignant tumors (**Fig. 9**). These investigators concluded that the ADC measurement could be helpful to distinguish malignant tumors from cellular degenerated leiomyomas.

Another application of DWI and ADC mapping within uterine fibroid tumors is related to identifying and monitoring ablated tissue. Within posttreatment MR imaging, areas of ablated fibroid tissue showed increased signal intensity on DWI and decreased ADC values, according to a report by Jacobs and colleagues.[25] This finding likely reflects restricted water motion because of infarction. At 6-month follow-up, ablated tissue showed increased ADC value, which was attributed to cell loss and necrosis.

Ovarian Tumors

There is increasing literature regarding the clinical application of DWI to distinguish benign from malignant ovarian masses, but further investigation is necessary to define the role of this functional technique within this context.

Fujii and colleagues[26] analyzed MR images of 123 ovarian lesions in 119 patients, obtaining axial DW images with b-values of 0 and 1000 s/mm^2, and reported that most malignant ovarian tumors (**Fig. 10**) and mature cystic teratomas as well as almost half of the endometriomas showed abnormal signal intensity on DWI distinct from other benign tumors. However, in this study, there were some malignant lesions that did not show high-signal intensity on DWI, including serous adenocarcinoma with massive ascites, solid portions in clear cell adenocarcinomas, septal solid portions in a metastatic tumor of appendiceal cancer, and septal solid portions in endometrioid borderline tumor. In contrast, some benign lesions such as mucinous adenomas, decidualized endometrioma, and polypoid endometriosis presented abnormal signal intensity on DWI. Furthermore, there was significant overlap between the ADC

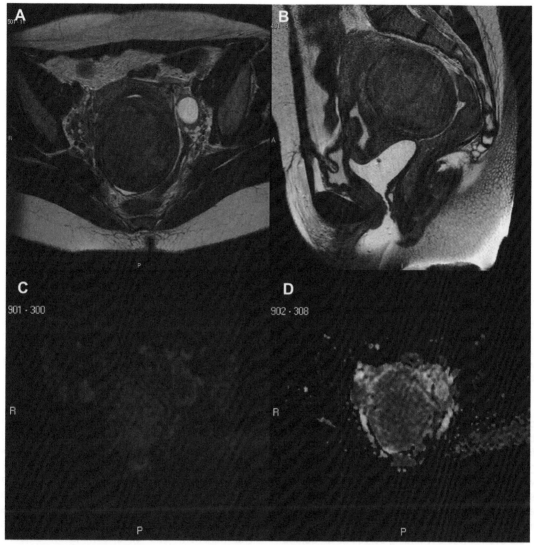

Fig. 8. 39-year-old asymptomatic woman. Axial (*A*) and sagittal (*B*) T2-weighted images showing a hypointense mass on the posterior wall of the uterus. The lesion shows low-signal intensity on DWI (b = 800) (*C*) and mild hypointensity on ADC map (*D*), consistent with no restricted diffusion. The mean ADC value was 1.8 × 10⁻³ mm²/s. Postresection pathologic examination confirmed the diagnosis of a benign leiomyoma.

values of the malignant and benign ovarian lesions, and the mean and lowest ADC values did not significantly differ between these 2 groups of ovarian lesions. Therefore, these investigators concluded that direct visual assessment of DW images of ovarian lesions and ADC measurement of solid components were not useful in differentiating benign from malignant ovarian masses.

With regard to cystic ovarian lesions, Nakayama and colleagues[27] assessed the potential usefulness of DWI by evaluating 131 lesions and also found that there was no significant difference in the ADC values between benign and malignant cystic neoplasms, concluding that the role of DWI in distinguishing between benign and

malignant ovarian cystic tumors may thus be limited. They also reported that the mean ADC of mature cystic teratomas was lower than that of endometrial cysts and malignant ovarian cystic tumors.

The high-signal intensity on DWI found within some mature cystic teratomas (**Fig. 11**), as well as its lower ADC values when compared with endometrial cysts and other ovarian neoplasms, is probably related to the presence of keratinoid substance within these tumors, as well as the fat content presented by the cystic components of these lesions.[27–30] Because DWI with EPI sequences usually uses a fat-saturation radio-frequency (RF) pulse, the low ADC values of the

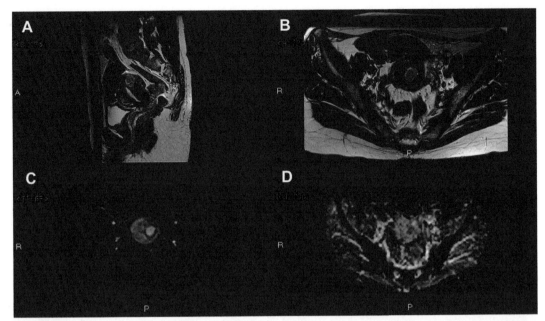

Fig. 9. 36-year-old asymptomatic woman. T2-weighted images on sagittal (*A*) and axial (*B*) images show an intermediate-signal intensity nodule in the posterior wall of the uterus. Note the early intense enhancement on the T1FS postcontrast image (*C*). The lesion showed low-signal intensity on ADC map (*D*), with a mean ADC value of 1.23×10^{-3} mm²/s. The constellation of findings is consistent with a cellular leiomyoma (pathologically proved).

cystic component of mature cystic teratomas have been attributed to artifacts caused by coexisting fat within the tumor.[28,29] Furthermore, the restricted Brownian movement of water molecules within the keratinoid substance results in a high signal on DWI and a low ADC value. This phenomenon has already been established as important information for the diagnosis of intracranial epidermoid cyst.[30] This DW finding serves as an adjunctive tool to ensure the diagnostic accuracy and may be especially useful in the diagnosis of mature cystic teratoma, which lacks macroscopic fat.[27]

Endometrial cysts also tend to show abnormal signal intensity on DWI because of their blood content, which tends to shorten T1 values, thereby resulting in a decrease in the ADC (**Fig. 12**).[28,29,31]

Among malignant ovarian tumors, many studies showed that the ADC value varied widely, a phenomenon attributable to their morphologic variety.[27,29,31]

Peritoneal Dissemination

The peritoneal cavity is a common site of metastatic spread for abdominopelvic malignancies, especially in patients with ovarian cancers. The detection of peritoneal dissemination is therefore important in preoperative imaging assessment of malignant tumors.

According to Fujii and colleagues,[32] the sensitivity and specificity of DW MR imaging with b-values of 0 and 1000 s/mm² for the detection of peritoneal dissemination were 90 and 95.5%, respectively (n = 26). Most peritoneal dissemination was easily shown on DWI as moderate or strong abnormal signal intensity, in contrast to mild intensity signal of surrounding organs. The minimum size of dissemination detected was 5 mm.

Other studies reported sensitivity and specificity to be 85% to 93% and 78% to 96%, respectively, on contrast-enhanced computed tomography (CT) imaging,[33,34] and 95% and 80%, respectively, on contrast-enhanced MR imaging.[35]

Therefore, Fujii and colleagues showed that DWI was of equal value to contrast-enhanced imaging for the evaluation of peritoneal dissemination (**Fig. 13**).

Rectal Cancer

Historically, endoluminal ultrasonography (ELUS) was the preferred modality to accurately depict the layers of the rectum to guide surgical planning and to assess the stage of rectal carcinoma.[36] Current MR imaging techniques using thin section T2-weighted imaging now allow for more accurate depiction of tumor margins and better assessment

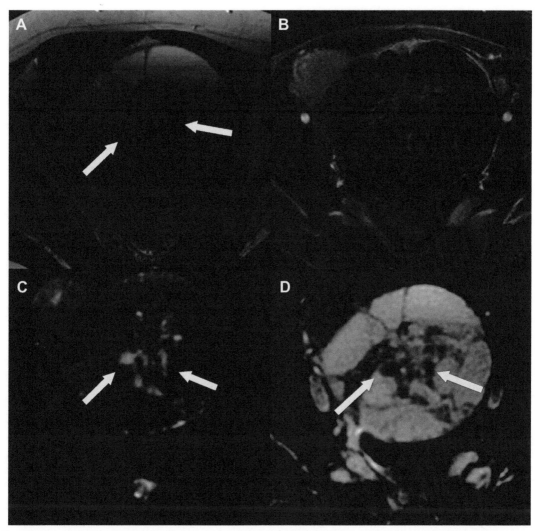

Fig. 10. T2-weighted axial (*A*), postcontrast T1-weighted axial (*B*), DWI (b = 600) (*C*), and ADC (*D*) maps in a large, complex septated mass within the pelvis (*arrow*). On T2-weighted imaging, there are thick and thin septations with nodularity throughout the ovary, all of which show enhancement (*B*). On DWI, many of these septations and nodules show hyperintensity (*C*), some of which show low signal on ADC (*D*) compatible with restricted diffusion. Findings on pathologic examination confirmed a diagnosis of ovarian carcinoma.

of depth of tumor invasion and extent of spread versus ELUS and digital rectal examination.[37] Unlike the remainder of the colon, the rectum is relatively fixed, allowing for high-resolution imaging (512 matrix) without the consequence of significant motion artifact. Endoluminal surface coils may also be used to further increase spatial resolution to better depict the layers of the rectal wall.[38] The addition of DWI is an emerging technique that improves the ability of MR imaging to detect rectal cancer and monitor its response to chemotherapy and radiotherapy (**Fig. 14**).[39–41]

Colorectal cancer is the third most common noncutaneous malignancy in men and women in the United States, and after lung cancer, is the second leading cause of cancer death when statistics on men and women are combined.[42] Rectal cancer comprises approximately 30% of all cases of colorectal cancers and carries with it a poorer prognosis vis-à-vis colon cancer because it is more prone to metastasize and have local recurrence.[43] Survival rates from rectal cancer are directly linked to tumor stage and are dependent on both local tumor extent and presence of lymph node involvement. T3 tumors have a higher recurrence rate than T2 tumors, and thus making a distinction between T2 and T3 tumor preoperatively by evaluating tumor involvement of the perirectal fat is an important role of imaging.

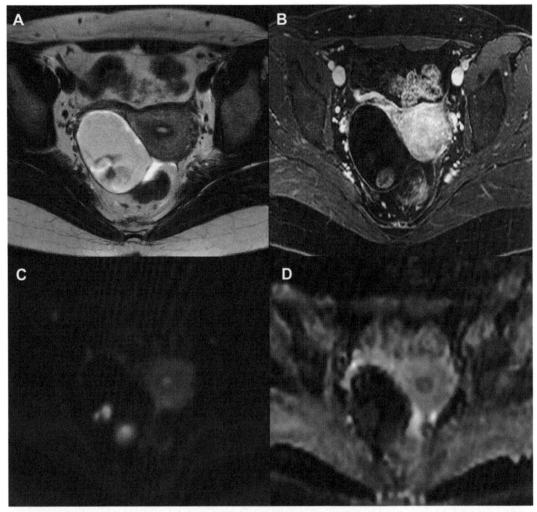

Fig. 11. 35-year-old woman with palpable right adnexal mass. MR imaging shows a T2 (*A*) hyperintense 6.5-cm mass with areas of macroscopic fat on T1-weighted fat-saturated images (*B*) and no significant enhancement. There are areas within the mass that show DWI bright foci (*C*) and ADC low-signal intensity (*D*). Pathologic examination confirmed a benign teratoma.

Advances in surgical technique, most notably the advent of total mesorectal excision (TME), and the use of preoperative neoadjuvant chemotherapy and radiation have led to improvement in disease-free survival.[44–46] However, careful patient selection is critical for preoperative radiotherapy and TME to be effective, specifically with regards to involvement of the circumferential resection margin (CRM) as involvement of the CRM has been shown to be a better predictor of local recurrence than T stage.[47] High-resolution MR imaging is effective in making this distinction and shows high specificity (92%) in its ability to predict curative resection of rectal carcinoma.[48,49] Moreover, the depth of extramural spread of tumor is accurately depicted by high-resolution MR imaging techniques.[50] The addition of DWI

sequences has recently been shown to further improve the diagnostic yield of MR imaging in both detecting rectal cancer and evaluating response to therapy.[51–54]

With specific regards to complete response (CR) after neoadjuvant chemotherapy and radiotherapy in patients with locally advanced rectal cancer, Kim and colleagues[40] showed improved diagnostic accuracy when DW images are viewed in addition to conventional MR imaging. However, these investigators note that DWI of the posttreatment patient with rectal cancer is limited by (1) the inability of DWI to accurately differentiate CR from near CR and discriminate between residual tumor and inactive mucin pools, (2) the limited threshold of even the highest spatial resolution ADC mapping because of the heterogeneity of the

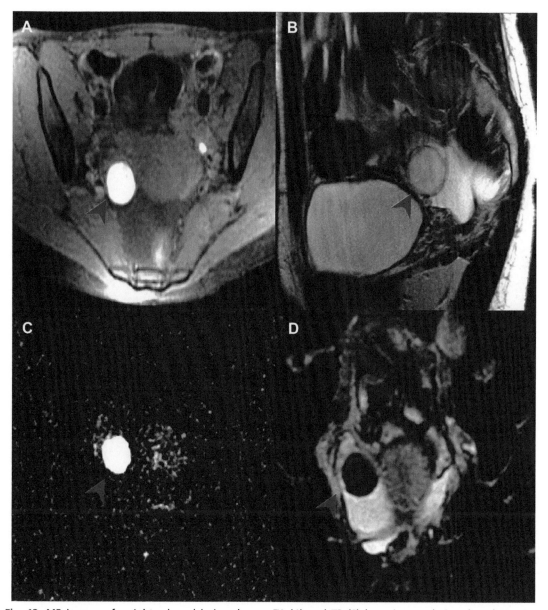

Fig. 12. MR images of a right adnexal lesion show a T1 (*A*) and T2 (*B*) hyperintense lesion that shows DWI hyperintensity and ADC hypointensity compatible with restricted diffusion. Pathologic diagnosis confirmed the diagnosis of a benign endometrioma (*C, D*).

tumor at the cellular level, and (3) the fact that high b-value DWI has poor SNR and limited spatial resolution.

MR imaging with DWI also shows benefit in noninvasively staging nodal involvement (**Fig. 15**). A recent study shows MR with DWI to be superior to fluorodeoxyglucose (FDG) positron emission tomography in detection of lymph node metastases (sensitivity 80% vs 30%, specificity 76.9% vs 100%, and accuracy of 78.3% vs 69.6%, respectively).[55] However, no study to date has shown any usefulness in DWI for

accurate prediction of lymph node involvement after treatment.

Rectal cancer imparts a poor prognosis when advanced (T3 stage and beyond). Advances in high-resolution thin-slice MR imaging have allowed for improved noninvasive anatomic localization of tumor. The addition of functional modalities such as DWI has further improved the ability of MR imaging to both preoperatively assess tumor extent and help better determine response to adjuvant therapy, an area in which conventional MR imaging has been lacking.[56]

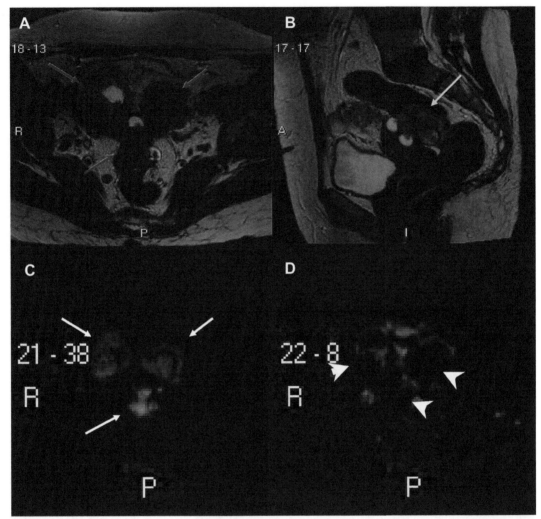

Fig. 13. 62-year-old woman with diffuse abdominal pain and history of contrast material allergy. Gadolinium intravenous administration could not be performed. T2-weighted images (*A, B*) show bilateral ovarian masses (*red arrows*) and a retrocervical lesion in intimate association with the anterior rectal wall (*yellow arrow*). (*C*) High-signal intensity on DWI (b = 1000) (*white arrows*) and (*D*) low-signal intensity on ADC map (*arrowheads*) indicate restricted diffusion. Pathologic diagnosis confirmed ovarian adenocarcinoma with a serosal implant.

Prostate Carcinoma

Advances in MR imaging and computing technology have resulted in the ability to detect disease within the male pelvis with a high degree of accuracy. Specifically, the use of endorectal coils and pelvic phased-array coils coupled with 3-T magnetic fields has resulted in improved signal-to-noise as well as improved spatial, temporal, and spectral resolution in the evaluation of the prostate gland for malignancy.[57–59] Further improvement in diagnostic accuracy in the detection of malignancy within the prostate gland can be achieved with the addition of DWI (**Fig. 16**).[60] Although more commonly used in the evaluation

of intracranial disease, the application of DWI in extracranial sites has increased in the last 20 years primarily because of improvements in the speed of acquisition of images using echo planar and parallel imaging, which helps diminish motion artifacts.[61] Moreover, DWI sequences can be added to standard imaging of the pelvis without the consequence of significant increases in imaging time or the need to administer exogenous contrast agents.[61] DWI images can provide both quantitative and qualitative information in the prostate gland, which coupled with standard sequences can aid in tumor detection and staging, guide biopsy, and allow for assessment of treatment response.[60]

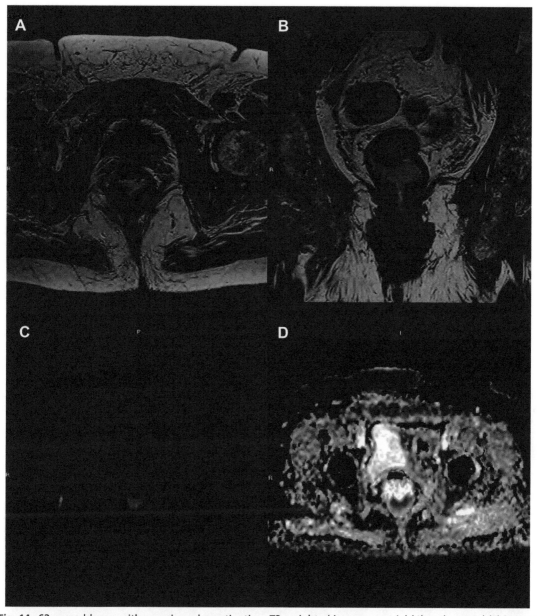

Fig. 14. 62-year-old man with anemia and constipation. T2-weighted images on axial (*A*) and coronal (*B*) images showing thickening of the posterior rectal wall. The lesion showed high-signal intensity on DWI (b = 1000) (*C*) and low-signal intensity on ADC map (*D*). These findings are consistent with restricted diffusion. Pathologic examination confirmed the diagnosis of adenocarcinoma of the rectum.

Prostate cancer is the most common noncutaneous malignancy in men and, after lung cancer, is the second leading cause of cancer death in men. The American Cancer Society estimates that 1 in 6 American men are diagnosed with prostate cancer during their lifetime and that an estimated 32,050 men will die of prostate cancer in 2010. Some studies estimate that as many as 80% of men older than 80 years and 50% of men older than 50 years harbor prostatic carcinoma.[62] However, what complicates the statistics on prostate cancer in men is that most prostatic carcinoma is latent. The aggressiveness of prostate adenocarcinoma is dependent on histologic grade (most commonly reported using the Gleason system) and tumor volume.[63] The role of imaging is to assist in both lesion detection, including extent of tumor (ie, extracapsular spread, invasion of neurovascular bundle, osseous metastasis, and lymph node involvement),

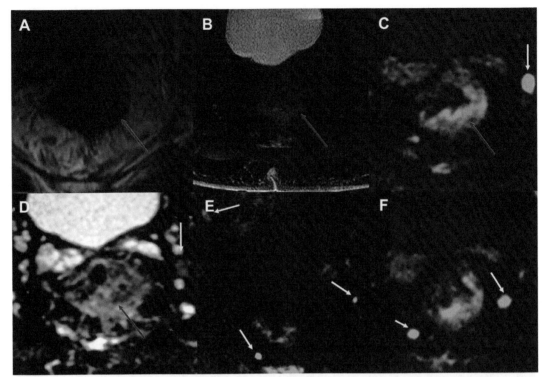

Fig. 15. Axial T2 (*A*), T1 postcontrast (*B*), DWI (*C*), and ADC (*D*) maps show a circumferential enhancing mass lesion (*red arrows*) in the rectum with a small adjacent lymph node (*yellow arrow*), which shows restricted diffusion on DWI and ADC maps. Also noted are multiple small pararectal and right iliac lymph nodes (*yellow arrow*), which also show restricted diffusion (*E, F*). All the lesions were positive for malignancy.

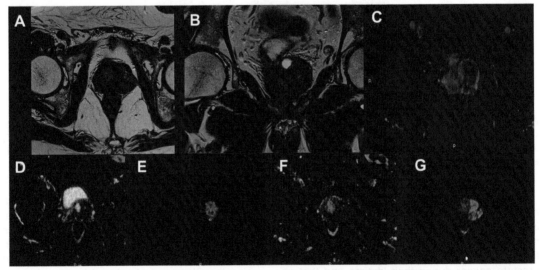

Fig. 16. 66-year-old man with abnormal digital rectal examination for prostate cancer screening. MR images show a large hypointense mass on the left peripheral zone of the prostate on T2-weighted images (*A, B*), with heterogeneous enhancement on T1FS after contrast (*C*). The mass is better delineated on DWI (b = 1000) (*E, G*) as a hyperintense lesion, with low-signal intensity on ADC map (*D, F*). These findings are consistent with restricted diffusion and malignancy.

and to help guide biopsy to reduce unnecessary morbidity.

Most prostatic adenocarcinomas (70%) arise from the glandular tissue of the peripheral zone. These tumors are more easily detected by their conspicuous low-signal intensity compared with the normal high T2 signal of the peripheral zone. However, low T2 signal within the peripheral zone is nonspecific and can be seen in other lesions such as hemorrhage, prostate infection, or as a result of posttreatment alterations. Moreover, when tumor is confined to the transitional or central zone, the lesions can be difficult to detect because of the often heterogeneous signal intensity of the central gland. The use of DWI and the subsequent calculation of ADCs helps differentiate between benign and malignant nodules in the prostate because malignant nodules show lower ADC values than normal tissue.[64] Recent studies have shown that the addition of DWI to standard T2 imaging can be effective in detecting aggressive disease within the peripheral zone and that DWI alone is superior to T2-weighted imaging alone.[65,66] A recent study from Kim and colleagues[67] for predicting tumor location in 68 patients notes an overall sensitivity and positive predictive value (PPV) of 84% and 86%, respectively, for T2-weighted images in addition to DWI. This exceeds T2-weighted imaging alone where the sensitivity and PPV were only 66% and 63%, respectively ($P<.05$). Several investigators have also shown that DWI aids in detection of tumor recurrence after treatment.[68,69]

Another diagnostic dilemma with regards to prostate cancer is the selection of high-yield sites for targeted biopsy. DWI when correlated with T2 imaging has been shown to help identify foci of aggressive tumor amenable to image-guided sampling in patients in whom prior transrectal ultrasound biopsy is negative despite rising prostate specific antigen.[70] DWI may also assist targeted sampling in regions with more aggressive tumor, as seen in a recent study showing correlation with biopsy samples and histologic grade.[71]

Although the addition of DWI to standard T2-weighted imaging protocols has the potential to significantly improve cancer detection in the prostate, there are limitations to its effectiveness. Kim and colleagues[60] note (1) that there is a general lack of standardization, with many different b-values being used at different institutions, (2) that there is a paucity of literature assessing the reproducibility of DWI MR imaging of the prostate, (3) that inherent flaws exist in DWI with regards to image distortion and susceptibility artifacts, and (4) that more in vivo studies are needed to assess how DWI relates to pathologic changes in the gland.

DWI is an effective adjunct to standard T2 imaging in the male pelvis for the assessment of prostate cancer. It allows for noninvasive cancer detection and staging, helps guide biopsy, and aids in posttreatment follow-up.

Bladder Cancer

Treatment options for urinary bladder cancer differ considerably depending on T-tumor staging. Distinguishing superficial tumors (stage T1 or lower) from invasive ones (stage T2 or higher) significantly alters therapeutic approach.

Many investigators have shown that bladder cancer shows higher-signal intensity on DWI when compared with normal surrounding tissues (**Fig. 17**), and that this functional technique could therefore be used to improve tumor staging.[72,73]

In a report by Matsuki and colleagues[74] evaluating the usefulness of DWI in the diagnosis of bladder tumors, all 17 carcinomas showed high-signal intensity relative to the surrounding structures, and the ADC values of the tumors were significantly lower compared with those of urine, normal bladder wall, prostate, and seminal vesicle. These investigators found no overlap between the ADC values of the tumors and the urine or bladder wall, but in some cases there was an overlap between the ADC values of the tumors and the prostate or seminal vesicles. They concluded that DW images could be useful in evaluating the tumor invading surrounding structures.

Takeuchi and colleagues[75] measured the correlation between the ADC and histologic grade of bladder cancers and evaluated the ability of DWI to determinate the T stage of these tumors. They highlighted the excellent specificity of DW images (97%) for enabling diagnosis of muscle invasion and concluded that the overall accuracy and specificity for diagnosing T2 or higher stages were significantly improved when DW images were viewed together with T2-weighted images. They also suggested that the presence of a low ADC ($<1 \times 10^{-3}$ mm^2/s) could indicate that the tumor is more likely to have a higher histologic grade (G3) (**Fig. 18**).

In another report, the data obtained at MR imaging with ultrasmall superparamagnetic particles of iron oxide (USPIO) combined with DWI suggested that this method could be useful for detecting pelvic lymph node metastases even in normal-sized nodes of patients with bladder cancer.[76]

OTHER LESIONS
Nodes

Until now, the differentiation between benign and malignant lymph nodes has been based mainly

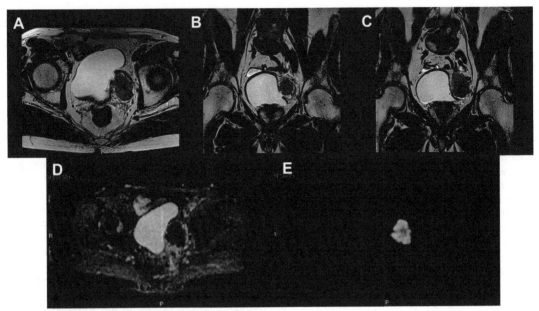

Fig. 17. 69-year-old man with hematuria. T2-weighted images on axial (*A*) and coronal (*B, C*) planes showing a mildly hypointense mass arising in a bladder diverticula. The lesions show marked hypointensity on ADC map (*D*) and hyperintensity on DWI (b = 800) (*E*), indicating restricted diffusion. Pathologic examination confirmed a diagnosis of transitional cell carcinoma arising in urinary bladder diverticula.

on the size of the short-axis axial diameter. However, this measure has been shown to be a poor discriminator in pelvic imaging.[77,78] The use of USPIO is a new technique which may help to improve the performance of MR, but it is not yet widely available.

Many studies have investigated the usefulness of DWI in evaluating lymph nodes in head and neck carcinomas and have found that the ADC value is significantly lower in lymphomatous nodes than in metastatic ones, but this conclusion is probably a result of the great prevalence of necrosis in squamous cell head and neck carcinomas.[79,80]

However, further studies are necessary to evaluate the role of DWI in discriminating malignant from benign pelvic nodes, because only a few papers have discussed this subject in patients with gynecologic malignancies, and discrepant results have been found between them.[81–83] Roy and colleagues[84] examined 79 patients with pelvic carcinoma and 180 controls using a diffusion MR imaging protocol including b-values of 0 and 1000 s/mm^2 and concluded that the addition of DW images to conventional MR imaging was useful in identifying small lymph nodes (see **Fig. 15**), because all nodes showed high-signal intensity on heavy DW images, thereby being clearly identified because of their high contrast against the low intensity of the surrounding

structures. However, the measurement of mean ADC values did not improve the differentiation of these nodes as having metastatic involvement over conventional measures.

In our experience, most pelvic lymph nodes appear bright on high b-value images, with corresponding low ADC values, regardless of their benign or metastatic nature, because the highly cellular tissue in reactive lymph nodes may also show increased intensity in DWI. This fact makes it difficult to accurately differentiate between these 2 categories based on ADC values and DWI (**Fig. 19**).

Assuming that lymph nodes invaded by tumor cells would display cellularity and/or microarchitecture similar to the primary tumor, one approach that can help in this difficult situation is to compare the signal intensity as well as the ADC value of a lymph node with those of the primary tumor (**Fig. 20**). Lin and colleagues[82] reported that the combination of size and relative ADC values was useful in detecting pelvic lymph node metastasis in patients with cervical and uterine cancers.

Endometriosis and Adenomyosis

There are only a few reports on the use of DWI in pelvic endometriosis. However, it is well known that because endometrial cysts tend to contain blood clots and hemosiderin, the T1 values are

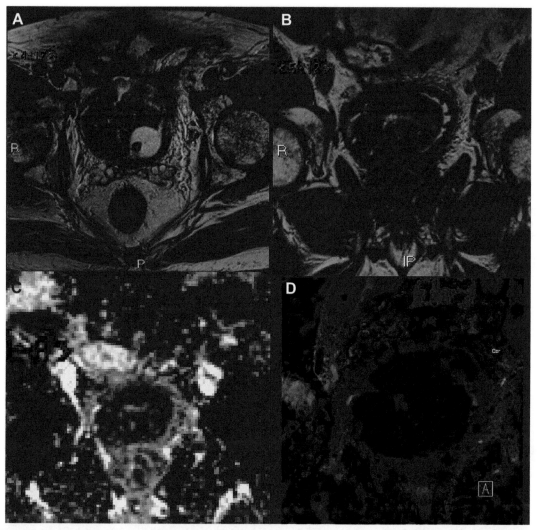

Fig. 18. 57-year-old man with chronic renal insufficiency and hematuria. MR images show a hypointense polypoid mass in the vesical lumen (*A, B*), which shows marked low-signal intensity on ADC map (*C*), with a mean ADC value of 0.97×10^{-3} mm²/s. Fused DW images/T2-weighted images (*D*) are consistent with restricted diffusion within the mass. A high histologic grade malignant tumor (G3) was confirmed on pathologic diagnosis after resection.

shortened, resulting in a decrease in the ADC.[26–29,31] Therefore, endometriomas, as well as ectopic endometrial gland with hemorrhagic products as seen in endometriosis and adenomyosis, may show restricted diffusion on DWI.

Adnexal Torsion

Adnexal torsion leads to circulatory stasis that is initially venous, but becomes arterial with progression of the torsion and resultant edema. When complete torsion occurs, the arterial blood supply is obstructed, causing hemorrhagic necrosis.[85]

Thickening of the fallopian tube is considered the most specific imaging finding of adnexal torsion, and it usually appears on conventional imaging as an amorphous solid masslike structure with a targetlike appearance, or as a beaklike protrusion extending from the uterus and partially covering the adnexal mass. However, visualization of the thickened tube is not always straightforward because it may be poorly differentiated from other surrounding organs, especially if the torsion is associated with a large adnexal mass.

Fujii and colleagues[86] analyzed the DWI findings in 11 patients with surgical confirmation of adnexal

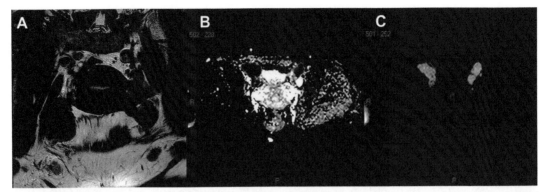

Fig. 19. Investigation of a 43-year-old woman with generalized lymphadenopathy. (*A*) Pelvic MR shows multiple pathologically enlarged lymph nodes along the common and external iliac chains. These nodes show high-signal intensity on DWI (*B*) and hypointensity on ADC map (*C*). These findings are consistent with restricted diffusion. Biopsy confirmed a diagnosis of diffuse large B-cell lymphoma.

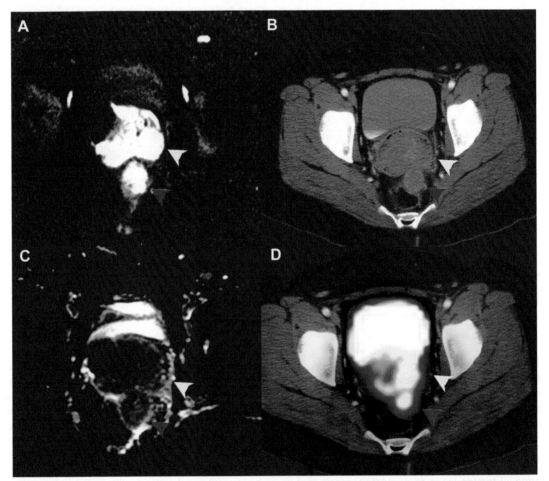

Fig. 20. 34-year-old woman with dyspareunia and suspicious Papanicolaou smear. DWI (b = 1000) (*A*) and ADC map (*C*) showing restricted diffusion within the cervical mass (*yellow arrowhead*) in the axial plane with a large lymph node (*red arrowhead*) in the mesorectal fascia. CT imaging (*B*) shows a large, bulky enhancing mass centered in the upper vagina and lower cervix with a large lymph node posterior to the mass and anterior to the rectum. There is FDG avidity (*D*) within the mass. Biopsy showed cervical adenocarcinoma.

torsion using b-values of 0 and 1000 s/mm² and reported that fallopian tube thickening showed inhomogeneous abnormal signal intensity on DWI. This finding may be a reflection of infarcted tissues and blood clots, thereby indicating that this functional technique could facilitate making this difficult diagnosis.

Other findings of adnexal torsion include wall thickening of the twisted adnexal cystic mass, ascites, uterine deviation to the twisted side, adnexal hemorrhage, and lack of contrast enhancement of the adnexal mass.[85,87,88]

Wall thickening of a cystic mass is presumed to be related to edematous wall congestion in the cystic mass or clots caused by hemorrhagic infarction. Fujii and colleagues[86] also found restricted diffusion on the walls of twisted cystic adnexal masses, probably because of the presence of infarcted tissues and blood cots similarly as that for tube thickening and to the T2 shine-through effect by congestive edema. The investigators then suggested that when abnormal signal intensity is found in the wall of a cystic adnexal mass, adnexal torsion should be considered.

Because clots show strong signal intensity on DWI, intracystic clots from adnexal hemorrhage may also show high-signal intensity on DW. However, this finding cannot be interpreted as a specific one for the diagnosis of adnexal torsion because the intracystic portions of some non-twisted ovarian lesions such as mature cystic teratomas and mucinous adenomas may also show abnormal intensity on DW images.

Because lack of contrast enhancement of the adnexal mass is also an important imaging finding for the diagnosis of adnexal torsion, DWI added to conventional MR imaging plays a special role as a useful technique in diagnosing this condition in those patients in whom contrast-enhanced imaging cannot be performed.

PITFALLS IN DWI INTERPRETATION
Tumors with Low Cellularity

Not all tumors are composed of high-cellular tissue. Therefore, malignant tumors with low cellularity, such as mixed tumors with large cystic components, may not show restricted diffusion.[77]

Restricted Diffusion in Normal Structures

DWI is based on the random motion of water molecules within the cytoplasm and is nonspecific in that any tissue with high cellular density appears bright on high b-value images. Therefore, some normal pelvic structures, such as normal endometrium, normal or reactive nodes, and bowel mucosal, may present with high-signal intensity on DWI.[77] This concept must be taken into consideration during interpretation of pelvic imaging.

T2 Shine-through

Because DW images are intrinsically T2 weighted, it is important to be aware that signal intensity on DWI can be influenced by the signal intensity on T2-weighted images (**Fig. 21**). Normal tissues with slow T2 relaxation rates might show hyperintensity on b-value images with a corresponding high ADC value.[89,90] Therefore, care should be taken when b-value images are interpreted in isolation without reference to corresponding ADC maps.

Based on this information, many investigators suggest that DWI with a higher b-value (eg, 800 or 1000 s/mm²) may be required for the female pelvic region.[28,77]

FUTURE DIRECTIONS OF DW PELVIC IMAGING

As MR imaging techniques continue to evolve in conjunction with improvements in pelvic imaging at higher field strengths (eg, 4 Tesla using better

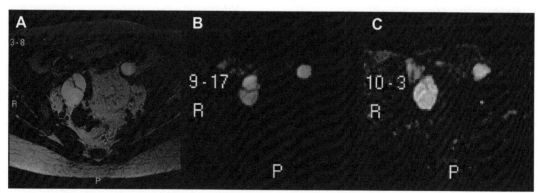

Fig. 21. 35-year-old asymptomatic woman. Both ovaries show high-signal intensity on DWI (b = 600) (*A, B*). However, signal intensity is also high on ADC map (*C*), consistent with no restricted diffusion (T2 shine-through effect).

gradient and RF coil designs), DWI will likely play an increasing role in both drug development and individual clinical practice management decisions. The potential of including DWI to early, phase-I/II studies to better understand the microscopic changes ongoing in various cancer systems, serially, may allow a go-no-go decision within these settings to occur before more costly phase-III trials occur.

Moreover, as further refinements occur, ADC measurements may surpass RECIST (Response Evaluation Criteria In Solid Tumors) criteria[91] in tumor response metrics. DWI has the potential to affect both drug development, by assessing at earlier time points whether a drug is efficacious, and the prediction of tumor response to therapy using ADC combined with dynamic contrast-enhanced parameters (eg, Ktrans). In the era of molecular medicine, techniques such as DWI may provide insight into novel, personalized approaches to oncologic care.

ACKNOWLEDGMENTS

The authors thank Claudio M.A.O. Lima, MD for valuable logistic and technical support for text edition and Susanna Lee MD (MGH) and Nagaraj Holalkere from Boston University for cases and figures.

REFERENCES

1. Qayyum Aliya. Diffusion-weighted imaging in the abdomen and pelvis: concepts and applications. Radiographics 2009;29:1797–810.
2. Sugahara T, Korogi Y, Kochi M, et al. Usefulness of diffusion-weighted MRI with echo-planar technique in the evaluation of cellularity in gliomas. J Magn Reson Imaging 1999;9:53–60.
3. Kim HS, Kim SH, Yang DM, et al. Unusual causes of tubo-ovarian abscess: CT and MR imaging findings. Radiographics 2004;24:1575–89.
4. Heverhagen JT, Klose KJ. MR imaging for acute lower abdominal and pelvic pain. Radiographics 2009;29:1781–96.
5. Bouman DE, Wiarda BM. Diffusion-weighted imaging of acute abdominal and pelvic pain [abstr]. In: Radiological Society of North America scientific assembly and annual meeting program. Oak Brook (IL): Radiological Society of North America; 2008. p. 845.
6. Tamai K, Koyama T, Saga T, et al. Diffusion-weighted MR imaging of uterine endometrial cancer. J Magn Reson Imaging 2007;26:682–7.
7. Szafer A, Zhong J, Gore JC. Theoretical model for water diffusion in tissues. Magn Reson Med 1995;33:697–712.
8. Koyama T, Togashi K. Functional MR imaging of the female pelvis. J Magn Reson Imaging 2007;25:1101–12.
9. Sato C, Naganawa S, Nakamura T, et al. Differentiation of noncancerous tissue and cancer lesions by apparent diffusion coefficient values in transition and peripheral zones of the prostate. J Magn Reson Imaging 2005;21:258–62.
10. Castillo M, Smith JK, Kwock L, et al. Apparent diffusion coefficients in the evaluation of high-grade cerebral gliomas. AJNR Am J Neuroradiol 2001;22:60–4.
11. Saremi F, Knoll AN, Bendavid OF, et al. Characterization of genitourinary lesions with diffusion weighted imaging. Radiographics 2009;29:1295–317.
12. Inada Y, Matsuki M, Nakai G, et al. Body diffusion-weighted MR imaging of uterine endometrial cancer: is it helpful in the detection of cancer in nonenhanced MR imaging? Eur J Radiol 2009;70:122–7.
13. Takahashi S, Murakami T, Narumi Y, et al. Preoperative staging of endometrial carcinoma: diagnostic effect of T2-weighted fast spin-echo MR imaging. Radiology 1998;206:539–47.
14. Manfredi R, Gui B, Maresca G, et al. Endometrial cancer: magnetic resonance imaging. Abdom Imaging 2005;30:626–36.
15. Rechich G, Galimberti S, Signorelli M, et al. Myometrial invasion in endometrial cancer: diagnostic performance of diffusion-weighted MR imaging at 1.5-T. Eur Radiol 2010;20:754–62.
16. Frei KA, Kinkel K, Bonel HM, et al. Prediction of deep myometrial invasion in patients with endometrial cancer: clinical utility of contrast-enhanced MR imaging—a meta-analysis and Bayesian analysis. Radiology 2000;216:444–9.
17. Nicolet V, Carignan L, Bourdon F, et al. MR imaging of cervical carcinoma: a practical staging approach. Radiographics 2000;20:1539–49.
18. Abe Y, Yamashita Y, Namimoto T, et al. Carcinoma of the uterine cervix: high-resolution turbo spin-echo MR imaging with contrast-enhanced dynamic scanning and T2-weighting. Acta Radiol 1998;39:322–6.
19. Tsuda K, Murakami T, Kurachi H, et al. MR imaging of cervical carcinoma: comparison among T2-weighted, dynamic, and postcontrast T1-weighted images with histopathological correlation. Abdom Imaging 1997;22:103–7.
20. McVeigh PZ, Syed AM, Milosevic M, et al. Diffusion-weighted MRI in cervical cancer. Eur Radiol 2008;18:1058–64.
21. Naganawa S, Sato C, Kumada H, et al. Apparent diffusion coefficient in cervical cancer of the uterus: comparison with the normal uterine cervix. Eur Radiol 2005;15:71–8.
22. Tamai K, Koyama T, Saga T, et al. The utility of diffusion-weighted MR imaging for differentiating

uterine sarcomas from benign leiomyomas. Eur Radiol 2008;18:723–30.

23. Murase E, Siegelman ES, Outwater EK, et al. Uterine leiomyomas: histopathologic features, MR imaging findings, differential diagnosis, and treatment. Radiographics 1999;19(5):1179–97.

24. Takeuchi M, Matsuzaki K, Nishitani H. Hyperintense uterine myometrial masses on T2-weighted magnetic resonance imaging: differentiation with diffusion-weighted magnetic resonance imaging. J Comput Assist Tomogr 2009;33(6):834–7.

25. Jacobs MA, Herskovits EH, Kim HS. Uterine fibroids: diffusion-weighted MR imaging for monitoring therapy with focused ultrasound surgery – preliminary study. Radiology 2005;236(1):196–203.

26. Fujii S, Kakite S, Nishihara K, et al. Diagnostic accuracy of diffusion-weighted imaging in differentiating benign from malignant ovarian lesions. J Magn Reson Imaging 2008;28(5):1149–56.

27. Nakayama T, Yoshimitsu K, Irie H, et al. Diffusion weighted echo-planar MR imaging and ADC mapping in the differential diagnosis of ovarian cystic masses: usefulness of detecting keratinoid substances in mature cystic teratomas. J Magn Reson Imaging 2005;22:271–8.

28. Namimoto T, Awai K, Nakaura T, et al. Role of diffusion-weighted imaging in the diagnosis of gynecological diseases. Eur Radiol 2009;19:745–60.

29. Moteki T, Ishizaka H. Diffusion weighted EPI of cystic ovarian lesions: evaluation of cystic contents using apparent diffusion coefficients. J Magn Reson Imaging 2000;12:1014–9.

30. Chen S, Ikawa F, Kurisu K, et al. Quantitative MR evaluation of intracranial epidermoid tumors by fast fluid attenuated inversion recovery imaging and echo-planar diffusion-weighted imaging. AJNR Am J Neuroradiol 2001;22:1089–96.

31. Katayama M, Masui T, Kobayashi S, et al. Diffusion-weighted echo planar imaging of ovarian tumors: is it useful to measure apparent diffusion coefficients? J Comput Assist Tomogr 2002;26:250–6.

32. Fujii S, Matsusue E, Kanasaki Y, et al. Detection of peritoneal dissemination in gynecological malignancy: evaluation by diffusion-weighted MR imaging. Eur Radiol 2008;18:18–23.

33. Tempany CM, Zou KH, Silverman SG, et al. Staging of advanced ovarian cancer: comparison of imaging modalities – report from the Radiological Diagnostic Oncology Group. Radiology 2000;215:761–7.

34. Coakley FV, Choi PH, Gougoutas CA, et al. Peritoneal metastases: detection with spiral CT in patients with ovarian cancer. Radiology 2002;223:495–9.

35. Ricke J, Sehouli J, Hach C, et al. Prospective evaluation of contrast enhanced MRI in the depiction of peritoneal spread in primary or recurrent ovarian cancer. Eur Radiol 2003;13:943–9.

36. Meyenberger C, Huch Boni RA, Bertschinger P, et al. Endoscopic ultrasound and endorectal magnetic resonance imaging: a prospective, comparative study for preoperative staging and follow-up of rectal cancer. Endoscopy 1995;27:469–79.

37. Brown G, Davies S, Williams GT, et al. Effectiveness of preoperative staging in rectal cancer: digital rectal examination, endoluminal ultrasound or magnetic resonance imaging? Br J Cancer 2004;91(1):23–9.

38. Schnall MD, Furth EE, Rosato EF, et al. Rectal tumor stage: correlation of endorectal MR imaging and pathologic findings. Radiology 1994;190(3):709–14.

39. Ichikawa T, Erturk SM, Motosugi U, et al. High-B-value diffusion-weighted MRI in colorectal cancer. AJR Am J Roentgenol 2006;187:181–4.

40. Kim SH, Lee JM, Hong SH, et al. Locally advanced rectal cancer: added value of diffusion-weighted MR imaging in the evaluation of tumor response to neoadjuvant chemo- and radiation therapy. Radiology 2009;253(1):116–25.

41. Dzik-Jurasz A, Domenig C, George M, et al. Diffusion MRI for prediction of response of rectal cancer to chemoradiation. Lancet 2002;360(32):307–8.

42. American Cancer Society Website. Available at: http://www.cancer.org/cancer/colonandrectumcancer/detailedguide/colorectal-cancer-key-statistics. Accessed July 17, 2010.

43. Sagar PM, Pemberton JH. Surgical management of locally recurrent rectal cancer. Br J Surg 1996;83(3):293–304.

44. Enker WE, Thaler HT, Cranor ML, et al. Total mesorectal excision in the operative treatment of carcinoma of the rectum. J Am Coll Surg 1995;181:335–46.

45. Camma C, Giunta M, Fiorica F, et al. Preoperative radiotherapy for resectable rectal cancer: a meta-analysis. JAMA 2000;284:1008–15.

46. Kapiteijn E, Marijnen CA, Nagtegaal ID, et al. Preoperative radiotherapy combined with total mesorectal excision for resectable rectal cancer. N Engl J Med 2001;345:638–46.

47. Quirke P, Durdey P, Dixon MF, et al. Local recurrence of rectal adenocarcinoma due to inadequate surgical resection. Histopathological study of lateral tumour spread and surgical excision. Lancet 1986;2(8514):996–9.

48. MERCURY Study Group. Diagnostic accuracy of preoperative magnetic resonance imaging in predicting curative resection of rectal cancer: prospective observational study. BMJ 2006;333(7572):779.

49. Brown G, Radcliffe AG, Newcombe RG, et al. Preoperative assessment of prognostic factors in rectal cancer using high-resolution magnetic resonance imaging. Br J Surg 2003;90(3):355–64.

50. Brown G, Richards CJ, Newcombe RG, et al. Rectal carcinoma: thin-section MR imaging for staging in 28 patients. Radiology 1999;211:215–22.

51. Rao SX, Zeng MS, Chen CZ, et al. The value of diffusion-weighted imaging in combination with T2-weighted imaging for rectal cancer detection. Eur J Radiol 2008;65(2):299–303.

52. Kilickesmez O, Atilla S, Soylu A, et al. Diffusion-weighted imaging of the rectosigmoid colon: preliminary findings. J Comput Assist Tomogr 2009;33(6): 863–6.

53. Hosonuma T, Tozaki M, Ichiba N, et al. Clinical usefulness of diffusion-weighted imaging using low and high b-values to detect rectal cancer. Magn Reson Med Sci 2006;5(4):173–7.

54. Soyer P, Lagadec M, Sirol M, et al. Free-breathing diffusion-weighted single-shot echo-planar MR imaging using parallel imaging (GRAPPA 2) and high b value for the detection of primary rectal adenocarcinoma. Cancer Imaging 2010;10(1):32–9.

55. Ono K, Ochiai R, Yoshida T, et al. Comparison of diffusion-weighted MRI and 2-[fluorine-18]-fluoro-2-deoxy-D-glucose positron emission tomography (FDG-PET) for detecting primary colorectal cancer and regional lymph node metastases. J Magn Reson Imaging 2009;29(2):336–40.

56. Barbaro B, Vitale R, Leccisotti L, et al. Restaging locally advanced rectal cancer with MR imaging after chemoradiation therapy. Radiographics 2010; 30(3):699–716.

57. Kim CK, Park BK. Update of prostate magnetic resonance imaging at 3 T. J Comput Assist Tomogr 2008; 32(2):163–72.

58. Cornfeld DM, Weinreb JC. MR imaging of the prostate: 1.5T versus 3T. Magn Reson Imaging Clin N Am 2007;15(3):433–48.

59. Hricak H, White S, Vigneron D, et al. Carcinoma of the prostate gland: MR imaging with pelvic phased-array coils versus integrated endorectal–pelvic phased-array coils. Radiology 1994; 193(3):703–9.

60. Kim CK, Park BK, Kim B. Diffusion-weighted MRI at 3 T for the evaluation of prostate cancer. AJR Am J Roentgenol 2010;194:1461–9.

61. Koh DM, Collins DJ. Diffusion-weighted MRI in the body: applications and challenges in oncology. AJR Am J Roentgenol 2007;188:1622–35.

62. Lovett K, Rifkin MD, McCue PA, et al. MR imaging characteristics of noncancerous lesions of the prostate. J Magn Reson Imaging 1992;2(1):35–9.

63. Helpap B, Egevad L. Correlation of modified Gleason grading with pT stage of prostatic carcinoma after radical prostatectomy. Anal Quant Cytol Histol 2008;30:1–7.

64. DeSouza NM, Reinsberg SA, Scurr ED, et al. Magnetic resonance imaging in prostate cancer: the value of apparent diffusion coefficients for identifying malignant nodules. Br J Radiol 2007;80:90–5.

65. Haider MA, van der Kwast TH, Tanguay J, et al. Combined T2-weighted and diffusion-weighted MRI for localization of prostate cancer. AJR Am J Roentgenol 2007;189:323–8.

66. Miao H, Fukatsu H, Ishigaki T. Prostate cancer detection with 3-T MRI: comparison of diffusion-weighted and T2-weighted imaging. Eur J Radiol 2007;61:297–302.

67. Kim CK, Park BK, Lee HM, et al. Value of diffusion-weighted imaging for the prediction of prostate cancer location at 3T using a phased-array coil: preliminary results. Invest Radiol 2007;42:842–7.

68. Kim CK, Park BK, Lee HM. Prediction of locally recurrent prostate cancer after radiation therapy: incremental value of 3T diffusion-weighted MRI. J Magn Reson Imaging 2009;29:391–7.

69. Kim CK, Park BK, Lee HM, et al. MRI techniques for prediction of local tumor progression after high-intensity focused ultrasonic ablation of prostate cancer. AJR Am J Roentgenol 2008;190:1180–6.

70. Park BK, Lee HM, Kim CK, et al. Lesion localization in patients with a previous negative transrectal ultrasound biopsy and persistently elevated prostate specific antigen level using diffusion-weighted imaging at three Tesla before rebiopsy. Invest Radiol 2008;43:789–93.

71. Tamada T, Sone T, Jo Y, et al. Apparent diffusion coefficient values in peripheral and transition zones of the prostate: comparison between normal and malignant prostatic tissues and correlation with histologic grade. J Magn Reson Imaging 2008;28:720–6.

72. Abou-El-Ghar ME, El-Assmy A, Refaie HF, et al. Bladder cancer: diagnosis with diffusion-weighted MR imaging in patients with gross hematuria. Radiology 2009;251:415–21.

73. Watanabe H, Kanematsu M, Kondo H, et al. Preoperative T staging of urinary bladder cancer: does diffusion-weighted MRI have supplementary value? AJR Am J Roentgenol 2009;192:1361–6.

74. Matsuki M, Inada Y, Tatsugami F, et al. Diffusion-weighted MR imaging for urinary bladder carcinoma: initial results. Eur Radiol 2007;17:201–4.

75. Takeuchi M, Sasaki S, Ito M, et al. Urinary bladder cancer: diffusion weighted MR imaging—accuracy for diagnosing T stage and estimating histologic grade. Radiology 2009;251:112–21.

76. El-Assmy A, Abou-El-Ghar ME, Mosbah A, et al. Bladder tumour staging: comparison of diffusion- and T2-weighted MR imaging. Eur Radiol 2009;19: 1575–81.

77. Whittaker CS, Coady A, Culver L, et al. Diffusion-weighted MR imaging of female pelvic tumors: a pictorial review. Radiographics 2009;29:759–78.

78. Tangjitgamol S, Manusirivithaya S, Jesadapatarakul S, et al. Lymph node size in uterine cancer: a revisit. Int J Gynecol Cancer 2006;16:1880–4.

79. Sumi M, Ichikawa Y, Nakamura T. Diagnostic ability of apparent diffusion coefficients for lymphomas and carcinomas in the pharynx. Eur Radiol 2007;17:2631–7.

80. Sumi M, Van Cauteren M, Nakamura T. MR microimaging of benign and malignant nodes in the neck. AJR Am J Roentgenol 2006;186:749–57.

81. Kim JH, Beets GL, Kim MJ, et al. High-resolution MR imaging for nodal staging in rectal cancer: are there any criteria in addition to the size? Eur J Radiol 2004; 52:78–83.

82. Lin G, Ho KC, Wang JJ, et al. Detection of lymph node metastasis in cervical and uterine cancers by diffusion-weighted magnetic resonance imaging at 3T. J Magn Reson Imaging 2008;28:128–35.

83. Nakai G, Matsuki M, Inada Y, et al. Detection and evaluation of pelvic lymph nodes in patients with gynecologic malignancies using body diffusion-weighted magnetic resonance imaging. J Comput Assist Tomogr 2008;32:764–8.

84. Roy C, Bierry G, Matau A, et al. Value of diffusion-weighted imaging to detect small malignant pelvic lymph nodes at 3 T. Eur Radiol 2010;20(8):1803–11.

85. Kimura I, Togashi K, Kawakami S, et al. Ovarian torsion: CT and MR imaging appearances. Radiology 1994;190(2):337–41.

86. Fujii S, Kaneda S, Kakite S, et al. Diffusion-weighted imaging findings of adnexal torsion: initial results. Eur J Radiol 2009. [Epub ahead of print].

87. Rha SE, Byun JY, Jung SE, et al. CT and MR imaging features of adnexal torsion. Radiographics 2002; 22(2):283–94.

88. Hiller N, Appelbaum L, Simanovsky N, et al. CT features of adnexal torsion. AJR Am J Roentgenol 2007;189(1):124–9.

89. Silvera S, Oppenheim C, Touzé E, et al. Spontaneous intracerebral hematoma on diffusion-weighted images: influence of T2-shine-through and T2-blackout effects. AJNR Am J Neuroradiol 2005;26:236–41.

90. Provenzale JM, Engelter ST, Petrella JR, et al. Use of MR exponential diffusion-weighted images to eradicate T2 "shine-through" effect. AJR Am J Roentgenol 1999;172:537–9.

91. Therasse P, Arbuck SG, Eisenhauer EA, et al. New guidelines to evaluate the response to treatment in solid tumors. J Natl Cancer Inst 2000;92(3): 205–16.

Diffusion-Weighted Magnetic Resonance Imaging for the Evaluation of Musculoskeletal Tumors

Flávia Martins Costa, MD*, Elisa Carvalho Ferreira, MD,
Evandro Miguelote Vianna, MD

KEYWORDS

- Diffusion-weighted imaging • Contrast enhancement
- Hyperintensity • Musculoskeletal tumor

MR imaging has become the diagnostic method of choice for preoperative and posttreatment staging of musculoskeletal (MSK) tumors because of the high resolution, tissue contrast, and multiplanar capability of this technique.

In addition, MR imaging offers several advantages when compared with other imaging methods in the evaluation and staging of soft tissue tumors. Several studies have demonstrated morphologic parameters such as size, margin demarcation, involvement of adjacent vital structures, homogeneity in signal intensity, and measurement of relaxation time as criteria to evaluate soft tissue tumors.[1] In accordance with these criteria, malignancy can be predicted with the following parameters (**Fig. 1**)[2]:

- Heterogeneous signal intensity in a T1 scan
- Tumor necrosis
- Bone or neurovascular involvement
- Mean diameter of more than 66 mm.

However, conventional MR imaging provides low specificity in the differential diagnosis of several MSK tumors because many of the lesions exhibit nonspecific characteristics. As a result, a correct histologic diagnosis is possible in only a quarter to one-third of cases.[2] Conventional MR imaging is unable to offer information about the extent of tumoral necrosis and the presence of viable cells, information that is crucial for the assessment of treatment response and prognosis. Therefore, advanced MR imaging techniques, such as diffusion-weighted imaging (DWI), are now used in association with conventional MR imaging with the objective of improving diagnostic accuracy and treatment evaluation. DWI allows quantitative and qualitative analyses of tissue cellularity and cell membrane integrity and has been widely used for tumor detection and characterization and to monitor treatment response (**Fig. 2**).[3]

The tumor tissue is usually more cellular when compared with other tissues and tends to appear at high signal intensities (restricted diffusion) when DWI is used (**Fig. 3**).[4]

The tissue contrast obtained using DWI is different from that obtained using conventional MR imaging, which facilitates the detection of soft tissue and bone tumors, particularly bone metastasis.[5] In fact, previous studies have concluded that DWI is an extremely sensitive method for identifying bone metastases and is

Clínica Multi Imagem e Ressonância, Clínica de Diagnóstico por Imagem, Av. das Américas, 4666, 325, 22640 - 902, Barra da Tijuca, Rio de Janeiro, Brazil
* Corresponding author.
E-mail address: flavia26rio@hotmail.com

Magn Reson Imaging Clin N Am 19 (2011) 159–180
doi:10.1016/j.mric.2010.10.007
1064-9689/11/$ – see front matter © 2011 Elsevier Inc. All rights reserved.

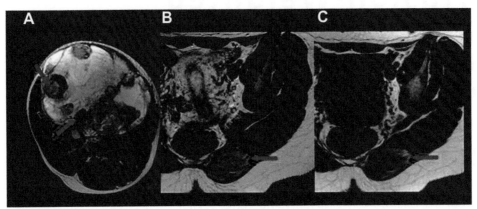

Fig. 1. The evaluation of soft tissue tumors with conventional MR imaging using morphologic parameters. (*A*) Axial T2-weighted image. A huge tumor inside the muscle with a necrotic center and many solid nodules on the wall (*arrows*), which suggests a malignant tumor. This is a synovial sarcoma. (*B*) Axial T2-weighted image. (*C*) Axial T1-weighted image. A solid tumor hyperintense on T2-weighed image (*B, arrow*) and isointense on T1-weighted image (*C, arrow*) inside the muscle, with fat surrounding it, which is highly suggestive of a hemangioma. However, in several cases, conventional MR imaging presents low specificity in the differential diagnosis because many of the lesions present nonspecific characteristics.

superior to both positron emission tomography (PET) and scintigraphy in terms of detection capability.[6] The detection of bone metastasis is important for cancer staging and in the determination of treatment strategy, and some reports have demonstrated whole body DWI to be highly sensitive and efficient for this purpose.

Tumors differ in cellularity characteristics, and this difference is useful in determining their histologic composition. It has been reported that DWI can differentiate benign from malignant soft tissue tumors (**Fig. 4**).

The malignant tumors have more cellularity than benign tumors and tend to have a more restricted diffusion (**Fig. 5**).[7]

In accordance with this finding, perfusion-corrected DWI has demonstrated potential in differentiating benign from malignant soft tissue

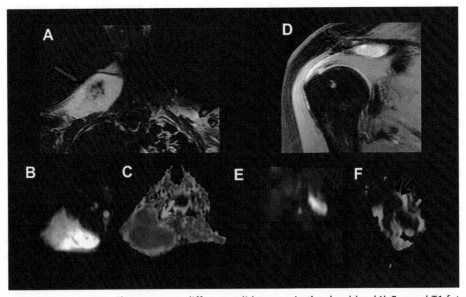

Fig. 2. Tumor characterization. There are two different solid tumors in the shoulder. (*A*) Coronal T1 fat suppression contrast-enhanced image. The bigger tumor has heterogeneous contrast enhancement with edema surrounding it (*arrow*). (*B*) Axial diffusion-weighted image. (*C*) In the axial ADC map, the tumor tissue presents facilitated diffusion (*arrow*) and PIDC value = 1.52×10^{-3} mm^2/s, suggesting benign tumor (desmoid tumor). (*D*) Coronal T1 fat suppression contrast-enhanced image. The smaller tumor has homogeneous contrast enhancement (*arrow*). (*E*) Axial diffusion-weighted image. (*F*) In the axial ADC map the tumor presents restricted diffusion (*arrow*) with a PIDC = 0.80×10^{-3} mm^2/s, suggesting malignant tumor (leiomyosarcoma grade 2).

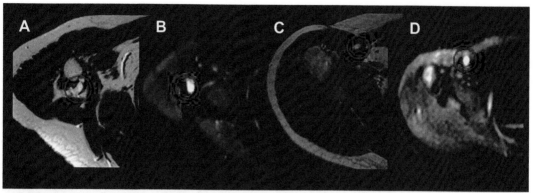

Fig. 3. Tumor detection. A grade 2 periosteal chondrosarcoma in the humeral shaft. (*A*) Axial T2-weighted image before surgery. There is a small lesion hyperintense on the image (*circle*) in the posterior periosteum of the humeral shaft. (*B*) Axial diffusion-weighted image. The tumor is hyperintense on DWI sequence (*circle*), easier to detect because of the high tissue contrast. (*C*) Axial T2-weighted image 6 months after the surgery. There is a very small recidive of the tumor in the surgical site (*circle*), which is difficult to find on conventional MR imaging. (*D*) Axial diffusion-weighted image. The tumoral recidive shows hyperintensity on diffusion-weighted image sequence (*circle*), which facilitates the detection.

masses.[8] In addition, DWI is also used for differentiating between chronic expanding hematomas (CEHs) and malignant soft tissue tumors.[9] CEHs are frequently misdiagnosed as malignant soft tissue tumors because of their morphologic characteristics, which include large size, slow progressive enlargement, and heterogeneous signal intensity on conventional MR imaging. DWI has also been shown to be an additional tool for differentiating vertebral fracture caused by osteoporotic collapse with bone marrow edema as well as pathologic collapse caused by tumor infiltration or metastatic disease.[10]

On the other hand, some investigators have reported overlapping apparent diffusion coefficient (ADC) values in benign and malignant soft tissue tumors, which consequently could not be used to differentiate them.[11] This overlapping is likely because of the fact that ADC values can be affected by cellularity and the extracellular matrix.[7] For example, myxoid matrix is widely seen in the interstitial spaces in many soft tissue tumors, and this presence can influence the ADC values (**Fig. 6**).

As a result, myxoid tumors will have significantly higher ADC values than nonmyxoid tumors. It makes no difference if the tumor is benign or malignant.[7]

DWI can also be used to monitor tumor response to treatment, most likely because effective anticancer therapy results in changes in the tumor microenvironment, resulting in an increase

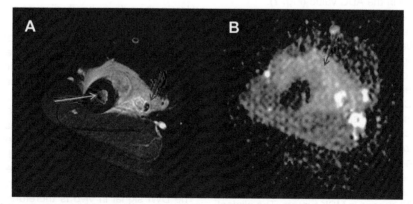

Fig. 4. An indeterminate palpable soft tissue mass for 2 months located inside the muscle in the right arm in a 16-year-old girl. (*A*) Axial T1-weighted fat suppression postcontrast image. The tumor presents diffuse enhancement encasing the neurovascular bundle (*red arrow*) and invading the periosteal surface with edema in the medullar region (*blue arrow*). (*B*) Axial ADC map. The tumor tissue has facilitated diffusion on the ADC map (*arrow*) with PIDC = 1.9×10^{-3} mm^2/s, suggesting a benign tumor (ossificans myositis).

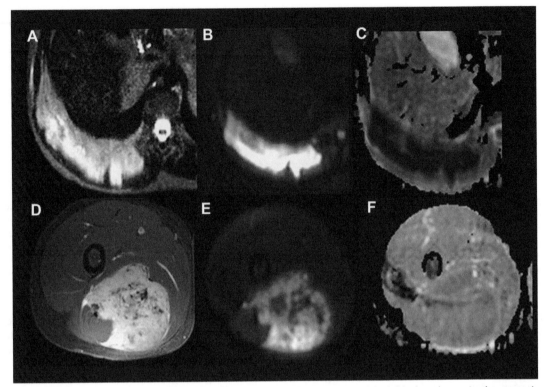

Fig. 5. The qualitative analysis of DWI. (*A*) Axial T2-weighted image. Non—Hodgkin lymphoma in the posterior ribs in a 52-year-old man, hyperintense on T2-weighted image. (*B*) Axial diffusion-weighted image. Tumor has high cellularity (non—Hodgkin lymphoma) and less extracellular space and presents very high signal intensity on diffusion-weighted image (b = 600 s/mm^2) sequence. (*C*) Very low signal intensity on the ADC map (restricted diffusion). (*D*) Axial T2 fat suppression image. A desmoid tumor inside the posterior muscle compartment of the thigh, hyperintense on T2-weighted fat suppression image. (*E*) Axial diffusion-weighted image. Tumor with less cellularity and more extracellular space shows high signal intensity on diffusion-weighted image (b = 600 s/mm^2) sequence. (*F*) Intermediate to high signal intensity on the ADC map (facilitated diffusion).

in the diffusion of water molecules and a consequent increase in the ADC value (**Fig. 7**).[4]

Furthermore, DWI has been used to provide information regarding cellular changes related to cytotoxic treatment in soft tissue sarcomas.[12] Some investigators have suggested that it could be possible to evaluate the response of osteosarcoma to chemotherapy using DWI, considering that the ADC values of viable tumor tissue and tumor necrosis differ significantly.[9,13] This information is a crucial prognostic factor for patients with osteosarcoma.

This article provides a short discussion of the technical aspects of DWI, particularly the quantitative and qualitative interpretation of diffusion-weighted (DW) images in MSK tumors. The clinical application of DWI for tumor detection, characterization, differentiation of tumor tissue from non-tumor tissue, and assessment of treatment response are emphasized.

TECHNICAL ASPECTS

Herein, the authors briefly discuss some important concepts regarding the specificity of DWI in the MSK system. However, for a detailed explanation of the physics of DWI see the article elsewhere in this issue. See the article by Figueiredo and colleagues elsewhere in this issues for further exploration of this topic.

DWI exploits the random motion of water molecules in the body, which is classically called the Brownian motion. In biologic tissues, the movement of water molecules is restricted because their motion is modified and limited by their interactions with cellular membranes and macromolecules.[14] The DWI signal in vivo is therefore derived from the motion of water protons in extracellular, intra-cellular, and intravascular spaces.[15]

DWI yields qualitative and quantitative information that reflects tissue cellularity and cell membrane

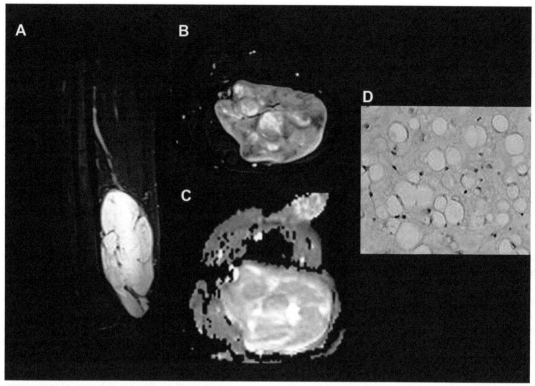

Fig. 6. A huge myxoid liposarcoma in the posterior muscular compartment of the thigh. (*A*) Sagittal short tau inversion recovery (STIR) image. The tumor looks like a cystic lesion on the STIR sequence, but (*B*) axial T1-weighted fat suppression postcontrast image shows contrast enhancement. (*C*) Axial ADC map. The tumor tissue has facilitated diffusion on the ADC map, with PIDC = 2.56×10^{-3} mm^2/s, probably because of the myxoid matrix in the extracellular space. These types of tumors will have significantly higher ADC and PIDC values than nonmyxoid malignant solid tumors. (*D*) On histologic evaluation, the final diagnosis was a myxoid liposarcoma (Hematoxylin-eosin [H&E], original magnification ×100).

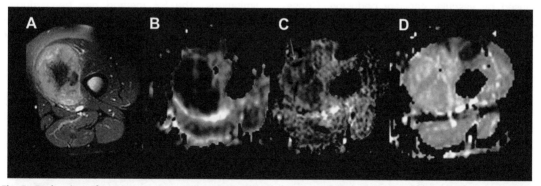

Fig. 7. Evaluation of response to mesenchymal chondrosarcoma using DWI. (*A*) Axial T1-weighted fat suppression postcontrast image. There is a big mass with heterogeneous contrast enhancement located inside the muscle in the thigh. (*B*) Axial ADC map (before treatment). The tumor presents very low signal intensity on the ADC map (restricted diffusion) and PIDC value = 0.89×10^{-3} mm^2/s. (*C*) Axial ADC map (3 months later). The tumor presents areas of intermediate to high signal intensity (facilitated diffusion) inside the tumor (*red arrow*) and a few areas of low signal intensity (restricted diffusion) (*blue arrow*) suggesting viable cells. (*D*) Axial ADC map (9 months later). The tumor presents high signal intensity on the ADC map (facilitated diffusion) and PIDC value = 2.8×10^{-3} mm^2/s suggesting good response to the treatment.

integrity, which complements the morphologic information obtained by conventional MR imaging.[3] Thus, the data obtained from DWI must be interpreted using qualitative and quantitative approaches.

Qualitative analysis is achieved via visual assessment of the relative tissue signal attenuation of both the DW image and the ADC parametric map. The visual assessment of DW image enables tissue characterization based on differences in water diffusion and is performed by observing the relative attenuation of the signal intensity of images obtained at different b values. In a heterogeneous tumor, for instance, the more cystic or necrotic fraction of the tumor will show greater signal attenuation on high−b value images because water diffusion is less restricted, whereas the more cellular solid tumor areas will continue to show a relatively high signal intensity (**Fig. 8**).

By contrast, on the ADC parametric map, visual assessment reveals a trend opposite to that of DW images: areas of restricted diffusion in highly cellular areas appear as low signal intensity areas compared with less cellular areas, which have a higher signal intensity (see **Fig. 5**).[4] Quantitative analysis is performed by calculating the conventional ADC value and/or perfusion-insensitive diffusion coefficient (PIDC) value. The conventional ADC value is calculated using a biexponential function from DWI, which includes low b values (b = 0−600 s/mm^2), or can be obtained alternatively by drawing regions of interest (ROIs) on the ADC map. However, an exponential function fitted only through the high b values (b = 300, 450, and 600s/mm^2) can be used to describe the PIDC value. This measurement excludes the initial reduction of signal intensity that is probably caused by vascular capillary perfusion. Consequently, for large b values, perfusion effects tend to be canceled out. The PIDC map may provide more accurate information about tumor tissue cellularity by minimizing vascular contributions, which are higher in malignant tumors (**Fig. 9**).[1]

The two most important components of signal attenuation on DWI in soft tissue tumors are diffusion of water molecules in the extracellular space and the perfusion fraction.[8] The latter tends to be higher in malignant tumors than in benign tumors and has more influence on the ADC values in malignant soft tissue tumors than in benign tumors. Based on this, the PIDC value is routinely calculated to differentiate benign from malignant solid soft tissue tumors, considering that the size of the extracellular space is the most important component influencing this measurement in soft tissue tumors.[8]

To maximize lesion visualization and characterization, diffusion-weighted MR imaging should be performed with sufficient degrees of diffusion weighting (by appropriate choices of b values), with consideration given to the anatomic region, tissue composition, and pathologic processes, which may require the customization of DW MR imaging protocols for different tumor types and locations. Indeed, in the MSK system, the geometric parameters of the imaging sequence must be flexible in terms of image positioning and field of view (FOV) to compensate for the great variety of tumor shapes and sites in the extremities and trunk.[11]

Several types of DW sequences have been described (**Table 1**). The range of imaging techniques includes conventional spin-echo (SE) and stimulated echo, fast SE, gradient-echo (eg, steady-state free precession), echo planar imaging (EPI), and line scan diffusion imaging. Each of these techniques has its advantages and limitations. The SE method has been studied extensively in phantom experiments, animal models, and brain imaging and allows for a precise

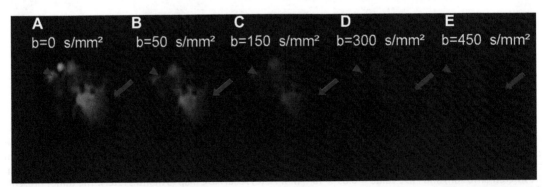

| A | B | C | D | E |
| b=0 s/mm^2 | b=50 s/mm^2 | b=150 s/mm^2 | b=300 s/mm^2 | b=450 s/mm^2 |

Fig. 8. (*A−E*) Signal attenuation of a heterogeneous tumor, with necrotic portion on axial diffusion images with different b values. The more cystic or necrotic fraction of the tumor (*long arrows*) shows greater signal attenuation on high−b value images because water diffusion is less restricted, whereas the more cellular solid tumor areas (*arrowhead*) will continue to show relatively high signal intensity.

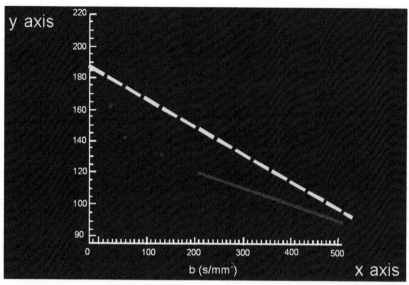

Fig. 9. DWI-Graph shows signal attenuation with increasing b values. Conventional ADC (*dashed line*) calculated with b values of 0 and 600 s/mm^2; PIDC (*solid line*) calculated with high b values (300, 450, and 600 s/mm^2); the initial reduction (*dots*) in signal intensity is probably caused by vascular capillary perfusion. For large b values, perfusion effects tend to be canceled out. The PIDC may provide more accurate information about tumor tissue cellularity by minimizing vascular contribution, which is higher in malignant tumors. y axis, logarithm of relative signal intensities; x axis, different b values.

calculation of the ADC value. The disadvantages of the SE method are long acquisition times and vulnerability to motion artifacts.[16] The most commonly used acquisition strategy for DWI is single or multishot EPI because of its efficiency in terms of scan time. The rapid acquisition of

this technique makes it less sensitive to patient motion while allowing for large volume coverage. EPI sequences usually achieve a comparably high signal-to-noise ratio. However, echo planar (EP) DW images are prone to artifacts, particularly magnetic susceptibility artifacts, especially at tissue interfaces such as those encountered between air and soft tissue or bone and soft tissue. The EP DW images are also prone to geometric distortions created by eddy currents, particularly in large FOVs.[17]

There are some practical aspects to be considered at the workstation when analyzing soft tissue tumors. First, depending on whether the tumor being evaluated is solid, cystic, or necrotic, there are some technical differences concerning the placement of the ROI for quantitative analysis. On predominantly solid tumors, the ROI must be placed in the most solid and homogeneous portion of the lesion, as selected from corresponding morphologic imaging, and cystic and necrotic areas should be avoided. The evaluation of cystic and necrotic lesions must be performed differently, taking into account the tumor content.

CLINICAL APPLICATION

Multiple studies have described the potential application of DWI in tumor detection, characterization, and assessment of treatment response. First, the authors emphasize the usefulness of this technique

Table 1 Summarized DWI protocol	
DWI Protocol	
TA	1:14/3:36
Field of view (cm)	250–180
TR (millisecond)	2200
Matrix size (voxel)	128 × 128
TE (millisecond)	75
Echo planar imaging factor	128
b factor (s/mm^2)	0, 50, 150, 300, 450, 600
Parallel imaging factor	2 GRAPPA
NEX (the number of excitations)	3
Section thickness (mm)	7–5
Directions of motion probing gradients	Phase, frequency, and slice

Abbreviations: TA, time acquisition; TE, echo time; TR, repetition time.

in tumor characterization, particularly in differentiating benign from malignant MSK tumors.

DWI has previously been used to differentiate benign from malignant soft tissue tumors by analyzing perfusion-corrected DW MR images, and a significant difference between the true diffusion coefficients of benign and malignant tumors was found ($P<.05$).[8] However, this study also noted that not all benign tumors have a large extracellular space and not all malignant soft tissue tumors are more cellular than benign soft tissue tumors.

The authors performed a study between January 2006 and August 2007, which was presented at the meeting of the Radiological Society of North America, 2007, in which 44 patients with MSK tumors (Table 2) with no previous surgical procedures or adjuvant treatment underwent MR examination, and the lesions were biopsied. The exclusion criteria were lesions with classic appearances on MR images (lipomas, hemangiomas, ganglions, and synovial cysts) and highly necrotic lesions surrounded by edema because edema likely contaminates the tumor tissue and consequently increases the diffusion coefficient value. Qualitative (ADC map) and quantitative analyses (PIDC value) of these tumors were obtained. A significantly increased PIDC value was obtained in benign tumors ([1.67 ± 0.18] × 10^{-3} mm²/s) compared with malignant tumors ([1.07 ± 0.46] × 10^{-3} mm²/s, $P = .0011$). These findings are consistent with previous work (Fig. 10).[8]

A type of border for PIDC values of approximately 1.1 × 10^{-3} mm²/s was observed, which separated malignant from benign solid tumors. Together with morphologic characteristics

analyzed using conventional MR imaging, this border has been useful in differentiating these tumors in the authors' clinical practice.

Based on the literature and their own clinical routine, the authors discuss the DWI characteristics of various types of MSK tumors.

Myxoid Tumors

In the authors' study, among benign and malignant tumors, the highest PIDC values were obtained from myxoid tumors (myxoma, myxoid liposarcoma, and low-grade myxofibrosarcoma), with a mean PIDC value of 2.92 × 10^{-3} mm²/s. These values reflect the high mucin and low collagen contents of the tumor, representing a lesion composed of a large amount of water, which has been confirmed by histologic analyses.[7] Many investigators have observed that the diffusion coefficients of these tumors are higher than those of nonmyxoid tumors because the myxoid matrix influences the diffusion coefficient in both benign and malignant soft tissue tumors.[5,7,8,18] Maeda and colleagues[7] concluded that ADC values overlap greatly between benign and malignant soft tissue tumors, so these values might not be useful for differentiating these tumors. Consequently, myxoid tumors, particularly myxoid liposarcomas, should be considered the main diagnostic hypothesis whenever an MSK tumor with the noncontrast conventional MR imaging characteristics of a cystic lesion is encountered and in which the contrast-enhanced MR images demonstrate a solid lesion and the DWI analyses show high PIDC values with facilitated diffusion on the ADC map.

Table 2
MR evaluation of 44 patients with histologically proven musculoskletal tumors

Malignant Tumors (n = 21)		Benign Tumors (n = 23)	
Malignant fibrohistiocytoma	1	Ossificans myositis	1
Nondifferentiated sarcoma (high grade)	3	Benign schwannoma	2
Myxoid liposarcoma (low grade)	1	Calcified fibrous tumor	1
Myxofibrosarcoma (low grade)	1	Hematoma (chronic)	1
PNET	1	Neurofibroma	2
Lymphoma non-Hodgkin	2	Myxoma	1
Clear cell sarcoma	1	Benign fibrous histiocytoma	1
Metastasis (prostate, stomach)	2	Benign leiomyoma	1
Ewing sarcoma	1	Desmoid tumor	7
Osteosarcomas	3	Hemangioma	4
Leiomyosarcoma	1	Fibrous dysplasia	1
Epithelioid sarcoma	1	Giant cell tumor	1
Synoviosarcoma	3	—	—

Abbreviation: PNET, primitive neuroectodermic tumor.

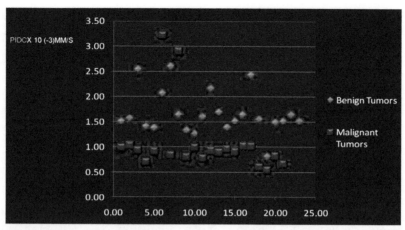

Fig. 10. Most malignant tumors have a PIDC value equal to or less than 1 mm²/s. There are only 2 exceptions of myxoid tumors, with a PIDC value greater than 2.5 mm²/s. Most benign tumors have a PIDC value ranging from 2.5 mm²/s down to 1.3 mm²/s. There is only one exception of a giant cell tumor with a PIDC value less than 1 mm²/s. PIDC values for benign tumors = $(1.67 \pm 0.18) \times 10^{-3}$ mm²/s and malignant tumors = $(1.07 \pm 0.46) \times 10^{-3}$ mm²/s (T test , $P = .0011$).

Myxoid liposarcomas account for 50% of all liposarcomas. Histologic evaluation has demonstrated that these tumors contain less than 10% mature fat, which accounts for their low signal intensity on T1-weighted sequences and differentiates them from the high signal intensity encountered in other liposarcomas.[19] From August 2007 until the present, the authors have performed quantitative and qualitative DWI analyses of several myxoid liposarcomas, and all of them demonstrated high PIDC values (mean PIDC value = 2.82×10^{-3} mm²/s) and high facilitated diffusion on the ADC map. An understanding of the MR image appearances and DWI characteristics of these tumors may permit it to be considered in the differential diagnosis of the indeterminate soft tissue mass (**Fig. 11**).

Small Round Blue Cell Tumors

Small round blue cell (SRBC) tumors are a group of undifferentiated aggressive embryonal tumors, which include neuroblastoma, rhabdomyosarcoma, non–Hodgkin lymphoma, and the Ewing family of tumors. These tumors have similar histologic features and immunohistochemistry, so alternative techniques are required to diagnosis them. Accurate diagnoses of these cancers is critical for the correct administration of therapy and for avoiding unnecessary patient procedures. At present, there is no readily available tool for real-time diagnosis.

Malignant lymphomas have characteristically low ADC values in the brain,[20] head and neck,

and retroperitoneal regions.[21] Nagata and colleagues[18] have shown that soft tissue tumors have this property as well. Because of their high cellularity and nucleocytoplasmic ratio, lymphomas have a high signal intensity on DW images. In addition, lymphomas have lower ADC values than other tumor types in different body regions (**Fig. 12**).[21–24]

In the authors' experience, these tumors also tend to have lower PIDC values and restricted diffusion on the ADC map than other malignant MSK tumors (**Fig. 13**).

The authors studied 15 patients with histologically proven SRBC soft tissue and bone tumors (trunk and extremities) and 15 patients with malignant non-SRBC (NSRBC) tumors with no previous surgical procedures or adjuvant treatment. All the patients underwent MR examination, and lesions were biopsied (**Table 3**). Malignant NSRBC tumors had significantly increased PIDC values (mean PIDC = $[0.98 \pm 0.21] \times 10^{-3}$ mm²/s) when compared with SRBC tumors (mean PIDC = $[0.64 \pm 0.18] \times 10^{-3}$ mm²/s). In addition, it was observed that SRBC tumors tend to contain tissue with a relatively uniform population of SRBCs, which have less extracellular space and typically smaller PIDC values than other NSRBC malignant tumors. In conclusion, in the differential diagnosis of a tumor with restricted diffusion on the ADC map and very low PIDC value, SRBC tumors should be the main diagnostic hypothesis. However, this conclusion must be corroborated by morphologic characteristics obtained using conventional MR imaging and other imaging methods.

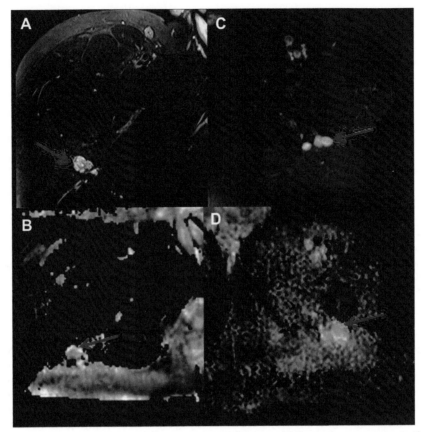

Fig. 11. Follow-up examinations of two different patients after myxoid liposarcoma surgery on the hip. (*A, C*) Axial T1-weighted fat suppression contrast-enhanced images. (*B, D*) Axial ADC map. There are two solid nodules on the surgical site in (*A, C; arrows*) with contrast enhancement. Analyzing the ADC map, both lesions have facilitated diffusion (*B, D; arrows*), but the PIDC value of the tumor in (*D*) is 3.1×10^{-3} mm²/s and in (*B*) is 1.9×10^{-3} mm²/s. The histopathologic analysis showed tumoral recidive in (*D*) and postsurgical neuroma in (*B*). The myxoid tumor had very facilitated diffusion with a PIDC more than 2.5×10^{-3} mm²/s.

Fibroblastic/Myofibroblastic and Fibrohistiocytic Tumors

Of the soft tissue tumors, benign fibrous and fibro-histiocytic tumors are the most commonly encountered tumors in clinical practice and are seen in all age groups.[2] These tumors usually have typical morphologic characteristics on conventional MR imaging. For example, MR imaging findings in aggressive fibromatosis typically include bands of low signal intensity across all sequences and uniform to moderate contrast enhancement after gadolinium administration, but sometimes a benign lesion can be misdiagnosed as a malignant tumor (**Fig. 14**).[25]

In a study that the authors conducted between January 2006 and January 2008, 21 patients with histologically proven fibroblastic/myofibroblastic and fibrohistiocytic soft tissue tumors (trunk and extremities), who had received no previous adjuvant treatment, underwent MR examination. In accordance with the World Health Organization classification, tumors were classified as benign (n = 5), intermediate (n = 9), or malignant (n = 8). The mean PIDC value of benign/intermediate tumors (mean ± standard deviation [SD] = [1.56 ± 0.25] $\times$ 10^{-3} mm²/s) was significantly different from that of malignant tumors (mean ± SD = [0.89 ± 0.15] $\times$ 10^{-3} mm²/s) (*P*<.001) (**Fig. 15**).

It was also found that there was no significant difference (*P*>.01) between the mean PIDC values of benign and intermediate tumors. Benign and intermediate tumors presented with facilitated diffusion, whereas malignant tumors presented with restricted diffusion on the ADC map. When used alongside conventional MR imaging, these parameters are useful in the differential diagnosis of an indeterminate mass

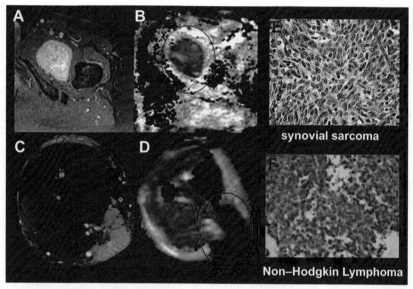

Fig. 12. Indeterminate soft tissues masses. Tumor characterization. (*A, C*) Axial T1-weighted fat suppression contrast-enhanced images of two different indeterminate soft tissue masses. (*B, D*) The respective axial ADC maps. There are two indeterminate soft tissue tumors with homogeneous contrast enhancement inside the adductor musculature in (*A*) and in the subcutaneous of the leg in (*C*). There is no specific characteristic on conventional MR imaging, and on analyzing the ADC map, both tumors present with restricted diffusion (*B, D; circles*) and PIDC = 0.92×10^{-3} mm²/s (*B*) and 0.58×10^{-3} mm²/s (*D*), suggesting malignant tumor. However, in (*D*) the PIDC value is less than 0.70×10^{-3} mm/s², which is commonly seen in hypercellular tumors, such as SRBC tumor. The histopathologic analysis showed synovial sarcoma in (*A*) and non–Hodgkin lymphoma in (*C*). (*E*, H&E, original magnification ×400; *F*, H&E, original magnification ×100)

with morphologic characteristics of a fibrous tissue tumor (**Fig. 16**).

Necrotic Lesions

Necrotic masses can either be malignant tumors or benign masses, such as abscesses and/or hematomas. Therefore, care must be taken during imaging to differentiate a hemorrhagic malignant soft tissue tumor from a hematoma. Previous work concluded that it is possible to differentiate CEHs from malignant soft tissue tumors using DWI.[9] The authors think that it is not possible to differentiate abscesses and/or hematomas from malignant tumors using PIDC values from the solid parts of tumors. This inability to differentiate is probably because of the edema that surrounds necrotic lesions, which likely contaminates the tumor tissue. Previous reports have shown that DWI analysis of brain abscesses usually reveals a markedly reduced ADC in the necrotic center.[26,27] For this reason, ADC maps are of great value in distinguishing abscesses from neoplasms. Neoplasms have more facilitated diffusion compared with abscesses, which tend to have more restricted diffusion in their necrotic portions. In addition, the authors have observed

that highly malignant tumors tend to have more restricted diffusion on the ADC map in the solid wall of the tumor, which has higher cellularity. On the other hand, acute and subacute hematomas have typical morphologic characteristics on conventional MR imaging and present with restricted diffusion on the ADC map in the central portion of the lesion. Therefore, the authors think that it is possible to differentiate abscesses and hematomas from malignant tumors using the ADC value from the necrotic portion of the tumor (**Fig. 17**).

Cartilaginous Lesions

Previous reports indicate that malignant cartilaginous tumors have higher ADC values than benign tumors.[18] The authors have found high PIDC values and facilitated diffusion on the ADC map in benign and malignant cartilaginous tumors, likely because of the high chondroid matrix content of these tumors (**Fig. 18**).

The authors have observed only one type of cartilaginous tumor, the mesenchymal chondrosarcoma, with a low PIDC value (0.89×10^{-3} mm²/s) and restricted diffusion on the ADC map (see **Fig. 7**). Histopathologically, this tumor has

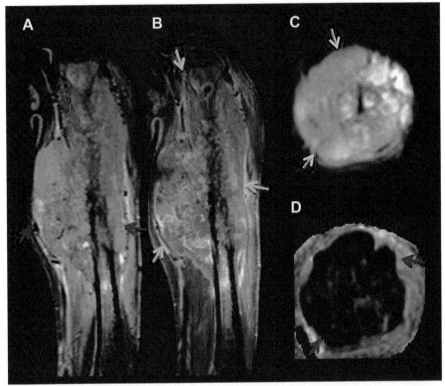

Fig. 13. Primitive neuroectodermal tumor (PNET) in the humerus in a 16-year-old boy. (*A*) Coronal STIR MR image shows a large heterogeneous hyperintense intraosseous mass (*arrows*). (*B*) Coronal T1-weighted fat suppressed image after contrast injection shows a large solid heterogeneous enhancing intraosseous mass (*arrows*). (*C*) Axial DWI shows hyperintense signal intensity tumor (*arrows*). (*D*) ADC map shows restricted diffusion of the tumor (*arrows*) and PIDC value = 0.67×10^{-3} mm²/s.

cellular zones composed of undifferentiated small cells and chondroid zones with a bimorphic appearance that is virtually pathognomonic in most cases.[28] However, the usefulness of

Table 3 MR evaluation of 30 patients with histologically proven SRBC and NSRBC soft tissue and bone tumors	
SRBC Tumors (n = 15)	
Ewing sarcoma	5
Non–Hodgkin lymphoma	6
Rhabdomyosarcoma	1
PNET	3
NSRBC Tumors (n = 15)	
Malignant fibrohistiocytoma	6
Nondifferentiated sarcoma (high grade)	3
Osteosarcoma	4
Synoviosarcoma	2

diffusion in the diagnosis of cartilaginous tumors requires further validation.

Giant Cell Tumors

Nagata and colleagues[5] found low ADC values in giant cell tumors (GCTs) of the tendon sheath and diffuse-type GCTs. GCTs of the tendon sheath contain histiocytic mononuclear cells, multinucleated giant cells, xanthoma cells, and collagenous strands. The diffuse-type GCT is characterized by synovial villonodular proliferation with hemosiderin pigmentation and stromal infiltration of histiocytes and giant cells.[29–31] In bone GCTs, histologic features include a moderately vascularized network of round, oval, or spindle-shaped stromal cells and multinucleated giant cells.[32,33] These characteristics probably contribute to reducing the extracellular space and the concomitant decrease in ADC value. In the authors' experience, soft tissue and bone GCTs tend to have low PIDC values and restricted diffusion on the ADC map. These

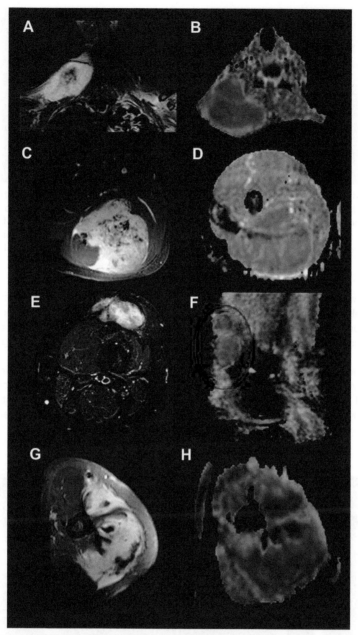

Fig. 14. Desmoid tumors. (*A*) Coronal T1-weighted fat suppression contrast-enhanced image. (*C, E, G*) Axial T1-weighted fat suppression contrast-enhanced image. (*B, D, H*) Axial ADC map. (*F*) Sagittal ADC map. A huge tumor with heterogeneous contrast enhancement with edema surrounding it (*A*), with facilitated diffusion (*B*) and a PIDC = 1.52×10^{-3} mm^2/s. There are no bands of low signal intensity across all sequences inside this tumor, which is characteristic of desmoid tumors. (*C, E, G*) Tumors with heterogeneous contrast enhancement and many bands of low signal intensity across all sequences, suggesting fibrous tumors. These tumors present facilitated diffusion in (*D, F, H*) and their PIDC = 1.65×10^{-3} mm^2/s (*D*), 1.55×10^{-3} mm^2/s (*F, circle*), and 1.40×10^{-3} mm^2/s (*H*).

parameters could be useful in the diagnosis of these tumors and in the management of local recurrence after surgery by allowing for the differentiation of postsurgical fibrosis from reciditive tumor (**Fig. 19**).

MALIGNANT BONE DISEASE

DWI performed regionally or as whole body imaging has been shown to have a high diagnostic accuracy for the identification of bone metastases

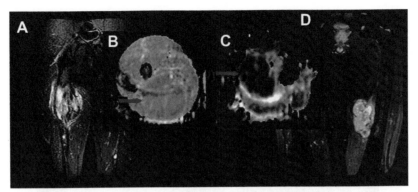

Fig. 15. Fibrous and fibrohistiocytic tumors. Tumor characterization. (*A, D*) Coronal T1-weighted fat suppression contrast-enhanced images and (*B, C*) axial ADC maps. There are two different fibrous tumors with similar characteristics on conventional MR imaging (*A, D*). The tumor on the left presents facilitated diffusion in (*B, arrow*) and a PIDC = 1.65×10^{-3} mm²/s, suggesting benign tumor (desmoid tumor). The tumor on the right presents restricted diffusion on the ADC map (*C, arrow*) and PIDC = 0.89×10^{-3} mm²/s (malignant fibrous histiocytoma).

when combined with conventional MR imaging. Goudarzi and colleagues[6] concluded that DWI could visualize more metastatic lesions and detect smaller metastases that PET or bone scintigraphy. The detection of bone metastasis is crucial for cancer staging and to determine the appropriate treatment strategy.[6]

Acute vertebral collapse is a common clinical problem in elderly patients and usually results from osteoporosis or metastasis.[16] Previous reports have concluded that both qualitative and quantitative DW MR imagings are effective additional tools for differentiating malignant from benign vertebral fractures.[16]

In osteosarcoma and Ewing sarcoma, the degree of necrosis after a course of induction chemotherapy is a prognostic factor for an event-free survival.[34] Consequently, a noninvasive

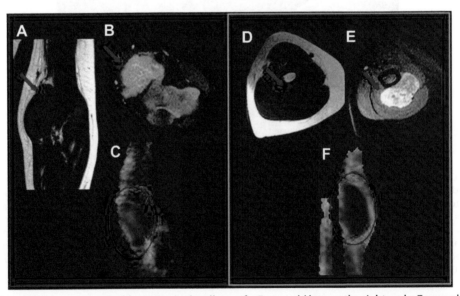

Fig. 16. Two similar painless palpable masses in the elbow of a 5-year-old boy on the right and a 7-year-old girl on the left. (*A*) Coronal and (*D*) axial T1-weighted images show intramuscular tumors isointense to muscle (*A, D; arrows*). (*B, E*) Axial T1-weighted contrast-enhanced images show homogeneous contrast enhancement in both tumors (*B, E; arrows*). (*C, F*) Sagittal ADC maps show that the tumor on the left presents facilitated diffusion (*C, circle*) and its PIDC = 1.6×10^{-3} mm²/s (desmoid tumor) and the tumor on the left presents restricted diffusion (*F, circle*) and its PIDC = 0.68×10^{-3} mm²/s (rhabdomyosarcoma).

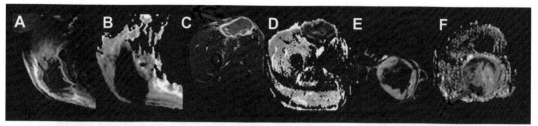

Fig. 17. Differentiation of necrotic lesions using DWI. (*A*) Axial T1-weighted fat suppression contrast-enhanced image. A necrotic lesion with peripheral contrast enhancement surrounded by edema. (*B*) Axial ADC map. The lesion presents restricted diffusion in the necrotic center (intramuscular abscess). (*C*) Axial T1-weighted image. A necrotic lesion with hyperintense peripheral rim (*arrow*) surrounded by edema. (*D*) Axial ADC map and restricted diffusion in the necrotic center (subacute hematoma). (*E*) Axial T1-weighted fat suppression contrast-enhanced image. A necrotic lesion with contrast enhancement on the wall. (*F*) Axial ADC map presents facilitated diffusion on the ADC map in the necrotic center and areas of restricted diffusion in the solid part of the tumor (*arrow*) (malignant schwannoma). Malignant tumors tend to have more facilitated diffusion in the necrotic center when compared with abscesses and hematomas.

method of assessing the presence of intracellular necrosis and viable cells is crucial for the evaluation of treatment response (**Fig. 20**).

In terms of osteosarcomas, tumor size does not diminish significantly with successful chemotherapy because therapy has a limited effect on the mineralized matrix of the tumors. In these tumors, the treatment response is considered effective if more than 90% of the tumor cells show necrosis histologically. The use of conventional MR imaging is limited to the assessment of tumoral viability because in T2-weighted images, both viable and necrotic tumor tissues show high signal intensities.[13] Morphologic changes induced by chemotherapy may be associated with hemorrhage, necrosis, edema, and inflammatory fibrosis without specific MR imaging patterns (**Fig. 21**).[34–36]

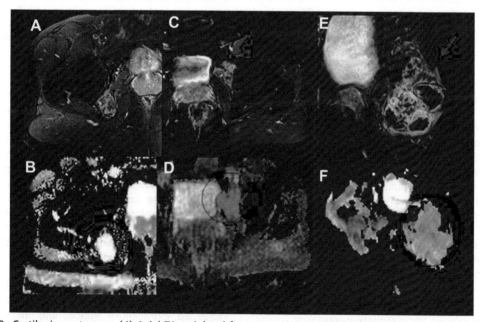

Fig. 18. Cartilaginous tumors. (*A*) Axial T1-weighted fat suppression contrast-enhanced image of a small lesion with heterogeneous contrast enhancement located in the ischiatic tuberosity (*arrow*). (*B, D, F*) Axial ADC map. The lesion presents facilitated diffusion in (*B, circle*) and a PIDC value of 2.1×10^{-3} mm^2/s (enchondroma). (*C*) Axial T1-weighted fat suppression contrast-enhanced image. A tumor with heterogeneous contrast enhancement, located in the left iliac bone (*arrow*), which shows facilitated diffusion in (*D, circle*) and PIDC = 1.9×10^{-3} mm^2/s (grade 2 chondrosarcoma). (*E*) Coronal T1-weighted fat suppression contrast-enhanced image. A huge tumor with heterogeneous contrast enhancement in the left hip (*arrow*) with facilitated diffusion in (*F, circle*) and a PIDC = 2.4×10^{-3} mm^2/s (grade 3 chondrosarcoma).

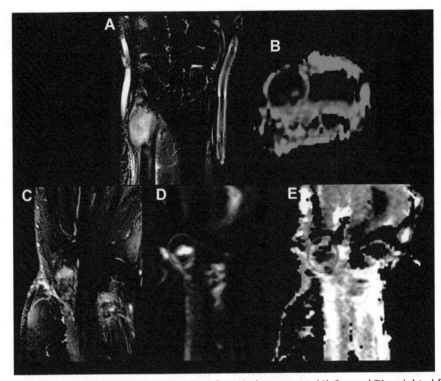

Fig. 19. A GCT in the ulnar epiphysis. The evaluation of surgical treatment. (*A*) Coronal T1-weighted fat suppression contrast-enhanced image of a tumor with homogeneous contrast enhancement, surrounded by edema (before treatment). (*B*) Axial ADC map. The lesion presents restricted diffusion and PIDC = 0.97×10^{-3} mm^2/s, 3 months after the surgery. (*C*) Coronal T1-weighted fat suppression contrast-enhanced image. (*D, E*) Coronal DW image and ADC map show many small areas of contrast enhancement in the surgical site (*C, arrows*), with high signal intensity on DWI (*D*), but just one lesion presents very high signal intensity on DWI (*D, circle*) and restricted diffusion on ADC map (*E, circle*), suggesting recidive tumor in the surgical site.

Considering that the ADC values of viable tumor tissue and tumor necrosis are significantly different, DWI could be used to evaluate treatment response by analyzing changes in the cellularity of the tumor with time.[13] Previous studies concluded that DWI is capable of providing earlier information about therapeutic results than those obtained from conventional MR imaging, considering that cellular changes usually precede reductions in tumor size.[13] Previous reports[9,13] concluded that DWI can be useful for evaluating the chemotherapeutic response of osteosarcomas and is considered to be a promising method for monitoring the therapeutic response of primary bone sarcomas.[34]

MONITORING TREATMENT RESPONSE

The use of conventional MR imaging on follow-up of treated MSK soft tissue masses is traditionally based on anatomic approaches, such as measurements of tumor size and the degree of contrast enhancement. However, anatomic imaging for this purpose has significant limitations,

including the presence of tumors that cannot be measured, poor measurement reproducibility, and mass lesions that persist after therapy.[37]

Because cellular death and vascular changes in response to treatment precede changes in lesion size, functional imaging such as DWI could provide earlier identification of patients with a poor treatment response or of those with tumor recurrence.[38] Therefore, DWI could provide an opportunity to adjust individual treatment regimens more rapidly, sparing patients the unnecessary morbidity, expense, and delays in the initiation of effective treatment.[39] Previous reports described an effective anticancer therapy that resulted in tumor lysis, loss of membrane integrity, increased extracellular space, and increase in water molecule diffusion. All these changes resulted in an increase in PIDC values.[3]

Preclinical and clinical studies have reported on the usefulness of DWI as a sensitive biomarker capable of detecting early cellular changes in treated tumors that precede morphologic response.[40,41] For instance, clinical studies

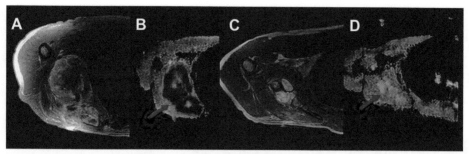

Fig. 20. Evaluation of response to Ewing sarcoma treatment by using DWI in a 28-year-old man. (*A*) Axial T1 contrast-enhanced image. (*B*) Axial ADC map. A huge tumor in the scapular region with heterogeneous contrast enhancement (*A*), restricted diffusion on the ADC map (*B, arrow*), and PIDC = 0.61×10^{-3} mm²/s in the pretreatment phase. (*C*) Axial T1 contrast-enhanced image. (*D*) Axial ADC map. The tumor got reduced after treatment (8 months later), with heterogeneous contrast enhancement (*C*), facilitated diffusion on the ADC map (*D, arrow*), and PIDC = 2.6×10^{-3} mm²/s, suggesting good response to the treatment. The histopathologic analysis showed more than 90% of necrosis, which indicates a good response to treatment.

of gliomas,[42] primary and metastatic liver cancers,[43–45] and breast cancers[46] have demonstrated an increase in ADC values in response to successful treatment.

In MSK tumors, several investigators have also demonstrated increasing ADC values with successful therapy (**Fig. 22**).[13,34,47]

In the study by Oka and colleagues,[9] which evaluated the chemotherapeutic response of osteosarcomas using the minimum ADC value in the solid components of tumors, a significant difference was demonstrated between patients with a good response to chemotherapy and those with a poor response.

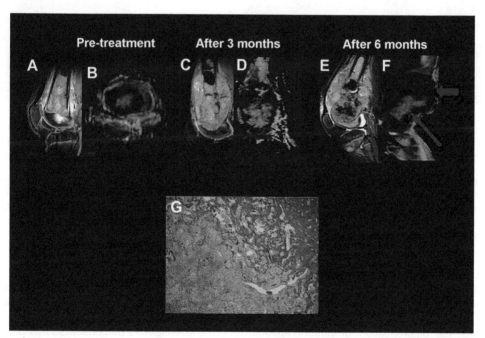

Fig. 21. Classic osteosarcoma in a 12-year-old boy. Evaluation of treatment response. (*A, C, E*) Sagittal T1-weighted fat suppression contrast-enhanced images. (*B*) Axial ADC map and (*D, F*) sagittal ADC map. Here there is a case of a huge osteosarcoma in the distal femur, with heterogeneous contrast enhancement before treatment (*A*) and areas of restricted diffusion in the ADC map (*B*) with PIDC = 0.89×10^{-3} mm²/s. During the treatment, the tumor grew (*C, E*) and presented restricted diffusion in the ADC map (*D, F*) in the peripheral portion (*F, short arrow*) with PIDC = 0.87×10^{-3} mm²/s and facilitated diffusion in the central part (*F, long arrow*) suggesting necrosis. There were no changes in the ADC map and in the PIDC value in the peripheral portion of the lesion, suggesting viable cells and consequently poor response to the treatment. The histopathologic analysis showed Huvos grade II necrosis (*G*, H&E, original magnification ×40).

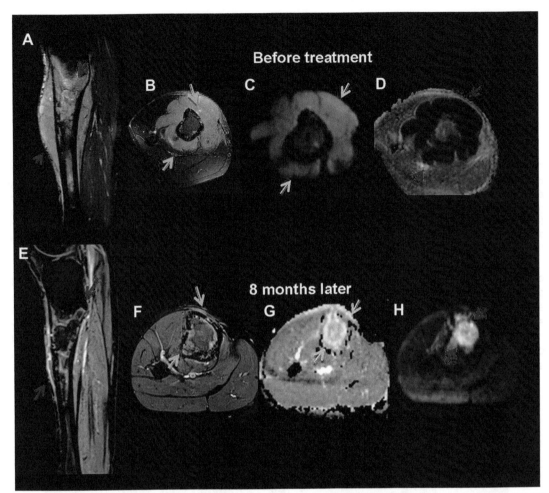

Fig. 22. Non–Hodgkin lymphoma in the tibia in a 27-year-old man. Before treatment (*A–D*). (*A*) Sagittal STIR MR image shows a large heterogeneous hyperintense intraosseous tumor extending in to the soft tissues (*arrows*). (*B*) Axial T1-weighted fat-suppressed image after contrast injection shows solid enhancing mass extending to the soft tissues (*arrows*). (*C*) Axial DWI shows hyperintense mass (*arrows*). (*D*) ADC map shows restricted diffusion of the tumor (*arrows*) and PIDC = 0.62×10^{-3} mm^2/s. Monitoring chemotherapy and radiotherapy 8 months later (*E–H*). (*E*) Sagittal T1-weighted fat-suppressed image after contrast injection shows heterogeneous enhancing intraosseous tumor that does not extend in to the soft tissues (*arrows*). (*F*) Axial T1-weighted fat-suppressed image after contrast injection shows heterogeneous enhancing intraosseous lesion (*arrows*). (*G*) Axial DWI shows hyperintense mass (T2 effect) (*arrows*). (*H*) ADC map shows facilitated diffusion of the tumor (*arrows*) and PIDC = 2.2×10^{-3} mm^2/s, suggesting tumor necrosis and good response to treatment.

DWI is also being used to assess the activity of residual disease after treatment and to detect early recurrence at a time when a salvage therapy might still be implemented (**Fig. 23**).[37]

Indeed, the differentiation of posttherapeutic soft tissue changes and residual or recurrent tumor is a common diagnostic problem because these abnormalities have the same appearance in morphologic imaging. Specifically, these pathologies are characterized by a high signal intensity on T2-weighted and short tau inversion recovery images and a low signal intensity on T1-weighted SE images.[48]

Baur and colleagues[48] evaluated the signal characteristics of recurring solid soft tissue tumors and posttherapeutic soft tissue changes with DWI (**Fig. 24**).

The investigators demonstrated that posttherapeutic soft tissue changes showed a significantly higher diffusion than viable recurrent tumors. This is an expected finding because solid tumors demonstrate high cellularity and intact cell membranes, whereas as antineoplastic therapy progresses successfully the cellularity within the tumor decreases and cell membranes lose their integrity.[17]

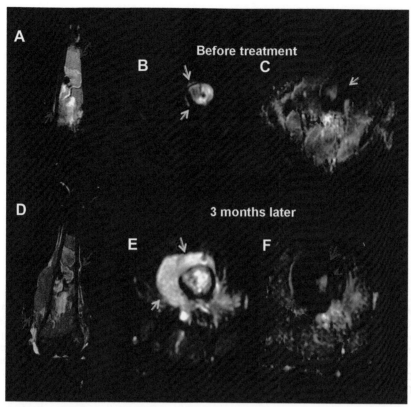

Fig. 23. Non–Hodgkin lymphoma in the femur in a 52-year-old woman (after biopsy and before treatment [A−C]). (A) Coronal STIR MR image shows a heterogeneous hyperintense intraosseous tumor (*arrows*). (B) Axial DWI shows hyperintense intraosseous mass (*arrows*). (C) Axial ADC map shows small areas of restricted diffusion (*arrow*) with PIDC = 0.62×10^{-3} mm²/s, suggesting viable tumor. Monitoring chemotherapy 3 months later). (D) Coronal STIR MR image shows a larger heterogeneous hyperintense intraosseous tumor involving soft tissues (*arrows*). (E) Axial DW image shows hyperintense intraosseous mass extending in to the soft tissues (*arrows*). (F) Axial ADC map shows a large area of restricted diffusion (*arrows*), with PIDC = 0.62×10^{-3} mm²/s, suggesting viable tumor and small areas of facilitated diffusion (*arrowhead*), with PIDC = 2.2×10^{-3} mm²/s, suggesting necrosis. All these findings suggest poor response to the treatment.

WHOLE BODY DW MR IMAGING

During the past decade, technological advances have led to the development of whole body MR imaging as well as whole body DW MR imaging. Now, within a single examination, it is possible to combine anatomic and functional information in whole body evaluation.[49]

Until recently, DWI performed with free breathing was considered to be impossible, because it was assumed that respiratory motion would lead to loss of DW image contrast.[49] However, in 2004, Takahara and colleagues[50] reported on the concept of DW whole body imaging with background body signal suppression (DWIBS). This technique intentionally uses free-breathing scanning rather than breath holding or respiratory triggering to visualize moving visceral organs and their lesions.[51]

DWIBS can be performed on most modern MR imaging scanners and is conducted in such a way as to suppress the signal of most tissues while highlighting potential malignancies or suspect lymph nodes in gray-scale inverted reformatted reconstructions.[52] The technique is characterized by heavy diffusion weighting (b values of up to 1000−1500 s/mm² are applied) and the application of excellent fat suppression in order to optimize background body signal suppression and improve lesion conspicuity.[49]

Several clinical applications for DWIBS are emerging in the literature, especially for oncological imaging.[53−55] Indeed, whole body DWI enables visualization of various primary and metastatic tumors exhibiting an impeded diffusion throughout the entire body.[49] This modality may also be useful in the detection of relatively small

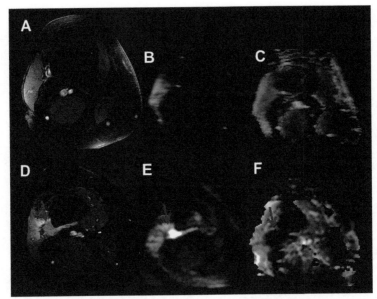

Fig. 24. Follow-up examination of a synovial sarcoma with postoperative myocutaneous flap. (*A*) Axial T1 fat suppression contrast-enhanced image. (*B*) Axial DWI and (*C*) axial ADC map. Two months after the surgery, there is a myocutaneous flap with a high signal intensity on DWI and facilitated diffusion on the ADC map (*C*) and PIDC = 2.1 × 10^{-3} mm^2/s. (*D*) Axial T1 fat suppression contrast-enhanced image. (*E*) Axial DW image, and (*F*) axial ADC map. Six months after the surgery, there is a small lump in the surgical site (*arrow in D*), with very high signal intensity on DW image (*arrow in E*) and restricted diffusion on the ADC map (*arrow in F*) and PIDC = 0.97 × 10^{-3} mm^2/s. There was a tumor recurrence.

lesions, for the identification and characterization of lymph nodes, and for monitoring response to cancer therapy.[51] Chen and colleagues[53] concluded that whole body DWI with ADC mapping can potentially be used for lesion detection. However, the true utility of whole body imaging requires further validation.

REFERENCES

1. Van der Woude HJ, Verstraete KL, Hogendoorn PC, et al. Musculoskeletal tumors: does fast dynamic contrast-enhanced subtraction MR imaging contribute to the characterization? Radiology 1998;208(3):821–8.
2. Kransdorf MJ, Murphey MD. Imaging of soft tissue tumors. In: Allister LM, Barrett K, editors. Imaging of soft tissue tumors. 2nd edition. Philadelphia: Lippincott Williams & Wilkins; 2006. p. 38–79.
3. Koh DM, Takahara T, Imai Y, et al. Practical aspects of assessing tumors using clinical diffusion-weighted imaging in the body. Magn Reson Med Sci 2007;6(4):211–24.
4. Koh DM, Collins DJ. Diffusion-weighted MRI in the body: applications and challenges in oncology. AJR Am J Roentgenol 2007;188(6):1622–35.
5. Nagata S, Nishimura H, Uchida M, et al. Diffusion-weighted imaging of soft tissue tumors: usefulness of the apparent diffusion coefficient for differential diagnosis. Radiat Med 2008;26(5):287–95.
6. Goudarzi B, Kishimoto R, Komatsu S, et al. Detection of bone metastases using diffusion weighted magnetic resonance imaging: comparison with (11)C-methionine PET and bone scintigraphy. Magn Reson Imaging 2010;28(3):372–9.
7. Maeda M, Matsumine A, Kato H, et al. Soft-tissue tumors evaluated by line-scan diffusion-weighted imaging: influence of myxoid matrix on the apparent diffusion coefficient. J Magn Reson Imaging 2007;25(6):1199–204.
8. Van Rijswijk CS, Kunz P, Hogendoorn PC, et al. Diffusion-weighted MRI in the characterization of soft-tissue tumors. J Magn Reson Imaging 2002;15(3):302–7.
9. Oka K, Yakushiji T, Sato H, et al. The value of diffusion-weighted imaging for monitoring the chemotherapeutic response of osteosarcoma: a comparison between average apparent diffusion coefficient and minimum apparent diffusion coefficient. Skeletal Radiol 2010;39(2):141–6.
10. Baur A, Dietrich O, Reiser M. Diffusion-weighted imaging of bone marrow: current status. Eur Radiol 2003;13(7):1699–708.
11. Einarsdóttir H, Karlsson M, Wejde J, et al. Diffusion-weighted MRI of soft tissue tumours. Eur Radiol 2004;14(6):959–63.

12. Schnapauff D, Zeile M, Niederhagen MB, et al. Diffusion-weighted echo-planar magnetic resonance imaging for the assessment of tumor cellularity in patients with soft-tissue sarcomas. J Magn Reson Imaging 2009;29(6):1355–9.

13. Uhl M, Saueressig U, van Buiren M, et al. Osteosarcoma: preliminary results of in vivo assessment of tumor necrosis after chemotherapy with diffusion- and perfusion-weighted magnetic resonance imaging. Invest Radiol 2006;41:618–23.

14. Stejskal EO, Tanner JE. Spin diffusion measurements: spin-echo in the presence of a time dependent field gradient. J Chem Phys 1965;42:288–92.

15. Le Bihan D, Breton E, Lallemand D, et al. Separation of diffusion and perfusion in intravoxel incoherent motion MR imaging. Radiology 1988;168:497–505.

16. Baur A, Reiser MF. Diffusion-weighted imaging of the musculoskeletal system in humans. Skeletal Radiol 2000;29(10):555–62.

17. Bley TA, Wieben O, Uhl M. Diffusion-weighted MR imaging in musculoskeletal radiology: applications in trauma, tumors, and inflammation. Magn Reson Imaging Clin N Am 2009;17(2):263–75.

18. Nagata S, Nishimura H, Uchida M, et al. Usefulness of diffusion-weighted MRI in differentiating benign from malignant musculoskeletal tumors. Nippon Igaku Hoshasen Gakkai Zasshi 2005;65(1):30–6.

19. Sundaram M, Baran G, Merenda G, et al. Myxoid liposarcoma: magnetic resonance imaging appearances with clinical and histological correlation. Skeletal Radiol 1990;19(5):359–62.

20. Guo AC, Cummings TJ, Dash RC, et al. Lymphomas and high-grade astrocytomas: comparison of water diffusibility and histologic characteristics. Radiology 2002;224:177–83.

21. Nakayama T, Yoshimitsu K, Irie H, et al. Usefulness of the calculated apparent diffusion coefficient value in the differential diagnosis of retroperitoneal masses. J Magn Reson Imaging 2004;20:735–42.

22. Sumi M, Ichikawa Y, Nakamura T. Diagnostic ability of apparent diffusion coefficients for lymphomas and carcinomas in the pharynx. Eur Radiol 2007; 17:2631–7.

23. King AD, Ahuja AT, Yeung DK, et al. Malignant cervical lymphadenopathy: diagnostic accuracy of diffusion-weighted MR imaging. Radiology 2007; 245:806–13.

24. Toh CH, Castillo M, Wong AM, et al. Primary cerebral lymphoma and glioblastoma multiforme: differences in diffusion characteristics evaluated with diffusion tensor imaging. AJNR Am J Neuroradiol 2008;29: 471–5.

25. Lee JC, Thomas JM, Phillips S, et al. Aggressive fibromatosis: MRI features with pathologic correlation. AJR Am J Roentgenol 2006;186(1):247–54.

26. Lai PH, Ho JT, Chen WL, et al. Brain abscess and necrotic brain tumor: discrimination with proton MR spectroscopy and diffusion-weighted imaging. AJNR Am J Neuroradiol 2002;23(8):1369–77.

27. Chang SC, Lai PH, Chen WL, et al. Diffusion-weighted MRI features of brain abscess and cystic or necrotic brain tumors: comparison with conventional MRI. Clin Imaging 2002;26(4):227–36.

28. Nakashima Y, Unni KK, Shives TC, et al. Mesenchymal chondrosarcoma of bone and soft tissue. A review of 111 cases. Cancer 1986;57(12): 2444–53.

29. Balsara ZN, Stainken BF, Martinez AJ. MR image of localized giant cell tumor of the tendon sheath involving the knee. J Comput Assist Tomogr 1989; 13(1):159–62.

30. Maheshwari AV, Muro-Cacho CA, Pitcher JD Jr. Pigmented villonodular bursitis/diffuse giant cell tumor of the pes anserine bursa: a report of two cases and review of literature. Knee 2007;14(5):402–7.

31. Somerhausen NS, Fletcher CD. Diffuse-type giant cell tumor: clinicopathologic and immunohistochemical analysis of 50 cases with extraarticular disease. Am J Surg Pathol 2000;24(4):479–92.

32. Goldenberg RR, Campbell CJ, Bonfiglio M. Giant-cell tumor of bone. An analysis of two hundred and eighteen cases. J Bone Joint Surg Am 1970;52(4): 619–64.

33. Koh DM, Thoeny HC. Evaluation of malignant bone disease using DW-MRI. In: Diffusion-weighted MR imaging. Springer Berlin Heidelberg; 2010. p. 207–26.

34. Hayashida Y, Yakushiji T, Awai K, et al. Monitoring therapeutic responses of primary bone tumors by diffusion-weighted image: Initial results. Eur Radiol 2006;16(12):2637–43.

35. Erlemann R, Reiser MF, Peters PE, et al. Musculoskeletal neoplasms: static and dynamic Gd-DTPA–enhanced MR imaging. Radiology 1989;171(3): 767–73.

36. Holscher HC, Bloem JL, Vanel D, et al. Osteosarcoma: chemotherapy-induced changes at MR imaging. Radiology 1992;182(3):839–44.

37. Padhani AR, Khan AA. Diffusion-weighted (DW) and dynamic contrast-enhanced (DCE) magnetic resonance imaging (MRI) for monitoring anticancer therapy. Target Oncol 2010;5(1):39–52.

38. Padhani AR, Liu G, Koh DM, et al. Diffusion-weighted magnetic resonance imaging as a cancer biomarker: consensus and recommendations. Neoplasia 2009;11(2):102–25.

39. Kwee TC, Takahara T, Klomp DW, et al. Cancer imaging: novel concepts in clinical magnetic resonance imaging. J Intern Med 2010;268:120–32.

40. Thoeny HC, De Keyzer F, Chen F, et al. Diffusion-weighted MR imaging in monitoring the effect of a vascular targeting agent on rhabdomyosarcoma in rats. Radiology 2005;234(3):756–64.

41. Roth Y, Tichler T, Kostenich G, et al. High-b-value diffusion-weighted MR imaging for pretreatment

prediction and early monitoring of tumor response to therapy in mice. Radiology 2004;232(3):685–92.

42. Chenevert TL, Stegman LD, Taylor JM, et al. Diffusion magnetic resonance imaging: an early surrogate marker of therapeutic efficacy in brain tumors. J Natl Cancer Inst 2000;92(24): 2029–36.

43. Kamel IR, Reyes DK, Liapi E, et al. Functional MR imaging assessment of tumor response after 90Y microsphere treatment in patients with unresectable hepatocellular carcinoma. J Vasc Interv Radiol 2007; 18:49–56.

44. Schraml C, Schwenzer NF, Martirosian P, et al. Diffusion-weighted MRI of advanced hepatocellular carcinoma during sorafenib treatment: initial results. AJR Am J Roentgenol 2009;193(4): W301–7.

45. Theilmann RJ, Borders R, Trouard TP, et al. Changes in water mobility measured by diffusion MRI predict response of metastatic breast cancer to chemotherapy. Neoplasia 2004;6:831–7.

46. Pickles MD, Gibbs P, Lowry M, et al. Diffusion changes precede size reduction in neoadjuvant treatment of breast cancer. Magn Reson imaging 2006;24:843–7.

47. Dudeck O, Zeile M, Pink D, et al. Diffusion-weighted magnetic resonance imaging allows monitoring of anticancer treatment effects in patients with soft-tissue sarcomas. J Magn Reson Imaging 2008;5: 1109–13.

48. Baur A, Huber A, Arbogast S, et al. Diffusion-weighted imaging of tumor recurrencies and posttherapeutical soft-tissue changes in humans. Eur Radiol 2001;11(5):828–33.

49. Kwee TC, Takahara T, Ochiai R, et al. Whole-body diffusion-weighted magnetic resonance imaging. Eur J Radiol 2009;70(3):409–17.

50. Takahara T, Imai Y, Yamashita T, et al. Diffusion weighted whole body imaging with background body signal suppression (DWIBS): technical improvement using free breathing, STIR and high resolution 3D display. Radiat Med 2004;22(4): 275–82.

51. Kwee TC, Takahara T, Ochiai R, et al. Diffusion-weighted whole-body imaging with background body signal suppression (DWIBS): features and potential applications in oncology. Eur Radiol 2008; 18(9):1937–52.

52. Dietrich O, Biffar A, Baur-Melnyk A, et al. Technical aspects of MR diffusion imaging of the body. Eur J Radiol 2010. [Epub ahead of print].

53. Chen W, Jian W, Li HT, et al. Whole-body diffusion-weighted imaging vs. FDG-PET for the detection of non-small-cell lung cancer. How do they measure up? Magn Reson Imaging 2010;28(5):613–20.

54. Lin C, Luciani A, Itti E, et al. Whole-body diffusion-weighted magnetic resonance imaging with apparent diffusion coefficient mapping for staging patients with diffuse large B-cell lymphoma. Eur Radiol 2010;20:2027–38.

55. Jacobs MA, Pan L, Macura KJ. Whole-body diffusion-weighted and proton imaging: a review of this emerging technology for monitoring metastatic cancer. Semin Roentgenol 2009;44(2):111–22.

Diffusion MR Imaging for Monitoring of Treatment Response

Anwar R. Padhani, MBBS, FRCP, FRCR[a],*,
Dow-Mu Koh, MD, MRCP, FRCR[b]

KEYWORDS

- Diffusion MR imaging • Biomarker • Cellularity
- Functional imaging • Response monitoring • Radiotherapy
- Antiangiogenics

Application of morphologic imaging to the evaluation of tumor response to treatment has led to the emergence of response criteria such as those proposed by the Response Evaluation Criteria in Solid Tumors (RECIST) committee.[1] However, there is increasing awareness that anatomic approaches have significant limitations, including tumors that cannot be measured, poor measurement reproducibility, and masses that persist following therapy.[2] Faced with these limitations, more sophisticated measurement criteria (such as tumor volume) and new morphologic approaches (such as changes in tumor computed tomography [CT] density values after contrast medium administration) have been applied to the evaluation of therapy response.[3,4]

However, with the increasing clinical use of cytostatic therapeutics, there is a recognition that anatomic evaluations are insensitive to changes that may inform on overall therapeutic success. This latter point has been exemplified by:

1. Numerous clinical studies showing survival advantages for antiangiogenic therapies with only modest anatomic responses for glioblastoma and hepatocellular, colorectal, and renal cancers[5–9]
2. Studies which, in contradistinction, that have shown improvements in progression-free survival (gauged morphologically) but with no subsequent benefits in overall survival, for colorectal and

breast cancer patients treated with the antiangiogenic drug bevacizumab[10–12]

Both of these observations suggest that the value of anatomic imaging as a surrogate marker of clinical efficacy for antiangiogenic therapies may be limited.

To overcome the limitations of anatomic evaluations, functional imaging techniques are increasingly being used to monitor response to therapies with novel mechanisms of action, which can predict the success of therapy before conventional measurements of size are altered.[13] In the latter setting, functional imaging methods are also being used as pharmacodynamic biomarkers of response in early phases of drug development of compounds with novel mechanisms of action, to see whether tumor physiology is correspondingly altered so as to provide confidence to proceed to more expensive efficacy studies.[14–16]

In this article the authors focus on diffusion-weighted magnetic resonance (DW-MR) imaging as a functional response imaging technique. The authors have assumed that readers are already familiar with the DW-MR imaging data acquisition techniques, including apparent diffusion coefficient (ADC) map generation (these aspects are discussed elsewhere in this issue and in the supporting medical literature).[17–20] For readers interested in imaging parameters used to acquire the

---

Financial disclosure: the authors have nothing to declare.
[a] Paul Strickland Scanner Centre, Mount Vernon Cancer Center, Rickmansworth Road, Northwood, Middlesex, HA6 2RN, UK
[b] Department of Radiology, Royal Marsden Hospital, Downs Road, Sutton, Surrey, SM2 5PT, UK
* Corresponding author.
E-mail address: anwar.padhani@stricklandscanner.org.uk

Magn Reson Imaging Clin N Am 19 (2011) 181–209
doi:10.1016/j.mric.2010.10.004

illustrative material in this text, refer to **Table 1**. The authors begin by demonstrating the link between ADC and tissue cellular density, reflecting tumor proliferation. Key data are then presented on changes in DW-MR imaging in response to therapies that cause tumor cell death and those that affect tumor vascularity. The article focuses on experience gained in extracranial human studies, seeking to use the more extensive animal literature for support and to point out new avenues for data exploration. The authors show that MR imaging—depicted water diffusivity can reflect the interaction between the mechanism of action of therapies and tissue micro-structural properties. It will become clear that therapy-induced changes in soft tissues and bone marrow differ when imaged by DW-MR imaging, depending on the mechanism of action of the treatments used; these differences are highlighted.

DW-MR IMAGING AS A BIOMARKER FOR THERAPY ASSESSMENTS

In a recent US National Cancer Institute sponsored consensus conference report, it was noted that there was "an extraordinary opportunity for DW-MRI to evolve into a clinically valuable imaging tool, potentially important for drug development."[17] Major advantages of DW-MR imaging include that no ionizing radiation is administered and that no injection of isotope or any other contrast medium is necessary for examinations. Data acquisition times are reasonably short in terms of patient comfort, and the method is easily repeated. The information obtained can be quantified and displayed as parametric maps, enabling spatial heterogeneity of tissues/tumors to be analyzed, before and in response to treatment. DW-MR imaging biomarkers such as ADC are theoretically independent of magnetic field strength (although in practice there may be variations due to technical reasons), and the relative simplicity of data acquisitions facilitates multicenter and longitudinal studies.

DW-MR imaging yields several potential biomarkers (signal intensity at different b-values, water diffusivity [D], perfusion fraction [F_p], apparent diffusion coefficient [ADC_{total}], fractionated ADC [ADC_{fast} and ADC_{slow}], and fractional anisotropy [FA]) that may act as therapy response parameters. ADC_{fast}, which is calculated using low b-values (0–100 s/mm^2), is dominated by the perfusion component of the total tissue diffusivity. At higher b-values (>100 s/mm^2), the perfusion component is largely extinguished, so ADC_{slow} measurements are more heavily determined by water diffusion within the cellular matrix. In most clinical studies only ADC_{total} is reported (usually simply written as ADC), so it is not possible to distinguish between the perfusion and nonperfusion components to the quoted diffusivity. This point is an important one to remember when interpreting clinical data with regard to therapy effects on tissues.

DW-MR IMAGING AS A MARKER OF CELLULAR DENSITY, PROLIFERATION, AND DEATH

DW-MR imaging is more able to detect and characterize the presence of tumors than morphologic

Table 1
Data acquisition parameters for whole body and abdominopelvic DW-MR imaging examinations

Machine Parameters	Free-Breathing Multiple Averaging: Abdomen	Free-Breathing Multiple Averaging: Pelvis	Whole Body DW-MR Imaging
Field of view	280–400 cm	260 cm	380–400 cm
Matrix size	128i	160–256	128i
TR	>2500 ms	>3500 ms	>6000 ms Multiple stations as required to the body
TE	min	min	min
NSA	4–7	6	6
Fat suppression	SPAIR/STIR	SPAIR/STIR	STIR
EPI factor	128	114	47
Parallel imaging factor	2	2	2
Section thickness	5–7 mm/1 mm gap	6 mm/1 mm gap	5 mm/0 mm overlap
b-values (s/mm^2)	3–4 b-values including 0, 100, 500, and 750	0, 100, 800	0–50 and 800–1000

Abbreviations: EPI, echo planar imaging; i, interpolated; NSA, number of signal averages; SPAIR, spectral selected attenuation inversion recovery; STIR, short-tau inversion recovery; TE, echo time; TR, repetition time.

sequences because it incorporates 2 contrast mechanisms into the images produced: (1) sensitivity to water content and (2) sensitivity to water movements within tissues. The basic biologic premise is that malignant tissues are generally more cellular than benign/normal tissues, so water diffusion is more impeded in tumors. However, when cystic, necrotic, and treated metastases are included, lesion characterization is less good, for example when evaluating focal liver lesions.[21] In fact, on closer observation there are several microscopic organizational features that affect tissue water diffusivity including cell density (number of cells/high-power field), nuclear-cytoplasmic ratio, distribution of cell sizes within a tissue, extracellular space tortuosity, integrity of cellular membranes, tissue organization (eg, glandular formation), and tissue perfusion. The relationships between these microscopic tissue properties and water diffusivity are important to know in order to understand changes in image contrast depicted by DW-MR imaging in response to therapies.

Inverse correlations between ADC and cell density in gliomas, metastatic brain tumors, renal cancers, and some childhood tumors can be found in the literature.[22–30] However, this is not a universal finding, and poorer correlations between ADC values and cell density have been noted in breast adenocarcinomas.[22] The latter may reflect the opposing effects of water movement in more than one tissue compartment (more limited in extracellular fluid space and relatively increased within glandular lumina in adenocarcinomas). ADC alterations in bone marrow as a consequence of disease merits separate consideration. The literature suggests that ADC correlations with cellularity of the bone marrow is biphasic, with initial increases in high b-value signal intensity and ADC, as fat cells of yellow marrow are progressively replaced by normal red marrow elements and/or tumor cells (**Fig. 1**).[31,32] The lower signal intensity on high b-value images and lower ADC values of yellow marrow is likely to be related to (1) reduced water content and (2) that larger sized fat cells may theoretically impede water movements to a greater extent than smaller hematopoietic cells. However, once all fat cells are lost, increasing bone marrow cellularity can then result in ADC decrease (but there are continued increases in signal intensity on high b-value images) (see **Fig. 1; Figs. 2** and **3**).

There are other important histologic properties that correlate with ADC, including tumor proliferation index,[33,34] tumor grade,[27,35] the presence of necrosis[29,36] and, in the therapy setting, tumor cell apoptosis.[36–38] Many of these histologic properties also determine the likelihood of a tumor responding to treatment; therefore, DW-MR imaging measurements of water diffusivity may also be used to predict treatment effectiveness, as is discussed in more detail in a later section.

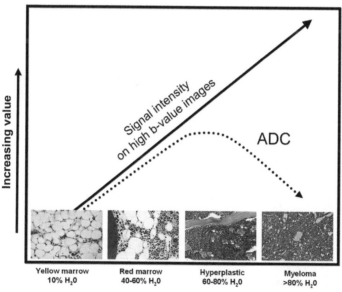

Fig. 1. DW-MR imaging relationships with bone marrow cellularity and water content. An abundance of fatty cells and low water content causes low signal intensity on high b-value images and low ADC values. Increasing bone marrow cellularity with replacement of fat cells and increases in water content causes initial increases in signal intensity and ADC values. Once fat cells are eliminated, increasing cell density may cause lowering of ADC values; however, persistent increases in signal intensity on high b-value images are seen.

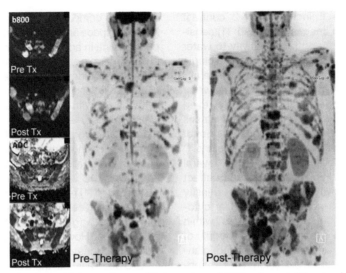

Fig. 2. Disease progression in multiple myeloma with lowering of ADC values. A 62-year-old man with multiple myeloma being treated with bortezomib (proteosome inhibitor). Two examinations performed 3 months apart are shown. Whole body DW-MR imaging (inverted gray scale, b800 s/mm²) show disease progression with increasing signal intensity and extent of the bony marrow disease. Extraosseous disease is also visible. ADC value decreases are seen in the sacrum and iliac bone. Please see Fig. 8 for details regarding the degree of ADC reductions in the sacrum and iliac bones. Tx, therapy.

ASSESSING DW-MR IMAGES IN THERAPY PARADIGMS

In the clinical therapy assessment setting, DW-MR imaging can be evaluated qualitatively as changes in signal intensity on high b-value images and/or quantitatively by noting changes in ADC values.

Qualitative Analysis

Visual assessments of signal intensity changes are clinically useful, particularly when global assessments of the changing tumor burden are being undertaken with whole body diffusion MR imaging techniques (see **Figs. 2** and **3; Fig. 4**). This method

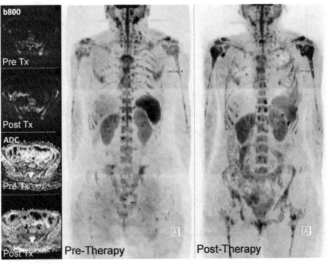

Fig. 3. Progressive disease in metastatic breast cancer with increasing ADC values. A 49-year-old woman with metastatic breast cancer. Two examinations performed 3 months apart are shown; whole body DW-MR imaging (inverted gray scale, b800 s/mm²) shows disease progression with increasing signal intensity and extent of the bony marrow disease. ADC increases are seen in the sacrum and iliac bones. The ADC of the right sacrum increased from 870 μm²/s to 990 μm²/s.

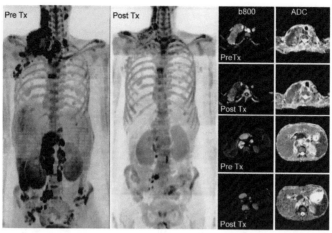

Fig. 4. Monitoring response to chemotherapy after ABVD chemotherapy (adriamycin, bleomycin, vinblastine, da-carbazine) for Hodgkin disease. A 29-year-old man with Hodgkin disease before and at day 8 after starting ABVD chemotherapy. The whole body DW-MR imaging (inverted scale, b800 s/mm^2) shows dramatic reduction in the signal intensity at all disease sites and corresponding increases in ADC values are seen in the nodal disease in the lower neck and upper abdomen (*arrows*). There are minor changes in tumor size at this early time point after commencing therapy.

of assessment is practically useful and clinically appealing for both radiologists and referring physicians because it enables "at-a-glance" assessments, in a manner similar to the data displayed by techniques such as scintigraphy and positron emission tomography (PET) scanning. With successful treatment, cell killing results in lowering of signal intensity on high b-value images (see **Fig. 4**). Disease progression is displayed as new areas of abnormal signal intensity or by changes in the extent, symmetry, and intensity of abnormalities (see **Figs. 2** and **3**). Ideally, when judging the intensity of abnormalities in whole body maximum intensity projection (MIP) reconstructions, normalization of images needs to be undertaken before the MIP reconstructions so as to enable comparisons of examinations. If normalization cannot be done, then window centering of MIP reconstructions should be with respect to organ(s) that has/have not changed (eg, kidney), maintaining window widths between the examinations being compared.

Intensity-based evaluations are successful because the increased signal intensity of tumors on high b-value images is related to both higher water content and impeded water diffusivity. The physiologic reasons for changes in tissue signal intensity with respect to the therapy given are detailed herein and summarized in **Table 2**. There are several potential confounding factors such as tissue edema during radiation therapy or following surgery that can increase tissue water, which demonstrates high signal intensity on the high b-value images. Increased lesion signal intensity on high b-value images (with corresponding increased ADC values)

in the face of inactive disease results from long T2-relaxation times of tissues and is termed T2 shine-through (**Fig. 5**). T2 shine-through is also a likely contributor to the visibility of normal salivary and prostate glands, gall bladder, liver hemangiomas, and normal breast parenchyma commonly seen on whole body DW-MR images. To avoid misinterpretations based on signal intensity assessments, it is necessary to always interpret signal intensity appearances with corresponding ADC maps, taking into account changes in morphology also.

Another confounding factor for increasing bone marrow signal intensity on high b-value images but without disease progression is the administration of granulocyte-colony stimulating factor (G-CSF).[39] G-CSF helps to moderate the degree of neutropenia occurring because of chemotherapy, thus enabling higher doses of chemotherapy to be given. G-CSF increases bone marrow cellularity and elevates the peripheral white cell count. Increased signal intensity is observed in normal adult red marrow areas (spine, vertebrae, pelvis, sternum, ribs). Reconversion of yellow marrow to red marrow is also seen in the proximal limb bones (**Fig. 6**). The effects on the bone marrow signal can occur within 2 weeks of the first G-CSF dose,[40] but it is unknown whether additional doses further alter the signal intensity or its extent, and whether these changes are reversed once therapy is stopped. The challenge for radiologists evaluating cancer patients being treated with G-CSF and chemotherapy is the differentiation of bone metastases or pathologic marrow infiltration from benign red marrow reconversion. As a general

Table 2
Summary of water diffusivity changes with therapies and possible biological explanations

ADC Change	Therapy Type	Dominant Biological Explanation	Onset and/or Duration of DW-MRI Changes	Organ or Tissues	Strength of Observations[a]
↑↑ (T2-shine through)	Radiation and chemotherapy	Massive liquefactive necrosis. Correlation with signal intensity appearances on high b-value images and on other techniques is essential in order to avoid this pitfall.	Persistent	Bone	Firm
↑	Chemotherapy	Tumor cell death. ADC reduces at a variable time as tumor cells are clear, with tissues remodeling, vascular normalisation and as mature fibrosis develops. Bony sclerosis and secondary chemotherapy induced marrow fibrosis also results in low ADC values. Residual active disease also results in low ADC values at the end of treatment.	Increases in ADC can be seen within a few days but duration of effects can be variable and maybe transient	Various	Firm
↑	Radiation	Tumor cell death, edema, inflammation and microvessel leak. Radiation induced increased ADC values dominates other processes attempting to normalise ADC such as those mention above resulting in prolonged ADC elevations.	Increases in ADC can be seen within 1–2 days but are more prolonged compared to chemotherapy	Bone, brain, other pelvic organs	Moderate to firm
↑	Embolization	Ischemic tumor cell death. Associated with non-enhancement due to vascular shutdown.	Transient	Liver	Moderate
↑↑	Radiofrequency ablation	Interstitial edema, hemorrhage, carbonization, necrosis and fibrosis. Time course of appearances within different organs and ability to predict outcomes are yet to be fully defined.	Early increases of ADC values but time courses of changes not well defined	Liver, lung	Preliminary
↑↑	Antiandrogens	Glandular atrophy. Decreased vascularity and microvessel permeability further reduces ADC values. Androgen deprivation in bone metastases can lead to initial ADC increases with cell killing with reductions later due to healing.	Persistent	Prostate gland	Preliminary
→	Antiangiogenics	Vascular normalisation. Appearance of necrosis can cause ADC increases. Vascular disruptive agents cause ADC increases via necrosis.	Onset at the time of reduced vascular permeability. Persistent	Brain tumors Primary liver malignancy	Moderate
→	Chemoradiation	Cell swelling prior to cell death. Cell swelling is observed in animal tumors but its presence in human studies has not been convincingly shown. Chemoradiation more often increases ADC values.	Transient	Brain tumors	Preliminary

[a] Based on authors own observations and evaluations of literature data.

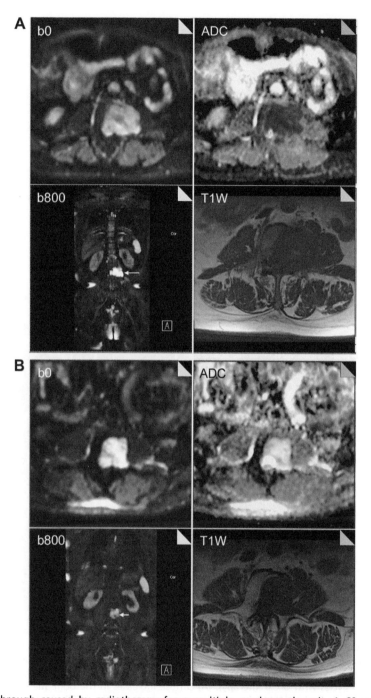

Fig. 5. T2 shine-through caused by radiotherapy for a multiple myeloma deposit. A 69-year-old man with multiple myeloma deposit in the L3 vertebral body before (*A*) and 5 months later after radiotherapy (*B*). b0, ADC map, coronal b800 reconstruction, and T1-weighted images are shown. Before therapy (*A*) the deposit shows the typical appearance of a high-cellularity lesion with high signal intensity on b800 images (*arrow*) and low ADC values; spinal canal narrowing is noted. Following radiotherapy (*B*), the lesion is a little smaller with no compromise of the thecal sac; yellow bone marrow atrophy is also noted on the T1-weighted image. ADC values have increased but the lesion remains bright on the b800 image (*arrow*; T2 shine-through). T2 shine-through suggests inactive disease.

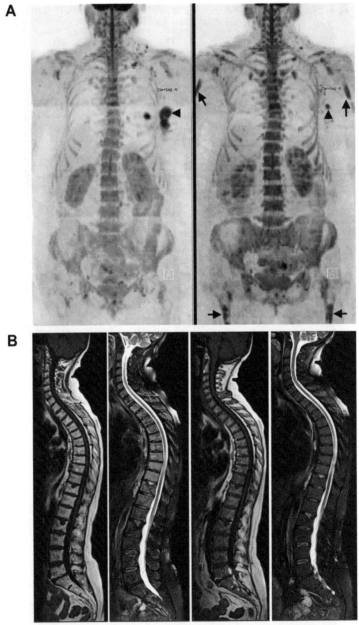

Fig. 6. Bone marrow hyperplasia following G-CSF therapy. A 63-year-old woman with a locally advanced left breast cancer with axillary nodal disease (*arrowhead*) before (*left panel*) and during neoadjuvant chemotherapy (*right panel*). The patient received FEC chemotherapy (5-fluorouracil, epirubicin, cyclophosphamide) (×3 cycles) and then taxotere (2 cycles with G-CSF therapy). (*A*) Diffuse increases in the bone marrow signal intensity are observable on the whole-body DW-MR imaging images (inverted scale, b800 s/mm² images) in normal red bone marrow areas (spine, pectoral and pelvic girdles). Increased signal intensity is also noted in yellow marrow areas (*arrows*). A good response to treatment is seen in the primary breast cancer and nodal disease, although residual active disease is still visible (*arrowhead*). (*B*) Sagittal T1- and T2-weighted images with spectral fat saturation show increased bone marrow cellularity in the normal spinal bone marrow on the T1-weighted images. (*C*) Diffuse increases in signal intensity of the sacral bone marrow on b800 images with corresponding decreases in ADC values after treatment (*bottom row*).

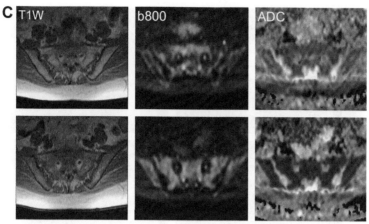

Fig. 6. (*continued*)

guide, disease progression may be suspected with new areas of focal abnormal signal intensity, or through changes in the extent, symmetry, and intensity of abnormalities. Signal intensity changes should be correlated with ADC values and with appearances on other MR imaging sequences, and by other imaging modalities. Note that G-CSF can also increase bone marrow ^{18}F-fluorodeoxy-glucose (FDG) uptake on PET scans.[41]

Quantitative Analyses

Quantitative response assessments are mostly undertaken by noting changes in ADC values. There are several approaches for analyzing ADC maps. Most studies report on single median or mean values of ADC using whole tumor regions of interest or on selected areas within tumors. However, visual inspection shows that tumors are often heterogeneous in their spatial ADC distributions. Simple measures of central tendency have limited abilities to detect treatment-related changes if there are both increases and decreases in ADC in response to treatment. In these cases the net mean or median change in ADC values are reduced, thus hiding treatment-related effects. Furthermore, if large cystic or necrotic areas are present before therapy, the ability to detect changes in response to therapy can become blunted. It is possible to capture some aspects of displayed heterogeneity in the descriptors of histograms such as range, standard deviation, centile values, skewness, and kurtosis. Changes in histogram descriptors can then be correlated with therapy response (**Fig. 7**). Of course the histogram approach need not be simplistic, and many sophisticated histogram analysis approaches have appeared in the literature; unfortunately relatively complex approaches such as principal component

descriptors remove them from clinical usability. Another major disadvantage of the histogram approach is that the spatial distribution of this information is lost, but it is known that spatial heterogeneity of functional imaging parameters does have significant diagnostic or predictive utility.[42,43]

A new analytical method for retaining spatial information in response to therapy is called the functional diffusion map (fDM) or the ADC parametric response map (PRM_{ADC}).[44] This method requires that pre- and post-therapy ADC volumes are spatially registered using sophisticated software. The procedure involves the initial registration of pre- and posttreatment morphologic/reference images and subsequent ADC volume registrations with data resampling as needed. Differences in the registered voxel data between the 2 examinations are determined and a threshold value for ADC change applied according to predetermined criteria (discussed later in the section on additional considerations). Statistically significant changes in voxels are color labeled (such as "red" for increase, "green" for no change, and "blue" for decrease) and overlaid onto anatomic images, enabling the spatial distribution of changed voxels to be appreciated. This approach allows for the quantification of the relative tumor volume in which ADC changes have occurred. The fractional tumor volume where ADC values have changed can then be correlated with therapy response (see **Fig. 7**).

PRM_{ADC} have been evaluated in studies of brain tumors,[45] head and neck,[46] and metastatic prostate cancer to bones,[47] with promising initial results (**Fig. 8**). Although there are preliminary data from brain tumors showing that changes in water diffusivity on PRM_{ADC} do correlate with patient outcomes,[45] it is not clear how this kind of approach will be useful in clinical practice,

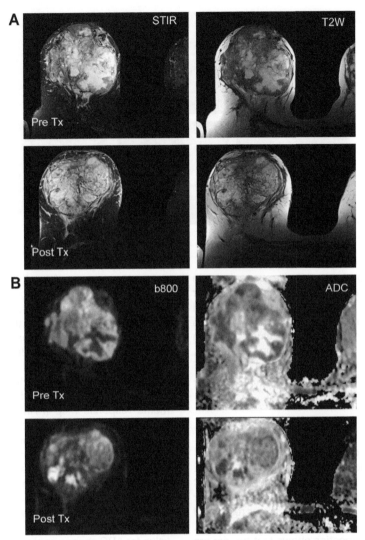

Fig. 7. DW-MR imaging changes of primary breast cancer treated with chemotherapy. A 42-year-old woman with a locally advanced left breast cancer treated with FEC chemotherapy. Examinations were performed before and after 3 cycles. (*A*) Axial T2-weighted (T2W) and short-tau inversion recovery (STIR) images show that there has been little change in tumor size (*top row*, pretherapy; *bottom row*, after 3 cycles of treatment). (*B*) b800 and ADC maps before and after therapy at the same time points shows some reduction in signal intensity on b800 images, but marked increases in global ADC values are noted. (*C*) Volume-rendered images shows that the tumor volume increases from 454.5 mL (designated as PRIOR) to 539.9 mL (designated as CURRENT). Histograms show increases in ADC values (mean 1450 µm²/s to 1779 µm²/s) with a greater proportion of pixels having ADC values greater than 2000 µm²/s. The mastectomy specimen showed tumor necrosis with macroscopic areas of invasive cancer.

particularly for tumors located in areas of the body with significant physiologic motions such as the thorax and abdomen, and for organs with significant tissue and tumor distortions such as the breast.[48] In addition, the technique cannot be easily applied when there is an observable change in tumor size or shape after treatment. The intrinsic assumption that there is little or no change in size and morphology between examinations being compared needs to be explicitly tested, by at the very least a comparative volume measurement.

PRETREATMENT PREDICTION OF THERAPY EFFECTIVENESS

Several preclinical and clinical studies have noted that pretherapy ADC values may indicate the outcome of therapies administered; most studies

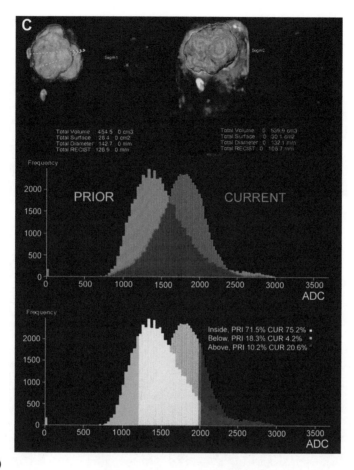

Fig. 7. (*continued*)

show that tumors with high ADC values respond less favorably to treatments,[49–52] although this not a universal finding.[53] The prognostic significance of pretreatment ADC values probably stems from the relationship between the presence of tumor necrosis and poorer patient outcomes.[54,55] The linking hypothesis appears to be low oxygen tension in tumors. Tumor hypoxia mediates resistance to chemotherapy, radiation, and photodynamic therapy, and leads to the selection of more aggressive tumor clones capable of evading the hostile tumor microenvironment.[56,57] As a caveat, it is conceivable that low-grade tumors with little necrosis could have similar mean ADC values to necrotic, high-grade tumors, so caution should be used when prognosticating on the basis of ADC values alone. Furthermore, caution should be also exercised in trying to assign prognostic significance to a mean or median tumor ADC value, particularly for tumors that are known to readily undergo necrosis (eg, squamous cell cancers and gliomas); for these tumor types, histogram approaches may be valuable when

evaluating the prognostic value of the pretherapy ADC values.[58,59]

Lemaire and colleagues[50] demonstrated that rat mammary tumors with a lower pretreatment ADC did not regrow 7 days after chemotherapy, unlike the tumors with higher initial ADC values where tumor regrowth was seen; they ascribed these observations to necrosis and suggested that hypoxia resulted in clonal selection of more aggressive, therapy-resistant tumor cells. Roth and colleagues[49] examined C26 colon tumors, and also demonstrated a similar correlation between high pretreatment ADC values and poor responsiveness to doxorubicin chemotherapy.

There have been a few studies in primary rectal cancer patients that assessed the prognostic value of pretreatment ADC measurements. Dzik-Jurasz and colleagues[60] found a strong negative correlation between pretreatment whole tumor mean ADC values and tumor response in 14 rectal cancer patients who received neoadjuvant chemotherapy followed by chemoradiation, with higher ADC value tumors responding more poorly. DeVries and

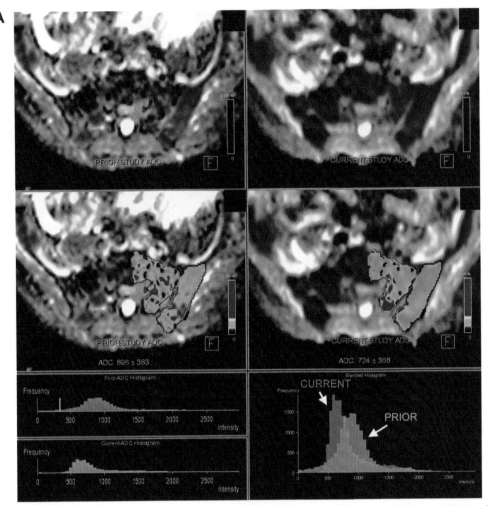

Fig. 8. Disease progression in multiple myeloma depicted by parametric response maps. Same patient as illustrated in **Fig. 2**. A 62-year-old man with multiple myeloma progressing on bortezomib (proteosome inhibitor) therapy. Two examinations performed 3 months apart are shown. (*A*) Top row: ADC maps before (*left*, designated as PRIOR) and after therapy (*right*, designated as CURRENT); the 2 examinations have been spatially coregistered. Middle row: Colored ADC maps before and after therapy within identical-sized regions of interest (ROIs) placed on left iliac bone and left sacrum. Reductions in mean ADC values are seen on visual inspection of the parametric maps and on combined ROI histogram on the bottom row. Mean ADC 896 $\mu m^2/s$ pretreatment to 724 $\mu m^2/s$ post-treatment. (*B*) Same ROIs used in (*A*) with parametric response maps of ADC (PRM_{ADC}) also called functional diffusion maps (fDM), where voxel-by-voxel differences between the 2 examinations shown in (*A*) are classified as decreased (*blue*), unchanged (*green*), or increased (*red*). The percentage of changed voxels is highly dependent on the ADC threshold that has been set. The thresholds used for illustration were 100, 200, 300, and 400 $\mu m^2/s$. Voxel-by-voxel differences can be illustrated as ADC change histograms (see 100 and 300 $\mu m^2/s$ plots) or as scatter plots (see 200 and 400 $\mu m^2/s$ plots). The greater the change in threshold used, the fewer are the pixels classified as unchanged (*green*).

colleagues[58] highlighted the potential pitfall of using mean tumor ADC values for prognostication in 34 rectal cancer patients undergoing chemoradiation. Unlike the Dzik-Jurasz study, they showed no differences between mean pretreatment ADC in the 18 patients who responded and the 16 patients who were nonresponders. However, histogram plots of tumor ADC values did reveal that the nonresponding group had a greater fraction of high ADCs than the responding group, implying that nonresponders had more necrosis.

Similar correlations between high pretherapy ADC values and poorer response to chemotherapy have also been shown in patients with metastatic cancer to the liver (**Fig. 9**).[51,52] Koh and colleagues[51] reported an inverse correlation between the

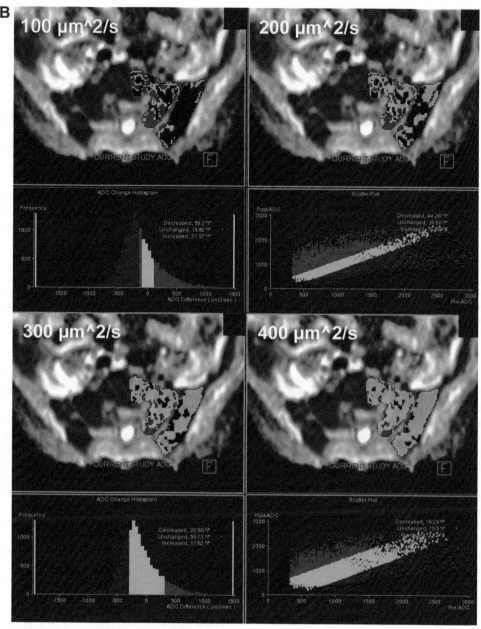

Fig. 8. (*continued*)

percentage size reduction of metastatic liver lesions from colorectal cancer and pretreatment ADC values ($r = -0.58$; $P = .03$). However, Cui and colleagues[52] (who studied liver metastases from colorectal and stomach cancers) found a weaker correlation ($r = -0.293$, $P = .006$) between tumor size reduction and pretreatment ADC values, suggesting that the type of tumor and chemotherapy given may play important roles in determining the

ability of baseline water diffusivity to predict response to therapy.

DW-MR IMAGING CHANGES IN RESPONSE TO THERAPIES THAT INDUCE CELL KILL

When considering the effects of treatment on tumors, it is important to consider tissue-specific responses and therapy effects separately. Thus,

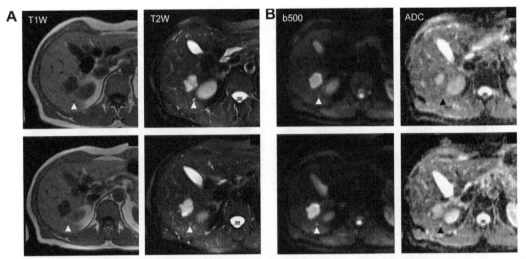

Fig. 9. High ADC values before therapy predict for poor response in metastatic colorectal cancer. A 62-year-old man undergoing examinations before (*top rows*) and after (*bottom rows*) chemotherapy for metastatic colorectal cancer. Two liver metastases are shown that are of high signal intensity on the T2-weighted images (*A*) and are of high signal intensity on ADC maps (*B*). Both lesions were shown to be metastases on contrast-enhanced scans (not shown). Neither the large nor the small (*arrowhead*) lesions show evidence of response after therapy.

there are differences in the way that DW-MR imaging appearances change in response to treatment between soft tissue tumors and bone metastases. When considering therapy effects on tumors, there appear to be differences in DW-MR imaging observations between cytotoxics and other treatments such as radiation, antivascular, embolization, and ablations (see **Table 2**). Differences are observed in the direction of signal intensity and ADC values depending on the therapy given. The data show that the onset and evolution of changes are also not comprehensively documented in the literature. In each case, (soft tissue vs bone) and/or (chemotherapy vs radiation vs antivascular) DW-MR imaging observations appear to reflect interactions between tissue microstructure and the mechanism of action of therapy given.

Soft Tissue Response

As a general rule any pharmacologic, physical, or radioactive process that causes necrosis or cellular lysis will lead to increases in extracellular space water diffusion, with lowering of signal intensity on high b-value images and corresponding increases in ADC values.[17,61] Because cellular death in response to treatment precedes changes in lesion size, changes in DW-MR imaging may be an effective early marker of response for therapies that induce apoptosis.[20,61] Thus, most studies have shown that successful treatment is reflected by increases in tumor ADC values (see **Figs. 4, 5** and **7; Fig. 10**). Rising ADC values with successful

therapy have been noted in several anatomic sites, including breast cancers,[62,63] primary and metastatic cancers to the liver,[51,52,64,65] primary bone sarcomas,[66,67] and brain malignancies.[24,45,68,69] In bone sarcomas, increased ADC values are associated with pathologic response gauged by the extent of necrosis in resection specimens.[66] In soft tissue sarcomas treated with chemotherapy, increases in ADC values are associated with reductions in tumor size and vice versa; as a result, strong negative correlations between tumor volume and ADC changes have been reported ($r = -0.925$, $P<.0001$).[70]

Both animal tumors[71,72] and some human cancer studies have shown that increases in ADC values can occur rapidly after the first dose of chemotherapy at a time consistent with the onset of apoptosis (see **Fig. 4**). A recent human study looked at the onset of changes in ADC in metastatic liver lesions from stomach and colorectal cancer, noting ADC increases as early as 3 to 7 days after the first dose of chemotherapy, and also observed that ADC increases correlated with therapy response.[52] Theilmann and colleagues[64] evaluated 13 women with breast cancer, evaluating 60 liver metastases before and after chemotherapy. Increases in ADC values were observed 4 to 11 days after the start of therapy, particularly in small lesions. Several studies have evaluated ADC changes in patients with primary breast cancer treated with neoadjuvant chemotherapy.[62,73] Stepwise increases in ADC values were shown with each therapy cycle in responding patients, with

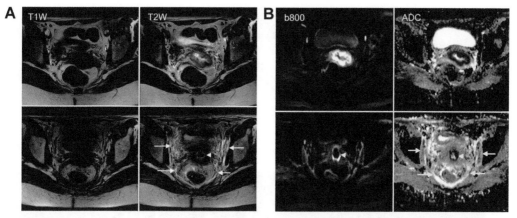

Fig. 10. Response of cervix carcinoma to chemoradiation. A 30-year-old woman undergoing examinations before and after chemoradiation for locally advanced squamous carcinoma of the cervix. (*A*) Anatomic T1- and T2-weighted images before (*top row*) and 6 months after therapy (*bottom row*). The tumor has responded well to therapy with a reduction in tumor size (*arrowhead*). There are new edematous changes in the pelvic fat and pelvic side walls (*arrows*) consistent with microvessel leakage and inflammation occurring after radiotherapy. Radiation-induced fatty marrow atrophy also appears. (*B*) Corresponding b800 and ADC images show a marked increase in ADC values in the cervical stroma and in the pelvic fatty tissues (*arrows*). However, persistent increases on high b-value images associated with decreased ADC values are seen at the edge of the excavated cervix tumor (*arrowhead*), raising the suspicion of residual active disease.

changes in diffusivity preceding changes in tumor size/volume (see **Fig. 7**).

Increases in ADC values as cells die are often transient, and ADC values do decrease subsequently as dead cells are removed by tissue macrophages, as tissues become remodeled, with vascular normalization, and as mature fibrosis develop. Of course if tumors become therapy-resistant then that too may lower ADC values to tumor levels, which is a potential pitfall. Reductions in ADC may not be seen or may be delayed when radiation is given either alone or in combination with chemotherapy. Indeed, when radiotherapy is given there is often a prolonged, persistent elevated ADC because of prolonged tissue edema. This situation appears to be related to ongoing microvascular hyperpermeability and tissue inflammation in normal soft tissues that have been treated with radiation (see **Fig. 10**).

Bone Marrow Response

Before considering bone marrow response to therapy, it is necessary to recall again the relationship between bone marrow cellularity and ADC as illustrated in **Fig. 1**. Changes in ADC values with increasing bone marrow cellularity are biphasic, with initial increases in ADC with increasing marrow cellularity as fat cells are replaced by myeloid and/or tumor cells. However, once fat cells are replaced then reductions in ADC may

be observed with further malignant progression (see **Figs. 2** and **3; Fig. 11**). It has also already been noted that signal intensity on high b-value images increases continually as bone marrow fat cells are progressively replaced with tumor cells.[74] When bone marrow disease is treated successfully, tumor cell death results in increased water diffusivity manifested as increased ADC values. Unlike soft tissue response to therapy, signal intensity changes on high b-value images of bone marrow are more variable; they can be patchy and difficult to interpret, requiring serial follow-up in order to appreciate the time course of changes (see **Fig. 11; Fig. 12**).

At this point it is important to recall that bone marrow disease responding successfully to therapy occurs through 2 dominant mechanisms: first, the appearance of bone sclerosis (ie, reconstitution and subsequent thickening of cancellous bony trabeculae) often promoted by the additional administration of bisphosphonates that are given to prevent skeletal related adverse events; second, by removal of dead tumor cells and the subsequent repopulation with normal marrow elements, predominantly the reemergence of yellow bone marrow.[74] Both of these processes (with or without secondary chemotherapy related myelofibrosis) often occur in proximity to each other within the same bone, particularly in patients with metastatic breast and prostate cancer for whom the sclerotic bony response to successful

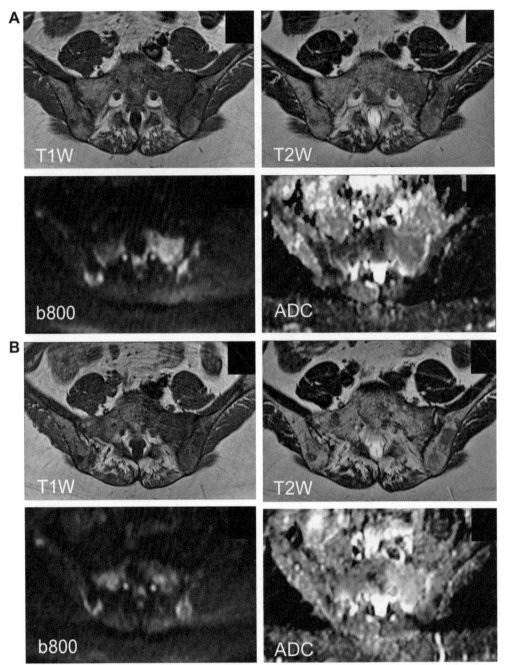

Fig. 11. Differential response of metastatic bone disease. A 41-year-old woman with metastatic breast cancer being treated with chemotherapy and bisphosphonates. Images show T1-weighted, T2-weighted, b800, and ADC maps of the sacrum before therapy (*A*) in April, during therapy (*B*) in June, and in September (*C*). Corresponding ADC spread plots from the left (*D*) and right sacrum (*E*) are also illustrated. These images should be studied bearing in mind **Fig. 1**. The left sacral metastasis has higher signal intensity on the b800 image in April (*A*) compared with the right sacrum. By June this metastasis shows increasing ADC values (*B*) which remain elevated in September (*C*). Note lowering of signal intensity on b800 images by September. These changes in ADC values are consistent with therapy response. The right sacrum is relatively normal on the T1-weighted image in April but shows mild increase in signal intensity on b800 images. By June there are increases in ADC values of the right sacrum with increases in signal intensity on b800 images. These DW-MR imaging findings with lowering of the signal intensity on T1-weighted image are consistent with new metastatic infiltration (no G-CSF therapy given). By September, the right sacrum shows lowering of signal intensity on T1-weighted images with lowering of ADC values. This appearance is consistent with increasing bone marrow infiltration.

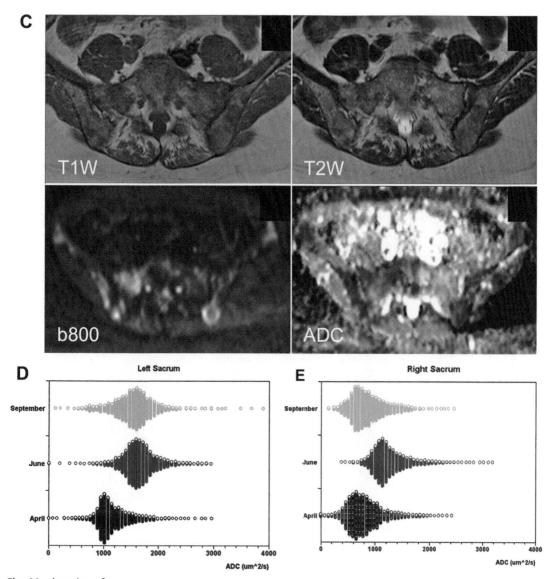

Fig. 11. (*continued*)

therapy can be pronounced. Radiologists should be aware that the emergence of focal sclerosis on CT scans or an increase in activity on bone scans, in a successfully treated breast or prostate cancer patient, should not be misinterpreted as disease progression, but should instead be considered as part of the "healing or flare response" of bone.[75] Tumor necrosis, removal of apoptotic tumor cells, bone sclerosis, reemergence of yellow marrow, loss of tissue water, and secondary myelofibrosis assist in reductions of signal intensity on high b-value images and in ADC values. DW-MR imaging–depicted changes

of water diffusivity occur slowly, becoming visible many months after starting therapy,[76] depending on the tumor type and type of therapy administered (see **Figs. 11** and **12**).

Reductions in signal intensity on high b-value images can also be observed in normal bone marrow, which is also sensitive to the effects of cytotoxic chemotherapy, responding with modest fatty marrow atrophy. However, the sequence and timing of normal bone marrow changes on DW-MR imaging in response to chemotherapy have not as yet been established. Normal bone marrow responds to radiotherapy with marked fatty marrow

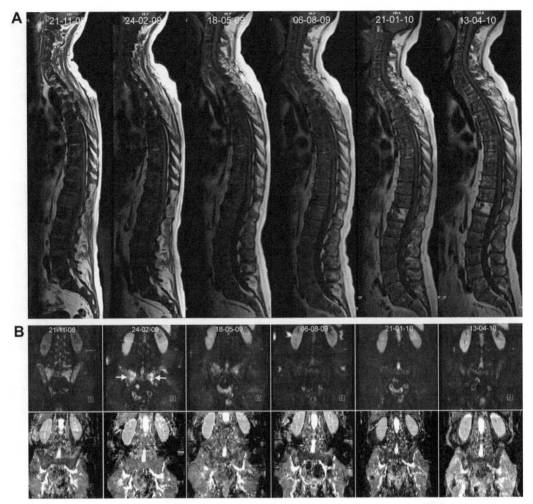

Fig. 12. Serial changes in metastatic prostate cancer responding to abiraterone acetate. A 69 year-old-man with advanced metastatic prostate cancer that was hormone refractory. The patient received abiraterone acetate, an inhibitor of 17α-hydroxylase that reduces testosterone production by both the testes and adrenal glands. (*A*) Serial changes on T1-weighted spinal images over 17 months. Gradual increases in signal intensity are seen consistent with tumor cell replacement by fatty bone marrow. Residual areas of lowed signal intensity represent areas of secondary myelofibrosis and sclerotic bone. (*B*) Serial changes on b800 (*top row*) and ADC maps (*bottom row*) of the sacrum on coronal reconstructions over the same time period. Note initial patchy increases in signal intensity on b800 images (*arrows*) with diffuse increases in ADC values. After February 2009, gradual decreases in signal intensity on b800 images and ADC values are observed, consistent with a healing response to treatment.

atrophy, which is also visible as areas of low signal intensity on high b-value images (**Fig. 13**).[77]

Occasionally within the malignant bone marrow, massive liquefactive necrosis occurs in response to successful treatment. This necrosis has been noted particularly in patients with multiple myeloma, lymphoma, and occasionally other solid metastatic neoplasms. In these cases, persistent high signal intensity is observed on high b-value images with high ADC values (so-called T2 shine-through) (see **Fig. 5; Fig. 14**), which can last for years. On close inspection, there are often lower ADC values at the edge of lesions or sometimes within lesions (forming geometric patterns). This combination of imaging findings suggests inactive disease, reemphasizing the need to always interpret DW-MR imaging by inspecting both the high b-value images and corresponding ADC maps, correlating with other imaging findings as necessary.

DW-MR IMAGING CHANGES IN RESPONSE TO THERAPIES TARGETING TUMOR BLOOD VESSELS

Several studies have shown that antiangiogenic treatments directed toward vascular endothelial

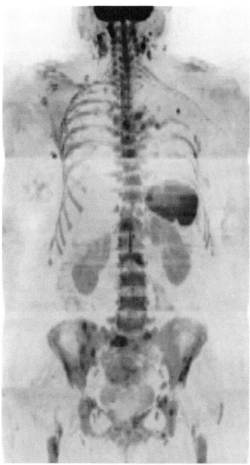

Fig. 13. Radiation atrophy of the bone marrow. A 56-year-old woman with metastatic breast cancer. Whole body DW-MR imaging scan (inverted scale, b800 s/mm^2) shows focal areas of increased signal intensity in the bone marrow of the spine and pelvis consistent with bony metastases. Focus on the left upper chest. Note that the left upper ribs, left clavicle, and scapular bone are not visible. The brachial plexus remains visible. This effect is caused by yellow marrow atrophy due to radiation, initially to the chest wall and then to the left supra-clavicular fossa, for recurrent nodal disease that is not visible.

growth factor (VEGF) causes reductions in tumor ADC values that coincide with reductions in contrast enhancement. This observation has been noted in brain glioblastomas treated with the anti-VEGF antibody bevacizumab[78] and with the small molecular weight tyrosine kinase inhibitor of the VEGF receptor cediranib.[79] Similar reductions in ADC values have been noted for sorafenib, an anti-angiogenic therapy used for treatment of hepatocellular carcinoma.[80] The mechanisms for this observation have been investigated in brain xenograft models and in patients with brain tumors who were given cediranib as a monotherapy.[81]

The principal explanation appears to be reductions of lesion extravascular-extracellular space secondary to vascular normalization and the lowering of vascular permeability.[79,82] Batchelor and colleagues[79] evaluated patients with recurrent glioblastomas treated with cediranib with multifunctional MR imaging examinations. Parameters assessed included contrast-enhanced tumor volume, vessel size index, microvessel permeability, extracellular leakage space, and water diffusivity. Using this panel of imaging tests, Batchelor and colleagues were able to show rapid reductions in microvessel permeability (inflow transfer constant), extracellular leakage space, and water diffusivity following treatment, which was interpreted as evidence of microvessel normalization.

The reader should be aware that reductions of ADC values are not always marked with antivascular therapies (Fig. 15). Indeed, the opposite (increased ADC) is observed if there is significant tumor necrosis caused by the antivascular treatment. This increase in ADC values been particularly noted for a distinct class of antivascular therapy called vascular disruptive agents (VDAs), which induce massive necrosis within tumor centers.[83,84] For example, Thoeny and colleagues[84,85] evaluated the effects of the vascular disruptive agent combretastatin-A4-phosphate on rat rhabdomyosarcoma, and showed that there were initial reductions in ADC values for 1 to 2 days after the administration of the drug. Reduction in ADC values coincided with reduced perfusion seen on dynamic contrast-enhanced MR imaging when no necrosis was seen histologically. Subsequently, increases in ADC values were observed that coincided with the onset of necrosis. Rising ADC values have also been seen in clinical studies by Koh and colleagues[83] when combretastatin-A4-phosphate was given with the anti-VEGF antibody bevacizumab. Like the studies of Thoeny and colleagues,[84,85] Koh and colleagues[83] found that increases in ADC were more likely to occur in tumors with higher pretreatment ADC values, indicating that necrotic tumors were more susceptible to the effects of combretastatin-A4-phosphate.

DIFFUSIVITY CHANGES INDUCED BY EMBOLIZATION AND ABLATIVE THERAPIES

Transarterial chemoembolization (TACE) is commonly used to treat unresectable hepatocellular carcinoma (HCC). The effects of TACE on animal liver tumors has been evaluated in several studies[36,86] showing that there is an early reduction of ADC values after therapy (within the first few hours), after which consistent rises in ADC values occur, coinciding with the development of

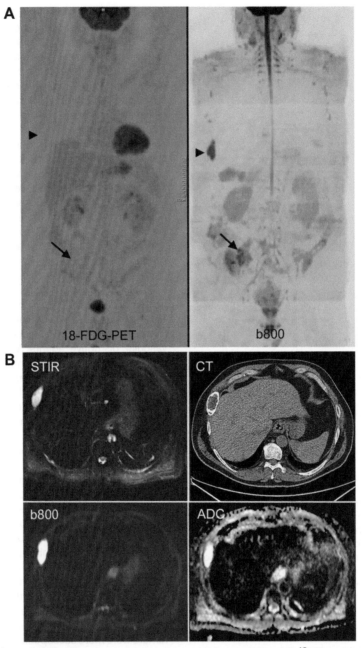

Fig. 14. T2 shine-through following chemotherapy for multiple myeloma. (*A*) ^{18}F-Fluorodexyglucose PET scan (*left*) and whole body DW-MR imaging image (inverted scale, b800 s/mm^2) on a 55-year-old man with multiple myeloma treated with chemotherapy alone. No areas of abnormal hypermetabolism are seen on the PET scan but 2 areas of increased signal intensity are seen on the DW-MR imaging image (right lower rib [*arrowhead*] and right iliac bone [*arrow*]). (*B*) Axial STIR, CT scan, b800 image, and ADC map through the rib lesion. The lesion is of high signal intensity on both the b800 image and the ADC map, indicating T2 shine-through. This appearance suggests inactive disease. Note low signal intensity of the liver on the b800 image and ADC map, consistent with iron overload.

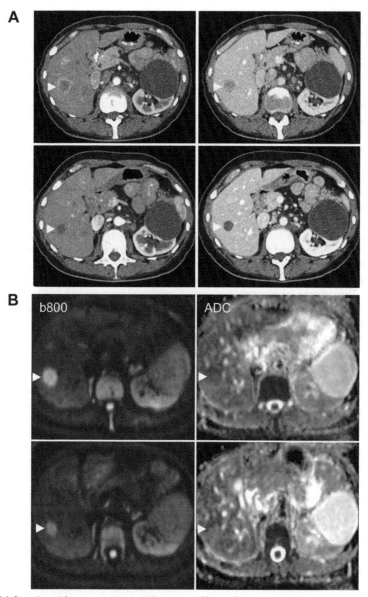

Fig. 15. 41 year old female with metastatic renal cancer. Effect of antiangiogenic therapy on renal carcinoma metastasis. (*A*) Axial CT scans of the liver in the arterial and portal phases of enhancement before (*top row*) and 6 weeks after commencing sorafenib therapy (*bottom row*). A modest reduction in tumor size is seen with marked reduction in enhancement, and CT density of large liver metastasis is noted (*arrowhead*). (*B*) b800 and ADC images at the same time points showing reduction in tumor size, but persistent high signal is visible on b800 images. There is a minimal increase in ADC values from 1410 $\mu m^2/s$ to 1460 $\mu m^2/s$.

cystic and necrotic changes.[87] Similar findings of increasing ADC values have also been seen when therapy with yttrium-90–labeled microspheres are used for radioembolization of hepatocellular carcinomas.[88,89]

Recently Kamel and colleagues[90] reported on a mechanistic imaging study that improved the understanding of temporal effects of TACE. These investigators evaluated serial changes on gadolinium contrast medium–enhanced MR imaging

and DW-MR imaging in patients with unresectable HCC after TACE. In this multiple time-point observational study, they assessed (1) tumor mass (by size changes on morphologic imaging), (2) underlying vascular properties of tissues (by qualitative relative arterial and portal phase enhancement assessments), and (3) cellular density and necrosis (by ADC values). Kamel and colleagues[90] observed that tumor size remained relatively unchanged for 4 weeks after TACE, whereas changes in dynamic contrast enhancement and tissue diffusivity had dissimilar time courses. Reductions in the degree of enhancement were seen immediately after chemoembolization and were sustained over the observation period. However, increases in ADC values became most apparent after 1 to 2 weeks but had returned to the baseline values by 4 weeks. Given the delivery mechanism of the therapy and prior knowledge that most primary and secondary liver malignancies are predominantly supplied by the hepatic artery, immediate reductions in arterial contrast enhancement after TACE were expected. There are also sound biologic mechanisms to explain ADC increases after treatment: treatment-induced necrosis and cell death. The transient period of increased ADC values followed by ADC normalization[90] could be explained by the removal of dead/dying cells and shifts of extracellular water with tissue compaction, fibrosis, and regeneration of native tissues. The effects of embolization on uterine fibroids have also been evaluated 6 months after therapy.[91] After embolization, fibroids are noted to have lower signal intensity on high b-value images and ADC values, confirming infarction and dehydration of fibroids following treatment. The time course of DW-MR imaging changes after uterine fibroid embolization has not been comprehensively investigated as far as the authors are aware.

The effects of ablative therapies on DW-MR imaging have been investigated. Jacobs and colleagues[92] evaluated the effects of high-intensity focused ultrasound (HIFU) therapy on uterine fibroids using contrast medium enhancement and DW-MR imaging. Initial reductions in ADC values within ablated tissues were observed (with decreasing contrast enhancement and high signal intensity on DW-MR images). These changes can be ascribed to decreasing water diffusivity due to ischemia, cellular swelling, and/or protein denaturation. At 6-month follow-up, areas of decreased contrast agent uptake persisted but the signal intensity on DW images appeared heterogeneous within treated regions. Increasing ADC values were presumed to reflect cell loss and liquefactive necrosis. These findings indicate the versatility of DW-MR imaging in helping to define the evolution of tissues treated with HIFU over time.

There are relatively few studies evaluating the DW-MR imaging effects of radiofrequency ablation (RFA)[93–95] on tumors and surrounding tissues. An animal study of VX2 rabbit tumors implanted into the back muscles of rabbits used DW-MR imaging and FDG-PET scans, showing modest increases in ADC values and reductions in glucose uptake 2 to 3 days after therapy,[95] indicating that both DW-MR imaging and FDG-PET are potentially useful

markers for monitoring the early effects of RFA. Okuma and colleagues[93] evaluated 17 patients with 20 lung lesions 3 days after treatment, and showed that all lesions regardless of outcome had higher ADC values after treatment ($P<.05$). These investigators also showed that nonprogressors had much greater increases in ADC compared with those lesions that did regrow over time. Schraml and colleagues[94] reviewed 54 patients treated by RFA for liver metastases. Ablation areas did not show any systematic changes in time course after treatment. Ablated areas did show heterogeneous appearances on ADC maps reflecting tissue damage following RFA, such as enlarged sinusoids, interstitial edema, hemorrhage, carbonization, necrosis, and fibrosis. Based on current data, it can be concluded that ADC changes may be useful for monitoring the response of tumors to RFA treatment, but the time course of appearances within organs and its ability to predict outcomes of RFA therapy are yet to be fully defined.

ADDITIONAL CONSIDERATIONS
Standardization

A major challenge to the widespread implementation of DW-MR imaging as response biomarker for the development of cancer therapies in the clinic is the lack of standard approaches to data collection and analysis.[17] This drawback creates challenges for support by commercial MR imaging and software vendors, and limits deployment of this technique to sites with significant experimental MR imaging expertise. Furthermore, the lack of standard approaches impairs multi-institutional validation and makes the ultimate qualification of DW-MR imaging as a response biomarker difficult. In large part, the lack of standardization is related to the technical challenges in performing examinations. In most practical situations performing "ideal" data acquisition is impractical, due to limits in technology and patient compliance. Approaches that accommodate technical limitations through compromises in acquisition and/or analysis are being developed to allow the practical implementation of this technique.

Region of Interest Drawing

The authors have noted that response assessments are generally undertaken by noting changes in signal intensity on high b-value images or by ADC changes, the latter allowing more objective assessments of therapy effectiveness. An important consideration when measuring ADC values is region of interest (ROI) placements. In general, ROIs should be placed just within tumor boundaries on high b-value images.[17] The b-value image chosen for this purpose should have the highest image contrast between the lesion and surrounding tissues, which will vary by anatomic site and treatment time point, which is why more specific recommendations are not given. ROIs should then be copied and placed onto corresponding ADC maps for diffusivity measurement readouts. It is not recommended that ROIs be drawn directly on ADC maps because lesion borders are often not well defined in soft tissue disease. On the other hand, bony lesions are often better defined on ADC maps compared with high b-value images after therapy because of increased ADC values compared with normal marrow, which has very low ADC values. Another point that merits consideration is that for the analysis of serial studies, it is helpful to delineate ROIs of all studies in the same image evaluation session to ensure close matching of imaging sections for the placement of ROIs.

Measurement Error and Reproducibility

To be able use quantitative DW-MR imaging kinetic parameters for the assessment of therapy response in individual patients, assessments of measurement error are needed. Estimates of measurement errors enable one to decide whether changes in ADC are "real" for both groups of patients and individuals. Test-retest assessments are facilitated by incorporating baseline repeated measurements to provide information directly relevant to the body sites being studied. It is important to also identify major sources of error leading to nonreproducible results, including the natural biologic variability of parameters such as ADC, the variability inherent in the measuring instruments (ie, the MR imaging scanner), and knowledge of additional errors induced by appraisers or analysis techniques. There have been relatively few published studies documenting measurement error in body applications for DW-MR imaging, and most published studies are from institutions with considerable technical expertise[80,91,92]; there are few larger-scale multicenter studies.[93] A threshold for ADC change in extracranial applications has not yet been safely established, but initial indications suggest that mean/median tumor reproducibility is likely to be somewhere in the range of 10% to 20%.[80]

Reproducibility information needs to be combined with the expected magnitude of therapeutic effects, so as to be able to determine the sensitivity of ADC as a useful tool for making therapeutic decisions at the individual patient level. The literature shows that ADC increases in response to therapeutic interventions are of small magnitude, particularly soon after starting therapy. So for

example, Cui and colleagues[52] studied liver metastases from stomach and colorectal cancers, observing changes in ADC values 3 and 7 days after the first dose of chemotherapy. Mean increases of ADC from baseline values were approximately 25% in responding patients (quartiles approximately +10% to +40%) and 8% to 10% (quartiles approximately −10% to +25%) in nonresponders. These changes are of relatively small magnitude compared with the expected reproducibility of the technique (which the authors have noted has yet to be firmly established!). Thus, the extent to which changes in ADC can be used in individual patients for the purpose of early therapeutic decision making has yet to be firmly established.

Thresholding of Parametric Response Maps

A basic assumption when undertaking PRM_{ADC} evaluations is that no change in tumor size/volume has occurred in the time elapsed between examinations (see section "Quantitative Analysis"). The authors have also noted that thresholds of individual voxel differences are needed to define the percentage of voxels that are changed in response to a therapeutic intervention (see **Fig. 8**) Defining actual PRM_{ADC} thresholds requires that test-retest examinations are performed in the organ/tumor of interest (ie, you cannot apply brain threshold values to liver studies). Such measurements should ideally be from tumor regions and not "surrogate" normal tissues because intrinsic variability is likely to be different. Furthermore, one cannot simply use reproducibility thresholds acquired at the "whole tumor" level, which is done on mean/median ADCs. Instead thresholds at the voxel level need to be defined, and these are likely to be much greater than those reported for mean/median reproducibility.

Defining PRM_{ADC} thresholds can be done on cancer patients using the so-called coffee-break examination approach. That is, patients are removed from the scanner and reexamined after a short period of time. In this way the variability inherent in the measuring instruments, setup errors, and additional errors induced by appraisers or analysis techniques can be accounted for. Paired pretherapy examinations can then be registered and a variety of thresholds established for no-change as appropriate. Such data are largely missing from the literature for both brain and visceral tumors, and are urgently needed if PRM_{ADC} is to become useful clinically.[30,48]

SUMMARY

We need to think of DW-MR imaging as an important means for biologic exploration because it

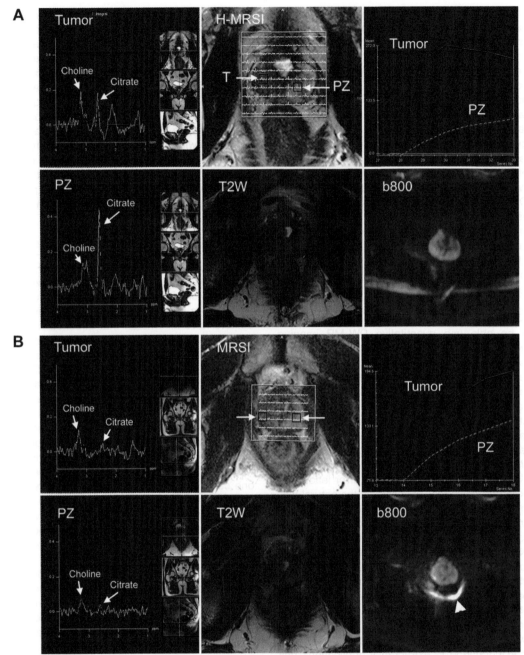

Fig. 16. 66 year old male with prostate cancer. Multiparametric imaging of primary prostate cancer treated with androgen deprivation. Locally advanced prostate cancer being treated with the antiandrogen goserelin acetate. Images were obtained 6 months apart. (*A*) Pretherapy T2-weighted (T2W), b800, and proton MR spectroscopic imaging (MRSI) images with selected spectra from normal peripheral zone (PZ) and tumor (T) depicted in separate panels; the spectra are scaled to the maximum peak (citrate) on the spectra. Dynamic-enhanced MR imaging curves from the region of the tumor and PZ are also shown. (*B*) Following therapy the gland is smaller (pretherapy gland volume 20.2 mL; posttreatment 10.6 ml) with poorer zonal differentiation on T2-weighted images, consistent with glandular atrophy. Reductions in citrate peaks are seen in tumor and PZ, also consistent with glandular atrophy. High choline levels indicate ongoing active disease in the tumor. Vascular shutdown in the tumor region is known to occur with androgen deprivation. There is no change in the b800 signal intensity. Curved artifact (*arrowhead*) does not interfere with the assessment of the prostate signal intensity appearances. (*C*) ADC histograms of the whole prostate showing reductions in number of pixels with ADC values greater than 1500 $\mu m^2/s$. The whole prostate ADC shows a minimal decrease from 1395 $\mu m^2/s$ to 1322 $\mu m^2/s$.

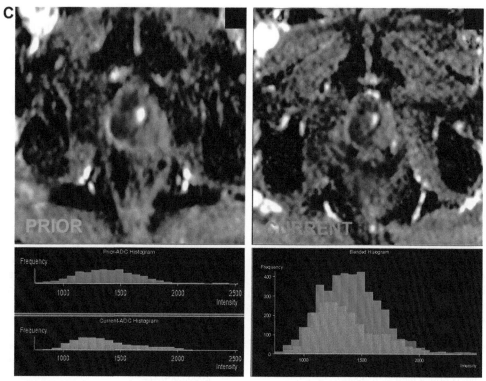

Fig. 16. (*continued*)

yields quantitative parameters that reflect specific aspects of the underlying tumor or tissue pathology relating to perfusion, cellularity, distribution of cell sizes, and necrosis. The direction, extent, and duration of ADC changes can vary depending on the type of treatment administered, tumor or tissue type, and the timing of imaging with respect to the treatment given. To be able understand these findings, DW-MR imaging needs to be correlated with other complementary anatomic and functional MR imaging techniques, which together provide a wealth of biologically relevant information concerning the nature of tumor response to therapy.[96] Observations from multiparametric MR imaging studies indicate that ADC changes are dependent on complex interplays of biophysical processes in response to therapy (**Fig. 16**), reemphasizing the need to better understand therapy-induced tissue changes that may be reflected in DW-MR imaging parameters.

DW-MR imaging data obtained is clinically useful in terms of disease detection and characterization, for tumor staging, and for the detection of relapsed disease. In the disease-response setting, many studies show that changes can be directly related to mechanism of treatments and that observations precede morphologic alterations. However, it has not been shown convincingly

that DW-MR imaging enables personalization of therapy response or that survival of cancer patients is improved by making use of DW-MR imaging response data. Potential economic benefits from DW-MR imaging response assessments are also largely missing. There is scope for considerable further investigations that will need to be done if DW-MR imaging is to take its place in the "roll-call" of functional imaging techniques of clinical relevance that are able to predict therapy response. It can therefore be said that DW-MR imaging is useful for assessing therapy response when applied together with other functional imaging techniques, but whether its use alone will result in a paradigm shift in clinical assessments is a question still open to debate.

REFERENCES

1. Eisenhauer EA, Therasse P, Bogaerts J, et al. New response evaluation criteria in solid tumours: revised RECIST guideline (version 1.1). Eur J Cancer 2009; 45(2):228–47.
2. Husband JE, Schwartz LH, Spencer J, et al. Evaluation of the response to treatment of solid tumours—a consensus statement of the International Cancer Imaging Society. Br J Cancer 2004; 90(12):2256–60.

3. Benjamin RS, Choi H, Macapinlac HA, et al. We should desist using RECIST, at least in GIST. J Clin Oncol 2007;25(13):1760–4.

4. Nathan P, Judson I, Padhani A, et al. A phase I study of combretastatin A4 phosphate (CA4P) and bevacizumab in subjects with advanced solid tumors. J Clin Oncol 2008;26(Suppl):3550.

5. Friedman HS, Prados MD, Wen PY, et al. Bevacizumab alone and in combination with irinotecan in recurrent glioblastoma. J Clin Oncol 2009;27(28): 4733–40.

6. Hurwitz H, Fehrenbacher L, Novotny W, et al. Bevacizumab plus irinotecan, fluorouracil, and leucovorin for metastatic colorectal cancer. N Engl J Med 2004; 350(23):2335–42.

7. Llovet JM, Ricci S, Mazzaferro V, et al. Sorafenib in advanced hepatocellular carcinoma. N Engl J Med 2008;359(4):378–90.

8. Escudier B, Pluzanska A, Koralewski P, et al. Bevacizumab plus interferon alfa-2a for treatment of metastatic renal cell carcinoma: a randomised, double-blind phase III trial. Lancet 2007;370(9605): 2103–11.

9. Motzer RJ, Hutson TE, Tomczak P, et al. Sunitinib versus interferon alfa in metastatic renal-cell carcinoma. N Engl J Med 2007;356(2):115–24.

10. Saltz LB, Clarke S, Diaz-Rubio E, et al. Bevacizumab in combination with oxaliplatin-based chemotherapy as first-line therapy in metastatic colorectal cancer: a randomized phase III study. J Clin Oncol 2008; 26(12):2013–9.

11. Miller K, Wang M, Gralow J, et al. Paclitaxel plus bevacizumab versus paclitaxel alone for metastatic breast cancer. N Engl J Med 2007;357(26): 2666–76.

12. Miller KD, Chap LI, Holmes FA, et al. Randomized phase III trial of capecitabine compared with bevacizumab plus capecitabine in patients with previously treated metastatic breast cancer. J Clin Oncol 2005;23(4):792–9.

13. Van den Abbeele AD, Badawi RD. Use of positron emission tomography in oncology and its potential role to assess response to imatinib mesylate therapy in gastrointestinal stromal tumors (GISTs). Eur J Cancer 2002;38(Suppl 5):S60–5.

14. Workman P, Aboagye EO, Chung YL, et al. Minimally invasive pharmacokinetic and pharmacodynamic technologies in hypothesis-testing clinical trials of innovative therapies. J Natl Cancer Inst 2006;98(9): 580–98.

15. Weber WA, Czernin J, Phelps ME, et al. Technology insight: novel imaging of molecular targets is an emerging area crucial to the development of targeted drugs. Nat Clin Pract Oncol 2008;5(1): 44–54.

16. Zweifel M, Padhani AR. Perfusion MRI in the early clinical development of antivascular drugs: decorations or decision making tools? Eur J Nucl Med Mol Imaging 2010;37(Suppl 1):S164–82.

17. Padhani AR, Liu G, Koh DM, et al. Diffusion-weighted magnetic resonance imaging as a cancer biomarker: consensus and recommendations. Neoplasia 2009;11(2):102–25.

18. Koh DM, Collins DJ. Diffusion-weighted MRI in the body: applications and challenges in oncology. AJR Am J Roentgenol 2007;188(6):1622–35.

19. Thoeny HC, De Keyzer F. Extracranial applications of diffusion-weighted magnetic resonance imaging. Eur Radiol 2007;17(6):1385–93.

20. Patterson DM, Padhani AR, Collins DJ. Technology insight: water diffusion MRI—a potential new biomarker of response to cancer therapy. Nat Clin Pract Oncol 2008;5(4):220–33.

21. Parikh T, Drew SJ, Lee VS, et al. Focal liver lesion detection and characterization with diffusion-weighted MR imaging: comparison with standard breath-hold T2-weighted imaging. Radiology 2008; 246(3):812–22.

22. Yoshikawa MI, Ohsumi S, Sugata S, et al. Relation between cancer cellularity and apparent diffusion coefficient values using diffusion-weighted magnetic resonance imaging in breast cancer. Radiat Med 2008;26(4):222–6.

23. Manenti G, Di Roma M, Mancino S, et al. Malignant renal neoplasms: correlation between ADC values and cellularity in diffusion weighted magnetic resonance imaging at 3 T. Radiol Med 2008;113(2): 199–213.

24. Hayashida Y, Hirai T, Morishita S, et al. Diffusion-weighted imaging of metastatic brain tumors: comparison with histologic type and tumor cellularity. AJNR Am J Neuroradiol 2006;27(7): 1419–25.

25. Humphries PD, Sebire NJ, Siegel MJ, et al. Tumors in pediatric patients at diffusion-weighted MR imaging: apparent diffusion coefficient and tumor cellularity. Radiology 2007;245(3):848–54.

26. Zelhof B, Pickles M, Liney G, et al. Correlation of diffusion-weighted magnetic resonance data with cellularity in prostate cancer. BJU Int 2009;103(7): 883–8.

27. Liu Y, Bai R, Sun H, et al. Diffusion-weighted magnetic resonance imaging of uterine cervical cancer. J Comput Assist Tomogr 2009;33(6): 858–62.

28. Sugahara T, Korogi Y, Kochi M, et al. Usefulness of diffusion-weighted MRI with echo-planar technique in the evaluation of cellularity in gliomas. J Magn Reson Imaging 1999;9(1):53–60.

29. Lyng H, Haraldseth O, Rofstad EK. Measurement of cell density and necrotic fraction in human melanoma xenografts by diffusion weighted magnetic resonance imaging. Magn Reson Med 2000;43(6): 828–36.

30. Ellingson BM, Malkin MG, Rand SD, et al. Validation of functional diffusion maps (fDMs) as a biomarker for human glioma cellularity. J Magn Reson Imaging 2010;31(3):538–48.

31. Nonomura Y, Yasumoto M, Yoshimura R, et al. Relationship between bone marrow cellularity and apparent diffusion coefficient. J Magn Reson Imaging 2001;13(5):757–60.

32. Tang GY, Lv ZW, Tang RB, et al. Evaluation of MR spectroscopy and diffusion-weighted MRI in detecting bone marrow changes in postmenopausal women with osteoporosis. Clin Radiol 2010;65(5):377–81.

33. Wang XZ, Wang B, Gao ZQ, et al. Diffusion-weighted imaging of prostate cancer: correlation between apparent diffusion coefficient values and tumor proliferation. J Magn Reson Imaging 2009;29(6):1360–6.

34. Calvar JA, Meli FJ, Romero C, et al. Characterization of brain tumors by MRS, DWI and Ki-67 labeling index. J Neurooncol 2005;72(3):273–80.

35. Arvinda HR, Kesavadas C, Sarma PS, et al. Glioma grading: sensitivity, specificity, positive and negative predictive values of diffusion and perfusion imaging. J Neurooncol 2009;94(1):87–96.

36. Geschwind JF, Artemov D, Abraham S, et al. Chemoembolization of liver tumor in a rabbit model: assessment of tumor cell death with diffusion-weighted MR imaging and histologic analysis. J Vasc Interv Radiol 2000;11(10):1245–55.

37. Kim H, Morgan DE, Zeng H, et al. Breast tumor xenografts: diffusion-weighted MR imaging to assess early therapy with novel apoptosis-inducing anti-DR5 antibody. Radiology 2008;248(3):844–51.

38. Liimatainen T, Hakumaki JM, Kauppinen RA, et al. Monitoring of gliomas in vivo by diffusion MRI and (1)H MRS during gene therapy-induced apoptosis: interrelationships between water diffusion and mobile lipids. NMR Biomed 2009;22(3):272–9.

39. Hartman RP, Sundaram M, Okuno SH, et al. Effect of granulocyte-stimulating factors on marrow of adult patients with musculoskeletal malignancies: incidence and MRI findings. Am J Roentgenol 2004;183(3):645–53.

40. Fletcher BD, Wall JE, Hanna SL. Effect of hematopoietic growth factors on MR images of bone marrow in children undergoing chemotherapy. Radiology 1993;189(3):745–51.

41. Yao WJ, Hoh CK, Hawkins RA, et al. Quantitative PET imaging of bone marrow glucose metabolic response to hematopoietic cytokines. J Nucl Med 1995;36(5):794–9.

42. Jackson A, O'Connor JP, Parker GJ, et al. Imaging tumor vascular heterogeneity and angiogenesis using dynamic contrast-enhanced magnetic resonance imaging. Clin Cancer Res 2007;13(12):3449–59.

43. Rose CJ, Mills SJ, O'Connor JP, et al. Quantifying spatial heterogeneity in dynamic contrast-enhanced MRI parameter maps. Magn Reson Med 2009;62(2):488–99.

44. Galban CJ, Chenevert TL, Meyer CR, et al. The parametric response map is an imaging biomarker for early cancer treatment outcome. Nat Med 2009;15(5):572–6.

45. Hamstra DA, Galban CJ, Meyer CR, et al. Functional diffusion map as an early imaging biomarker for high-grade glioma: correlation with conventional radiologic response and overall survival. J Clin Oncol 2008;26(20):3387–94.

46. Galban CJ, Mukherji SK, Chenevert TL, et al. A feasibility study of parametric response map analysis of diffusion-weighted magnetic resonance imaging scans of head and neck cancer patients for providing early detection of therapeutic efficacy. Transl Oncol 2009;2(3):184–90.

47. Reischauer C, Froehlich JM, Koh DM, et al. Bone metastases from prostate cancer: assessing treatment response by using diffusion-weighted imaging and functional diffusion maps - initial observations. Radiology 2010;257(2):523–31.

48. Ma B, Meyer CR, Pickles MD, et al. Voxel-by-voxel functional diffusion mapping for early evaluation of breast cancer treatment. Inf Process Med Imaging 2009;21:276–87.

49. Roth Y, Tichler T, Kostenich G, et al. High-b-value diffusion-weighted MR imaging for pretreatment prediction and early monitoring of tumor response to therapy in mice. Radiology 2004;232(3):685–92.

50. Lemaire L, Howe FA, Rodrigues LM, et al. Assessment of induced rat mammary tumour response to chemotherapy using the apparent diffusion coefficient of tissue water as determined by diffusion-weighted ^{1}H-NMR spectroscopy in vivo. MAGMA 1999;8(1):20–6.

51. Koh DM, Scurr E, Collins D, et al. Predicting response of colorectal hepatic metastasis: value of pretreatment apparent diffusion coefficients. AJR Am J Roentgenol 2007;188(4):1001–8.

52. Cui Y, Zhang XP, Sun YS, et al. Apparent diffusion coefficient: potential imaging biomarker for prediction and early detection of response to chemotherapy in hepatic metastases. Radiology 2008;248(3):894–900.

53. Niwa T, Ueno M, Ohkawa S, et al. Advanced pancreatic cancer: the use of the apparent diffusion coefficient to predict response to chemotherapy. Br J Radiol 2009;82(973):28–34.

54. Brizel D, Scully S, Harrelson J, et al. Tumor oxygenation predicts for the likelihood of distant metastases in human soft tissue sarcoma. Cancer Res 1996;56(5):941–3.

55. Swinson DE, Jones JL, Richardson D, et al. Tumour necrosis is an independent prognostic marker in

nonsmall cell lung cancer: correlation with biological variables. Lung Cancer 2002;37(3):235–40.

56. Gray LH, Conger AD, Ebert M, et al. The concentration of oxygen dissolved in tissues at the time of irradiation as a factor in radiotherapy. Br J Radiol 1953;26:638–48.

57. Leek RD, Landers RJ, Harris AL, et al. Necrosis correlates with high vascular density and focal macrophage infiltration in invasive carcinoma of the breast. Br J Cancer 1999;79(5–6):991–5.

58. DeVries AF, Kremser C, Hein PA, et al. Tumor microcirculation and diffusion predict therapy outcome for primary rectal carcinoma. Int J Radiat Oncol Biol Phys 2003;56(4):958–65.

59. Pope WB, Kim HJ, Huo J, et al. Recurrent glioblastoma multiforme: ADC histogram analysis predicts response to bevacizumab treatment. Radiology 2009;252(1):182–9.

60. Dzik-Jurasz A, Domenig C, George M, et al. Diffusion MRI for prediction of response of rectal cancer to chemoradiation. Lancet 2002;360:307–8.

61. Hamstra DA, Rehemtulla A, Ross BD. Diffusion magnetic resonance imaging: a biomarker for treatment response in oncology. J Clin Oncol 2007;25(26):4104–9.

62. Pickles MD, Gibbs P, Lowry M, et al. Diffusion changes precede size reduction in neoadjuvant treatment of breast cancer. Magn Reson Imaging 2006;24:843–7.

63. Yankeelov TE, Lepage M, Chakravarthy A, et al. Integration of quantitative DCE-MRI and ADC mapping to monitor treatment response in human breast cancer: initial results. Magn Reson Imaging 2007;25:1–13.

64. Theilmann RJ, Borders R, Trouard TP, et al. Changes in water mobility measured by diffusion MRI predict response of metastatic breast cancer to chemotherapy. Neoplasia 2004;6(6):831–7.

65. Kamel IR, Rayes DK, Liapi E, et al. Functional MR imaging assessment of tumor response after 90Y microsphere treatment in patients with unresectable hepatocellular carcinoma. J Vasc Interv Radiol 2007;18:49–56.

66. Hayashida Y, Yakushiji T, Awai K, et al. Monitoring therapeutic responses of primary bone tumors by diffusion-weighted image: initial results. Eur Radiol 2006;16(12):2637–43.

67. Uhl M, Saueressig U, van Buiren M, et al. Osteosarcoma: preliminary results of in vivo assessment of tumor necrosis after chemotherapy with diffusion- and perfusion-weighted magnetic resonance imaging. Invest Radiol 2006;41:618–23.

68. Moffat BA, Chenevert TL, Lawrence TS, et al. Functional diffusion map: a noninvasive MRI biomarker for early stratification of clinical brain tumor response. Proc Natl Acad Sci U S A 2005;102:5524–9.

69. Mardor Y, Pfeffer R, Spiegelmann R, et al. Early detection of response to radiation therapy in patients with brain malignancies using conventional and high b-value diffusion-weighted magnetic resonance imaging. J Clin Oncol 2003;21(6):1094–100.

70. Dudeck O, Zeile M, Pink D, et al. Diffusion-weighted magnetic resonance imaging allows monitoring of anticancer treatment effects in patients with soft-tissue sarcomas. J Magn Reson Imaging 2008;27(5):1109–13.

71. Jennings D, Hatton BN, Guo J, et al. Early response of prostate carcinoma xenografts to docetaxel chemotherapy monitored with diffusion MRI. Neoplasia 2002;4:255–62.

72. Jordan BF, Runquist M, Raghunand N, et al. Dynamic contrast-enhanced and diffusion MRI show rapid and dramatic changes in tumor microenvironment in response to inhibition of HIF-1alpha using PX-478. Neoplasia 2005;7(5):475–85.

73. Sharma U, Danishad KK, Seenu V, et al. Longitudinal study of the assessment by MRI and diffusion-weighted imaging of tumor response in patients with locally advanced breast cancer undergoing neoadjuvant chemotherapy. NMR Biomed 2009;22(1):104–13.

74. Messiou C, deSouza NM. Diffusion weighted magnetic resonance imaging of metastatic bone disease: a biomarker for treatment response monitoring. Cancer Biomark 2010;6(1):21–32.

75. Messiou C, Cook G, deSouza NM. Imaging metastatic bone disease from carcinoma of the prostate. Br J Cancer 2009;101(8):1225–32.

76. Messiou C, Collins D, Morgan V, et al. ADC changes with time in focal and diffuse myeloma bone disease as indicators of disease response and progression [Abstract no 1716]. In: Proceedings of the joint meeting of International Society of Magnetic Resonance in Medicine and the European Society of Magnetic Resonance in Medicine and Biology. Stockholm: 2010.

77. Bydder M, Liang Y, Yu H, et al. Monitoring bone marrow changes during chemoradiotherapy using MRI fat quantification [Abstract no 2822]. In: Proceedings of the joint meeting of International Society of Magnetic Resonance in Medicine and the European Society of Magnetic Resonance in Medicine and Biology. Stockholm: 2010.

78. Jain R, Scarpace LM, Ellika S, et al. Imaging response criteria for recurrent gliomas treated with bevacizumab: role of diffusion weighted imaging as an imaging biomarker. J Neurooncol 2010;96(3):423–31.

79. Batchelor TT, Sorensen AG, di Tomaso E, et al. AZD2171, a pan-VEGF receptor tyrosine kinase inhibitor, normalizes tumor vasculature and alleviates edema in glioblastoma patients. Cancer Cell 2007;11(1):83–95.

80. Schraml C, Schwenzer NF, Martirosian P, et al. Diffusion-weighted MRI of advanced hepatocellular

carcinoma during sorafenib treatment: initial results. AJR Am J Roentgenol 2009;193(4):W301–7.

81. Kamoun WS, Ley CD, Farrar CT, et al. Edema control by cediranib, a vascular endothelial growth factor receptor-targeted kinase inhibitor, prolongs survival despite persistent brain tumor growth in mice. J Clin Oncol 2009;27(15):2542–52.

82. Batchelor TT, Duda DG, di Tomaso E, et al. Phase II study of cediranib, an oral pan-vascular endothelial growth factor receptor tyrosine kinase inhibitor, in patients with recurrent glioblastoma. J Clin Oncol 2010;28(17):2817–23.

83. Koh DM, Blackledge M, Collins DJ, et al. Reproducibility and changes in the apparent diffusion coefficients of solid tumours treated with combretastatin A4 phosphate and bevacizumab in a two-centre phase I clinical trial. Eur Radiol 2009;19(11):2728–38.

84. Thoeny HC, De Keyzer F, Chen F, et al. Diffusion-weighted magnetic resonance imaging allows noninvasive in vivo monitoring of the effects of combretastatin a-4 phosphate after repeated administration. Neoplasia 2005;7(8):779–87.

85. Thoeny HC, De Keyzer F, Vandecaveye V, et al. Effect of vascular targeting agent in rat tumor model: dynamic contrast-enhanced versus diffusion-weighted MR imaging. Radiology 2005;237(2):492–9.

86. Yuan YH, Xiao EH, Liu JB, et al. Characteristics and pathological mechanism on magnetic resonance diffusion-weighted imaging after chemoembolization in rabbit liver VX-2 tumor model. World J Gastroenterol 2007;13(43):5699–706.

87. Yuan YH, Xiao EH, Liu JB, et al. Characteristics of liver on magnetic resonance diffusion-weighted imaging: dynamic and image pathological investigation in rabbit liver VX-2 tumor model. World J Gastroenterol 2008;14(25):3997–4004.

88. Kamel IR, Bluemke DA, Eng J, et al. The role of functional MR imaging in the assessment of tumor response after chemoembolization in patients with hepatocellular carcinoma. J Vasc Interv Radiol 2006;17(3):505–12.

89. Deng J, Miller FH, Rhee TK, et al. Diffusion-weighted MR imaging for determination of hepatocellular carcinoma response to yttrium-90 radioembolization. J Vasc Interv Radiol 2006;17(7):1195–200.

90. Kamel IR, Liapi E, Reyes DK, et al. Unresectable hepatocellular carcinoma: serial early vascular and cellular changes after transarterial chemoembolization as detected with MR imaging. Radiology 2009;250(2):466–73.

91. Liapi E, Kamel IR, Bluemke DA, et al. Assessment of response of uterine fibroids and myometrium to embolization using diffusion-weighted echoplanar MR imaging. J Comput Assist Tomogr 2005;29(1):83–6.

92. Jacobs MA, Herskovits EH, Kim HS. Uterine fibroids: diffusion-weighted MR imaging for monitoring therapy with focused ultrasound surgery—preliminary study. Radiology 2005;236(1):196–203.

93. Okuma T, Matsuoka T, Yamamoto A, et al. Assessment of early treatment response after CT-guided radiofrequency ablation of unresectable lung tumours by diffusion-weighted MRI: a pilot study. Br J Radiol 2009;82(984):989–94.

94. Schraml C, Schwenzer NF, Clasen S, et al. Navigator respiratory-triggered diffusion-weighted imaging in the follow-up after hepatic radiofrequency ablation-initial results. J Magn Reson Imaging 2009;29(6):1308–16.

95. Ohira T, Okuma T, Matsuoka T, et al. FDG-MicroPET and diffusion-weighted MR image evaluation of early changes after radiofrequency ablation in implanted VX2 tumors in rabbits. Cardiovasc Intervent Radiol 2009;32(1):114–20.

96. Padhani AR, Miles KA. Multiparametric imaging of tumor response to therapy. Radiology 2010;256(2):348–64.

Index

Note: Page numbers of article titles are in **boldface** type.

Magn Reson Imaging Clin N Am 19 (2011) 211–214
doi:10.1016/S1064-9689(10)00130-3

mri.theclinics.com